Maternity Services and Policy in an International Context

This book is the first comprehensive international overview of maternity services and policy. Drawing on concepts of risk and social citizenship, it explores the relationship between welfare regimes and health policy by comparing and contrasting provision for childbearing women in eleven countries.

Each substantive chapter focuses on a different country, presenting detailed contextual information on health care provision, maternity interventions and birth outcomes there. They discuss key issues such as birth rates and fertility patterns, the role of patient choice, attitudes to place of birth and maternity entitlements among others, and the countries covered represent diverse welfare regimes, including New Zealand, Ireland, the United States of America, Australia, Scotland, Canada, Japan, Italy, Germany, the Netherlands and Sweden.

It is an important reference for students and academics interested in comparative social policy, health services research, and maternity services and policies.

Patricia Kennedy is a writer and researcher. She was a Senior Lecturer in Social Policy at the School of Applied Social Science, University College Dublin, Ireland from 1995 until 2014. She has written extensively on motherhood and maternity policies in Ireland. Her areas of interest include: conceptual and theoretical approaches to social policy; health policy; consumers' involvement in maternity policy; sexual and reproductive health; migration; comparative social policy; and evidence-based policy. Her books include: *Welcoming the Stranger: Irish Migrant Welfare in Britain from 1957* (2015); *Key Themes in Social Policy* (2013); *Motherhood in Ireland: Creation and Context* (2004); and *Maternity in Ireland: a Woman-centred Perspective* (2002). She has co-edited several books, including: *Ageing and Social Policy* (2008); *Theorizing Irish Social Policy* (2004); *Contemporary Irish Social Policy* (2005, 1999); and *Irish Social Policy in Context* (1999). She has undertaken research and published on domestic violence, the maternity needs of refugee and asylum seekers, gender-based violence, women's health, the Irish Emigrant Chaplaincy Scheme and evidence-based policy.

On an international level she is a founding member of the *European Network for the Promotion of Sexual and Reproductive Health Rights of Refugees and Asylum Seekers* EnHera organisation sponsored by the European Refugee Fund. She was the Irish partner in the Daphne-funded research project *Frame of Reference in Prevention of Sexual and Gender-based Violence Against and Among Young Refugees, Asylum Seekers and Unaccompanied Minors in the European Reception and Asylum Sector*. From 2000 to 2001 she represented the National Women's Council of Ireland on the Kinder Review of Maternity Services and from 2001 to 2011 on the North East Health Services Executive Maternity Services Task Force, which led to the development of Maternity Led Units and Maternity Liaison Committees in Ireland for the first time.

Naonori Kodate is a Lecturer in Social Policy at the School of Applied Social Science, University College Dublin, Ireland. He holds a PhD in Political Science from the London School of Economics and Political Science. During his previous position as a Research Associate at King's College London/the NIHR Patient Safety and Service Quality Research Centre, he published several papers (for example, in the *Journal of Public Policy, BMJ Quality & Safety, International Journal of Nursing Studies*) relating to patient safety and risk decision-making in various clinical settings. He was part of the research team evaluating the effectiveness of a simulation-based training programme for nursing staff in elder care. He is also affiliated to the University of Tokyo and Hokkaido University. He has worked on projects funded by the Japanese Ministry of Health, Labour and Welfare, and the Japan Cancer Society. His main area of expertise is comparative social policy, in particular risk and safety regulation in health care.

Routledge advances in health and social policy

New titles

Health Care Reform and Globalisation
The US, China and Europe in comparative perspective
Edited by Peggy Watson

Power and Welfare
Understanding citizens' encounters with state welfare
Nanna Mik-Meyer and Kaspar Villadsen

International Perspectives on Elder Abuse
Amanda Phelan

Mental Health Services for Vulnerable Children and Young People
Supporting children who are, or have been, in foster care
Michael Tarren-Sweeney and Arlene Vetere

Providing Compassionate Health Care
Challenges in policy and practice
Edited by Sue Shea, Robin Wynyard and Christos Lionis

Teen Pregnancy and Parenting
Rethinking the myths and misperceptions
Keri Weed, Jody S. Nicholson and Jaelyn R. Farris

The Invisible Work of Nurses
Hospitals, organisation and healthcare
Davina Allen

Domestic Violence in Diverse Contexts
A re-examination of gender
Sarah Wendt and Lana Zannettino

Maternity Services and Policy in an International Context

Risk, citizenship and welfare regimes

**Edited by
Patricia Kennedy and
Naonori Kodate**

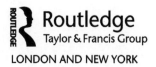

Routledge
Taylor & Francis Group

LONDON AND NEW YORK

First published 2015 by Routledge

2 Park Square, Milton Park, Abingdon, Oxfordshire OX14 4RN
52 Vanderbilt Avenue, New York, NY 10017

Routledge is an imprint of the Taylor & Francis Group, an informa business

First issued in paperback 2019

Copyright © 2015 selection and editorial matter, Patricia Kennedy and
Naonori Kodate; individual chapters, the contributors

The right of the editors to be identified as the authors of the
editorial matter, and of the authors for their individual chapters, has
been asserted in accordance with sections 77 and 78 of the
Copyright, Designs and Patents Act 1988.

All rights reserVed. No part of this book may be reprinted or reproduced or
utilised in any form or by any electronic, mechanical, or other means, now
known or hereafter inVented, including photocopying and recording, or in
any information storage or retrieVal system, without permission in writing
from the publishers.

Notice:
Product or corporate names may be trademarks or registered trademarks,
and are used only for identification and explanation without intent to
infringe.

British Library Cataloguing-in-Publication Data
A catalogue record for this book is available from the British Library

Library of Congress Cataloging in Publication Data
Maternity services and policy in an international context : risk,
citizenship and welfare regimes / edited by Patricia Kennedy and
Naonori Kodate.
    p. ; cm. – (Routledge advances in health and social policy)
    Includes bibliographical references and index.
    I. Kennedy, Patricia, 1963– , editor. II. Kodate, Naonori, editor.
    III. Series: Routledge advances in health and social policy.
    [DNLM: 1. Maternal Health Services. 2. Health Policy. 3. Maternal
    Welfare. WA 310.1]
    RG940
    362.1982–dc23   2014032465

ISBN: 978-0-415-73894-1 (hbk)
ISBN: 978-0-367-34142-8 (pbk)

Typeset in Baskerville
by Wearset Ltd, Boldon, Tyne and Wear

Contents

Illustrations

Contributors

Borman, Barry (PhD), Associate Professor, is the Associate Director of the Centre for Public Health Research, Massey University-Wellington and Director of the National Programme for Monitoring the Environmental Health of New Zealand. He has extensive experience in applied epidemiology, the establishment and operation of health surveillance systems and the analysis of national health data sets, record linkage, the use of epidemiological evidence in the development of health policy, health surveillance, and birth defects epidemiology. He has been Director of the New Zealand Birth Defects Registry since 1987. He teaches under-graduate and post-graduate courses in epidemiology and biostatistics and environmental epidemiology. He was previously the Manager of Public Health Intelligence, the epidemiology group of the Ministry of Health, New Zealand.

Cheyne, Helen (PhD, MSc (Med Sci) RM RGN) is the Royal College of Midwives (Scotland) Professor of Midwifery. She is based in the Nursing Midwifery and Allied Health Professions Research Unit, one of the research units funded by the Scottish Government's Chief Scientist's Office, where she leads a programme of research in maternity care and health care decision-making. Helen began her career as a nurse in Glasgow's Western Infirmary before training as a midwife in Glasgow's Royal Maternity Hospital (Rottenrow) in 1980, going on to work as a midwife in Glasgow and in a rural maternity unit in the north-east of Scotland. Her current research is primarily concerned with decision-making in early labour and the delivery of maternity services. Working closely with practising midwives and mothers is a key aspect of all her research. Helen has published widely and advises the Scottish Government on matters relating to maternity research. She is Chair of the Iolanthe Midwifery Trust.

Ellison-Loschmann, Lis (PhD) belongs to the people of Ngai Tahu, Te Atiawa, Ngati Raukawa and Ngati Toa Rangatira. She originally trained and worked as a nurse and midwife during the 1980s and 1990s. Lis completed a PhD in epidemiology in 2004 through Massey

University in Aotearoa/New Zealand. Her current and recent research activity involves investigations on the health and well-being of *Māori*, the epidemiology of chronic disease, particularly cancer and respiratory conditions, the social determinants of chronic diseases, occupational health, women's health and health system performance. A key component of this work involves supporting and promoting *Māori* research capacity and workforce development by working with *Māori* providers on developing and building research infrastructure within their organisations.

Firestone, Riz (PhD) is a Pacific Public Health researcher at the Centre for Public Health Research, Massey University, New Zealand. She is currently the Principal Investigator for an online birth cohort study (the first of its kind in New Zealand), examining early life risk factors for a wide range of non-communicable diseases. Riz's work also involves improving the health and well-being of Pacific peoples in New Zealand. This includes developing predictive lung function values for Pacific children and investigating metabolic risk among Pacific children and adolescents. Much of this work commenced when Riz received a Health Research Council of New Zealand Post-doctoral Fellowship (2006–2009).

Fukuzawa, Rieko Kishi (PhD) is an Assistant Professor in Nurse-Midwifery and Family Nursing at the University of Tokyo. She pursued her graduate study at the University of Illinois at Chicago and earned her doctoral degree in Nursing Science in 2009. Having had clinical experience as a nurse-midwife, she currently teaches graduate students in the university. Her focus of research has mainly been in doula support and, since 2005, she has brought information about doula support from Western countries to Japan, where there was no formal system for doula services. Her recent research has mainly been focused on the attitudes, values and experiences of maternal health care providers in Japan, while continuing her doctoral study on the refinement of the Japanese version of the 'Listening to Mothers' questionnaires to enable cross-national comparisons of women's perinatal experiences. She collaborates with international researchers, mainly in the USA and Ireland.

Henley, Megan M. is a PhD candidate in Sociology at the University of Arizona. She earned her BA in Sociology at the University of California, Irvine in 2007 and her MA in Sociology at the University of Arizona in 2010. Her research interests include gender, reproduction and the sociology of knowledge. Her dissertation research focuses on doula work and alternative knowledge. She is using data from the Maternity Support Survey, in addition to interviews with doulas and mothers, to look at the roles that certification, science and personal experiences or philosophies play in doulas' attitudes and approaches to childbirth and to doula work itself.

Hildingsson, Ingegerd (PhD) is Professor in Nursing/Midwifery at Mid Sweden University and is also affiliated with the Karolinska Institutet and Uppsala University. She has long experience as a clinical midwife working in prenatal and intrapartum care. She teaches on the Midwifery Program and is a member of the Scientific Board of the Swedish Association of Midwives. She has supervised seven PhD students who have completed their PhD exams and is currently supervising eight PhD students. Her focus of research has mainly been in women's birth preferences, such as planned home birth and caesarean sections on maternal request. Recent research has mainly been about fear of childbirth, fathers' experiences, parenting and the emotional well-being of midwives. Hildingsson collaborates with international researchers, mainly in Australia, the USA and Iceland.

Howe, Laura D. (PhD) is a statistical epidemiologist at the University of Bristol, UK. Her research focuses on child health, with a particular emphasis on early life determinants of patterns and trajectories of health across childhood. A particular focus has been on examining how socio-economic inequalities in health emerge and change across childhood and what processes mediate these inequalities. Much of her research utilises birth cohort studies, including the Avon Longitudinal Study of Parents and Children, Born in Bradford and the Pelotas cohorts in Brazil. Laura is funded by the UK Medical Research Council through a Population Health Scientist fellowship.

Kaminska, Monika Ewa (PhD) from the Centre for Social Policy Research (Zentrum für Sozialpolitik) and the Collaborative Research Centre 597 'Transformations of the State' (both at the University of Bremen) has researched on employment relations, social policies and health care reforms, and post-communist transition. She was previously based at the School of Slavonic and East European Studies (University College London), the Amsterdam Institute for Advanced Labour Studies and the Centre for Social Science and Global Health (both at the University of Amsterdam). At the Zentrum für Sozialpolitik she is leading a research project on 'Healthcare reforms and state desertion in East-Central Europe: privatising health care, privatising risks' and teaching on the welfare state in post-communist countries.

Kennedy, Patricia (PhD) is a researcher and writer. She was a Senior Lecturer in Social Policy at the School of Applied Social Science, University College Dublin, Ireland from 1995 to 2014. She has written extensively on motherhood and maternity policies in Ireland. Her areas of interest include: conceptual and theoretical approaches to social policy; health policy; consumers' involvement in maternity policy; sexual and reproductive health; migration; comparative social policy; and evidence-based policy. Her books include: *Welcoming the Stranger: Irish Migrant Welfare in*

Britain from 1957 (2015); *Key Themes in Social Policy* (2013); *Motherhood in Ireland: Creation and Context* (2004); and *Maternity in Ireland: a Woman-centred Perspective* (2002). She has co-edited several books, including: *Ageing and Social Policy* (2008); *Theorizing Irish Social Policy* (2004); *Contemporary Irish Social Policy* (2005, 1999); and *Irish Social Policy in Context* (1999). She has undertaken research and published on domestic violence, the maternity needs of refugee and asylum seekers, gender-based violence, women's health, the Irish Emigrant Chaplaincy Scheme and evidence-based policy. On an international level she is a founding member of the *European Network for the Promotion of Sexual and Reproductive Health Rights of Refugees and Asylum Seekers* EnHera organisation sponsored by the European Refugee Fund. She was the Irish partner in the Daphne-funded research project *Frame of Reference in Prevention of Sexual and Gender-based Violence Against and Among Young Refugees, Asylum Seekers and Unaccompanied Minors in the European Reception and Asylum Sector.* From 2000 to 2001 she represented the National Women's Council of Ireland on the Kinder Review of Maternity Services and from 2001 to 2011 on the North East Health Services Executive Maternity Services Task Force, which led to the development of Maternity Led Units and Maternity Liaison Committees in Ireland for the first time.

Kodate, Naonori (PhD) is a Lecturer in Social Policy at the School of Applied Social Science, University College Dublin, Ireland. He holds a PhD in Political Science from the London School of Economics and Political Science. During his previous position as a Research Associate at King's College London/the NIHR Patient Safety and Service Quality Research Centre, he published several papers (for example, in the *Journal of Public Policy, BMJ Quality & Safety, International Journal of Nursing Studies*) relating to patient safety and risk decision-making in various clinical settings. He was part of the research team evaluating the effectiveness of a simulation-based training programme for nursing staff in elder care. He is also affiliated to the University of Tokyo and Hokkaido University. He has worked on projects funded by the Japanese Ministry of Health, Labour and Welfare, and the Japan Cancer Society. His main area of expertise is comparative social policy, in particular risk and safety regulation in health care.

Lubold, Amanda M. (PhD) is an Assistant Professor of Sociology at the Indiana State University in Terre Haute. She received her PhD in Sociology from the University of Arizona in 2014. Her dissertation examined the effects of national policies and public health initiatives on breastfeeding rates and breastfeeding duration in OECD countries. She has also studied the effects of organizational policies on breastfeeding duration for new mothers that enter the workplace shortly after giving birth, and plans to compare policy effects on breastfeeding in the US and Canada.

Matheson, Anna (PhD) is a social scientist at the Centre for Public Health Research, Massey University and is the Coordinator of the Post-Graduate Diploma of Public Health and Masters of Public Health programmes. As well as teaching and supervision, Anna is involved in research relating to how to effectively reduce health inequalities for *Maori* and Pacific peoples and other groups with low socio-economic status. Her research in this area to date has focused on housing and health, access to cancer services, access to screening services, food security in the Pacific Islands and the social barriers globally to achieving universal health coverage. Anna is especially interested in the social determinants of health and the application of theories of complex systems to improve the outcomes of health and social policy interventions.

McIntyre, Meredith (PhD) is Associate Professor at the School of Nursing and Midwifery, Monash University and has been an active member of the Australian College of Midwives, serving as President and Vice President of the Victorian branch over a number of years. This role necessitated a close working relationship with the Maternity Services Policy Division of the Department of Health, Victoria. She was also instrumental in the formation of the Victorian Midwives Academic group, an academic lobby group committed to improving maternity services for women. Dr McIntyre has developed a reputation as an expert in the field of maternity care policy in Australia through her widely published PhD research, providing the Australian Government with a policy briefing paper on the safety of non-medical-led maternity care in 2012. She served as a founding member of the Werna Naloo Bachelor of Midwifery course consortium in Victoria, established in 2001. Meredith is committed to the professional advancement of midwifery in Australia in the interests of improving the experience of women having babies.

Mischke, Monika (PhD) studied sociology in Groningen (the Netherlands) and Berlin (Germany) and received her doctorate from the University of Mannheim (Germany). Currently, she holds a position as a post-doctoral research fellow and lecturer at the University of Siegen (Germany). At Siegen University she is working as a Senior Researcher in the research project 'Healthcare-seeking by Older People' funded by the German Research Foundation. This project analyses the social and institutional context of decision-making in the case of sickness. Previous responsibilities include research positions at Siegen University (2009–2012) and the Mannheim Center for European Social Research at the University of Mannheim (2006–2009). Mischke's research interests include international comparisons of welfare states and family policy systems, health care, public attitudes, social inequality and research methods in the social sciences.

Molinari, Chiara (MD) graduated from the Università Vita-Salute in Milan (Italy) in 2009. She is currently completing her fellowship in

Endocrinology and Metabolic Diseases at the San Raffaele Scientific Institute in Milan. During her fellowship she has developed a specific expertise in the intensive management of patients with type 1 diabetes using new technologies (e.g. external insulin pumps for continuous subcutaneous insulin infusion and continuous glucose monitoring) and she is involved in the care of women with type 1 diabetes during pregnancy. Her research interest is focused on the epidemiology of gestational diabetes – including compliance to screening, maternal and foetal outcomes of pregnancy, access to care of first-generation immigrant women and compliance with the postpartum screening of glucose tolerance – through the analysis of health care data in the Lombardy region in Northern Italy.

Morton, Christine H. (PhD) is a research sociologist at Stanford University's California Maternal Quality Care Collaborative, an organization working to improve maternal quality care and reduce preventable maternal death and injury. Her current research interests include maternal mortality and morbidity, maternity care advocacy and quality improvement in the US. She is co-investigator of two current projects: 'The Maternity Support Survey, a cross-national survey of doulas, childbirth educators and maternity nurses in the US and Canada' and 'Severe Maternal Events: Narratives of Women, their Partners and Health Care Practitioners'. In 1998, she founded an online listserve for social scientists studying reproduction, ReproNetwork.org, with more than 300 subscribers. She is the author of *Birth Ambassadors: Doulas and the Re-emergence of Woman-Supported Birth in the United States* (Praeclarus Press, 2014).

Reibling, Nadine (PhD cand.) is currently a postdoctoral researcher at the University of Siegen working on decision-making processes in the case of illness. In 2012–2013 she was a Harkness Fellow in Healthcare Policy and Practice at the Harvard School of Public Health. Reibling's research interests are comparative health systems, welfare state attitudes, health inequalities and health care utilisation. For her doctoral research, Reibling won the European Network for Social Policy Analysis/*Journal of European Social Policy* Doctoral Researcher Prize, as well as the most prestigious PhD merit scholarship in Germany from the German National Academic Foundation. Reibling has published eight peer-reviewed articles in journals such as *Health Expectations* and *Health Policy*.

Roth, Louise Marie (PhD) is an Associate Professor of Sociology at the University of Arizona. She earned her BA in Sociology at McGill University in Montreal and her PhD at New York University. Her research interests include gender inequality in organizations, organizational and legal effects on maternity care, and maternity support work. Her publications include a book, *Selling Women Short: Gender Inequality on Wall Street* and many articles related to gender inequality and reproduction, including an article on health disparities in American maternity care with Megan M. Henley and a chapter on the effects of organizational policies on breastfeeding initiation and duration with Amanda M. Lubold. Her current research examines gender differences in pay-for-performance among physicians, the effects of malpractice laws on maternity care practices, and the maternity support work of doulas, childbirth educators, and labour and delivery nurses. With Christine H. Morton, Megan M. Henley, and other collaborators, she designed and implemented the Maternity Support Survey in the United States and Canada.

Scavini, Marina (MD, PhD) graduated from the Università degli Studi di Milano in 1983, completed her fellowship in Diabetes and Metabolic Diseases in 1986 and earned her PhD in Clinical Pathophysiology in 1994. In the 1980s and 1990s she worked at the San Raffaele Scientific Institute in Milan on clinical research projects for the replacement of beta-cell function in patients with type 1 diabetes, with external or implantable programmable insulin pumps. She developed her expertise in epidemiology and outcome research while working at the University of New Mexico in the USA in 2000–2004. At the San Raffaele Scientific Institute in Milan, she is currently involved in the care of pregnant women with either pre-gestational or gestational diabetes, many of whom are first-generation immigrants from Northern Africa, the Middle East and the Far East. Her clinical research interests focus on access to antenatal care in under-served groups, preconceptional care, pregnancy outcomes and reproductive health in women with diabetes.

Thomas, Jan (PhD) is Associate Provost and Professor of Sociology at Kenyon College (Ohio, USA). Before coming to Kenyon in 1996, Thomas worked as a counsellor, educator and administrator at women's health centres in Chicago, Illinois and Denver, Colorado and operated her own health counselling practice in Denver. The focus of her scholarly work has been primarily in the area of women's health. She teaches classes on the US and Swedish health care systems, global women's health issues, gender inequality, inequality in America, gender and the welfare state, and research methods. Her early research was on the legacies of feminist women's health centres in the USA. Recent research projects have been looking beyond women's experiences with maternity services to include fathers' experiences and parenting in the first year. In her current position as an administrator, she is particularly interested in the experiences and development of faculty women and women in leadership in higher education.

Acknowledgements

The editors thank each of the contributors to this book and all those who have provided us with assistance, guidance and support, particularly the Routledge editorial team, our colleagues at the School of Applied Social Science, University College Dublin, and our families.

Introduction

Despite the fact that 150 million women give birth annually throughout the world, maternity services and policy have received very little attention in the academic literature. This book is the first comprehensive international study of maternity services and policy. It straddles three important areas: comparative social policy; health services research; and maternity services and policy. This book addresses fundamental questions relating to maternity care within welfare regimes in eleven countries across four continents. The particular countries chosen here reflect a range of welfare regimes, including liberal, conservative–corporatist, social democratic, Southern European and East Asian, and, in so doing, will contribute to scholarship on the classification of welfare regimes.

This book specifically addresses issues of risk and rights at individual and societal levels. It provides the most up-to-date statistical data on demographic patterns, including fertility patterns and birth rates. It presents detailed statistics on maternity interventions and birth outcomes in a diverse range of countries across several continents, including New Zealand, Ireland, the USA, Australia, Scotland, Canada, Japan, Italy, Germany, the Netherlands and Sweden. It is interdisciplinary and comparative and allows for micro-level (from the perspective of individual service users) and macro-level (across countries) analyses.

Maternity provision is a neglected area in comparative research on welfare states and yet it is a microcosm of the wider health services. Health services have received some attention in the comparative literature on welfare states (e.g. Moran 1999; Bambra 2005; Riebling 2010). Focusing on maternity provision illuminates the context of health services in each country. The complexity of issues such as health provision, the views of consumers, individual and collective choice, equity and birth outcomes in different economic, cultural and political regimes are addressed. The book sheds light on the inequalities of access to maternity services for groups such as new immigrants, young mothers, ethnic minorities and those at risk of diabetes as well as geographical and economic inequalities. It casts the consumer experience of maternity policies against quantitative data on outcomes.

This book considers convergence and divergence across welfare regimes. It adds insights to puzzles, neglected issues and unanswered questions in relation to consumers' experiences of maternity services. It contributes to our knowledge of social citizenship and access to maternity services in different regimes and by different groups.

Opening with an examination of what maternity services and policies encompass, the first chapter locates the topic within the literature on comparative welfare regimes. The vast literature on welfare regimes has exposed the importance of citizenship as a tool of analysis in understanding rights and access to health services, which are often organised and distributed according to differential rights in terms of prior payments, legal status, and age and membership of a community. Social/welfare citizenship relates to economic welfare and security and 'the right to share to the full in the social heritage and to live the life of a civilized being according to the standards prevailing in the society' (Marshall 1950: 10–11). This is very important when it comes to accessing maternity services.

As with social policy debates, the discourse around maternity provision is a discourse on risk. Risk is central to the formation and delivery of social policy. Technology expands the range of personal choice and also expands uncertainties and risk. This is very relevant to maternity services in which there is an increased emphasis on technology and old risks have been replaced by new risks. In this context, personal anxiety stakes rise. Beck (1992) suggests that the socially disadvantaged are most likely to experience risk while not having the resources to deal with it. This is true for maternity services. For those living in remote rural areas, a non-local birth can entail long-distance travel in early labour, relocating temporarily to be near an obstetric unit prior to labour, separation from family and social support networks at a vulnerable time and the logistical difficulties and financial costs associated with being far from friends or family and organising care for existing children. All of these factors can cause stress and anxiety for families and lead to health inequalities.

There is a dearth of published information on maternity services and policies at the national level. This book addresses this neglected topic. Each chapter, incorporating rights and risk, provides substantive information on the country under study. It locates each country as a welfare regime type and describes its health service, covering the following areas: demographics; maternity provision; maternity entitlements; antenatal, intrapartum and postnatal care; intervention rates; birth outcomes; breastfeeding; consumer involvement; risk and rights; and a discussion.

The individual authors are all experts on maternity services in the country under study. The first chapter introduces the book and the literature on welfare regimes, health regimes and maternity provision. Focusing on rights and risk, this book is concerned with how maternal and infant health care are perceived in a given society, whether service users are perceived as deserving or undeserving, and the extent to which service users have rights. It investigates the conflicts between the professions involved in maternal and infant health in specific regimes and whether these professions have differential rights to practise. It also explores the role of technology and the medicalisation of maternal and infant health in industrially advanced economies.

The book will be of interest to students and readers from a wide range of disciplines, including social policy, nursing and midwifery, health policy and management, public policy and political science.

References

Bambra, C. (2005) 'Worlds of welfare and the health care discrepancy', *Social Policy and Society* 4 (1): 31–41.
Beck, U. (1992) *Risk Society: Towards a New Modernity*. London: Sage.
Marshall, T.H. (1950) *Citizenship and Social Class, and other Essays*. Cambridge: Cambridge University Press.
Moran, M. (1999) *Governing the Healthcare State: a Comparative Study of the United Kingdom, the United States and Germany*. Manchester: Manchester University Press.
Riebling, N. (2010) 'Healthcare systems in Europe: towards an incorporation of patient access', *Journal of European Social Policy*, 20 (1), 5–18.

1 Welfare regimes, health care regimes and maternity services and policy

A comparative perspective

Patricia Kennedy, Naonori Kodate and Nadine Reibling

This chapter locates maternity services and policy within the literature on comparative welfare regimes. It identifies risk and rights as two important concepts that straddle the combined literature on welfare regimes, health regimes and scholarship on maternity policy and practice. It discusses the centrality of the social and medical models of health to the understanding of maternity policy. It strives for a greater understanding of the complexities of maternity policy.

We begin by introducing the comparative literature on welfare regimes that has emerged over the last two decades and explore the scholarship on health regimes and the emerging literature on 'maternity regimes'. We investigate how childbirth is perceived at the macro-, micro- and meso-levels, a framework developed by De Vries *et al.* (2001) in *Birth by Design: Pregnancy, Maternity Care and Midwifery in North America and Europe.* These authors claimed that their goal was 'to "decenter" the study of maternity care from particular national contexts, to move it analytically in a direction in which any and all contexts are perceived as problematic' (De Vries *et al.* 2001: xiii). They questioned how maternity care has been shaped by political systems, state organisations, the organisation of the professions, educational systems, stratification systems and inequality, and attitudes towards and uses of technology. They indicated the lack of a framework for the organisation of comparative studies of maternity care. They offered an analysis of the differences and similarities in the organisation of maternity care in a sample of high-income countries. Using a multi-country, multi-level method, they demonstrated that maternity care has not followed the same evolutionary path in different countries and suggested 'the social and cultural diversity of societies cannot be separated from the organisational arrangement of maternity care' (De Vries *et al.* 2001: xv).

Welfare regimes

The development of modern welfare states is rooted in the motivation and capacity of states to deal with 'social risks' (Pierson 2011; Taylor-Gooby

2004). Individual welfare programmes are generally organised around a specific risk, e.g. the risk of illness, disability, unemployment or old age. The welfare regime literature that originated from the seminal work *The Three Worlds of Welfare Capitalism* (Esping-Andersen 1990) argues that there are distinct ways in which welfare states deal with all these risks. For instance, it was argued that 'when we focus on the principles embedded in welfare states, we discover distinct regime-clusters, not merely variations of "more" or "less" around a common denominator' (Esping-Andersen 1990: 32). In his original work, Esping-Andersen identified three distinct welfare regimes: liberal, conservative–corporatist and social democratic welfare capitalism.

A vast scholarship on families of nations and welfare state regimes has developed since that publication (Arts and Gelissen 2010; Ferrera 1996; Huber and Bogliaccini 2010; Peng and Wong 2010). Castles and Mitchell (1993), for instance, suggest the existence of a fourth 'radical' world, composed of the Australian and New Zealand welfare states, which combines high-level minimum wage policies and more generous means-tested welfare programmes than the American and British systems. Ferrera (1996) has proposed the Southern European countries as another family of welfare states. Another new category contains the former Communist welfare states in Central and Eastern Europe, which do not fit the standard Esping-Andersen typology. Comparative social policy literature has paid limited attention to former Communist welfare systems, which are generally characterised as 'authoritarian–paternalist', including elements of both 'Continental' and 'Nordic' regimes – e.g. 'status-reinforcement' deriving from occupation-based social insurance systems and 'universality of certain services' (Kornai 1992). Finally, beyond the Europe–America focus, scholars have pointed out the distinct characteristics of welfare states in East Asia (Peng and Wong 2010), as well as in the developing world (Arts and Gelissen 2010).

Aside from this ongoing debate on the correct number of welfare regimes and the attribution of individual countries to these regimes, a more fundamental critique has been raised about the conceptual outline of Esping-Andersen's classification (Arts and Gelissen 2010), which excludes important dimensions of welfare policy, most importantly the role of social services and in-kind benefits (Alber 1995; Kautto 2002) and the role of gender or, more generally, how welfare states deal with new social risks.

Both of these lines of critique are directly linked with the 'risk of childbirth' and maternity care services because: (1) maternity care consists mostly of services and less of monetary payments; and (2) the way welfare states deal with gender relations and the role of women is crucial for how the transition to motherhood is perceived and enacted by citizens. The gendered analysis of welfare regimes has focused on the institutional organisation of social services for children and the elderly. Depending on whether or not these services are provided by the state, the market, or within families shapes women's 'capacity to form and maintain an autonomous household' by participating in the labour market (Orloff 1993a: 319). Esping-Andersen himself provided a revised typology in 1999 in which he added social services and extended his welfare regime typology by adding the dimension of de-familialisation. Although this work has mostly looked at the role of women and the provision of services in the welfare state globally, in this book our focus is on the time frame surrounding childbirth. Therefore we predominately look at maternity entitlements, while childcare services, which are of central importance later in life, are beyond the scope of this book. Nevertheless, following the welfare regime literature, we expect that the gender values that influence the institutional setup of all welfare programmes (e.g. childcare, elderly care, widows' pension) will also shape the different ways in which childbirth and the transition to motherhood is organised in the nations that we compare in this book.

Welfare or health care regimes: is health care different?

One of the major critiques of Esping-Andersen's welfare regimes has been his focus on income maintenance programmes and the omission of social services (Alber 1995) and, most importantly, the fact that health care, one of the most important (and expensive) fields of welfare state provision, was excluded (Bambra 2005). A primary example for this critique has been the UK, which – despite its liberal welfare regime – has a National Health Service that provides free access to health care for all residents.

A number of scholars have provided typologies and classifications of health care systems. Their results reveal both similarities and differences between 'welfare' and 'health care regimes'. The Nordic countries usually form a cluster and the USA is an outlier in all accounts. However, the liberal, conservative and Southern countries show differences in their welfare and health care arrangements. Differences across typologies are often based on their focus on different parts of the health care system

Bambra (2005) uses information on the public–private mix in spending and provision as an indicator of the degree of universality to create a health decommodification index that reveals many similarities with Esping-Andersen's welfare regimes. However, a number of liberal countries (the UK, Canada and New Zealand) provide a much higher level of decommodification in health care than in their general welfare provision. The typology of Moran (1995) of health care states adds the dimension of governance as the role of the state in the areas of consumption, production and technology. He distinguishes four ideal types: command and control states; supply states; corporatist states; and insecure command and control states. In this mainly conceptual work, individual countries are used to illustrate the types. However, Moran's analysis is mainly theoretical and so it is not possible to assess the extent to which welfare regimes and health care states overlap and in which cases they are distinct.

In contrast, Wendt (2009) provides an empirically based differentiation of health care systems. Based on a cluster analysis, three types of health care system were constructed: health service provision-oriented type; universal coverage–controlled access type; and low budget–restricted access type. Reibling (2010) develops a typology of health care regimes using indicators of patient access regulations, thereby providing a comparison of various systems from the perspective of service recipients. This classification shows that patient access regulations vary considerably from other aspects of health care systems (e.g. the public–private mix). Thus her results underscore another line of work showing that specific institutional regulations in welfare fields can considerably deviate from identified health care or welfare regimes (Burau and Blank 2006). Welfare and health care regimes can provide a useful framework of reference, but need to be complemented by the analysis of specific institutional arrangements, which is exactly what this book is about.

Aside from the empirical differences in countries' attachment to certain groups or regimes, there are a number of theoretical arguments about why health care systems can be detached from their general welfare regime. We would like to highlight three of these arguments.

1   Esping-Andersen's core argument for the formation of different worlds of welfare has been the power resources of the working class (Esping-Andersen 1990). Thus the conflict between capital and labour has played a core role in the formation (and generosity) of income maintenance programmes. Cultural accounts of welfare states have also stressed the variation in 'deservingness categories' as causes or results of varying welfare support (van Oorschot 2007). Health care, however, differs both culturally and institutionally from income maintenance programmes. For instance, studies on welfare attitudes repeatedly show an exceptionally high support for health care based on the idea that ill people are seen as highly deserving (Blekesaune und Quadagno 2003). Unlike poverty, illness is perceived less as a person's own fault, but rather as an unpredictable event. Thus social solidarity with respect to illness seems to be much higher in European countries than other forms of welfare provision. However, in the USA, the only advanced industrialised country without a universal system, public opinion is much less supportive of socialised solutions to individual health problems. Moreover, the fact that lifestyle risks are increasingly identified as major causes for disease has, and may in the future, undermine the high degree of solidarity present for health care in European countries. Nevertheless, the high degree of cross-national consensus around health care makes this field different from other parts of welfare provision. This has been shown empirically as spending on health care is much more stable and convergent in European countries than spending on other social services (Jensen 2008).

2   Another distinct characteristic of health care systems is the important role of the professions. Unlike in other fields of welfare provision, the major line of conflict is not between capital and labour, but between payers (states, companies, sickness funds) and providers (hospitals, doctors) or between providers (professions). The sociology of the professions as well as the institutional analysis of health care reforms have demonstrated the important role of the medical professions in the formation and reform of health care systems (Immergut 1992; Wilsford 1994; Hacker 1998; Tuohy 1999; Hassenteufel and Palier 2007; Kuhlmann *et al.* 2009; Kodate 2010). This perspective underlines the continuity of health care systems ('path dependency') in this pre-dominantly profession-driven policy sector. The medical profession has retained a considerable level of autonomy in its decisions for a long time. The medical profession has also succeeded in extending its field of activity by medicalising a number of physiological changes and social behaviours (e.g. attention-deficit hyperactivity disorder), including childbirth (Conrad 1992). However, in recent years, this auto-nomy has been challenged from two sides. On the one hand, policy-makers are increasingly concerned about health care costs that conflict with professional autonomy and profit-seeking. On the other hand, the availability of large amounts of data has demonstrated the wide variability of practice, quality and outcomes, resulting in a stronger reliance on 'evidence' for medical decision-making (Rosenthal 2008). As a result, although governments are keen to advocate patients' rights by increasing transparency and collaborating closely with the medical professions, tensions arise between the two actors.

McIntyre *et al.* (2012), in their paper 'Primary maternity care reform: whose influence is driving the change?', explore develop-ments in the Australian system, referring to developments in New Zealand, Canada and the UK and suggest that, although the Austral-ian government has strong support for primary maternity care, reform is backed by a strong key stakeholder alliance involving consumers, midwives and rural doctors. The obstetric profession has been unable to provide the government with solutions to escalating costs and work-force deficits in the delivery of safe and sustainable maternity services. Consumers, rural doctors, midwives and the government all agree on the need to safeguard the excellent safety and quality standards, while at the same time reducing high levels of medical intervention and pro-viding options for care in a reformed maternity service designed to meet the needs of all Australian women.

3   Welfare states are vulnerable towards external developments, espe-cially economic development, e.g. high unemployment puts pressure on unemployment insurance systems. Unlike other fields of welfare, health care systems are not only subject to exogenous factors in terms

of demand (e.g. the ageing of the population), but also in terms of the supply. The most important factor here is the constant development of medical knowledge and technology (Mechanic and Rochefort 1996). Health policy-makers face significant challenges in evaluating the usefulness and cost-effectiveness of medical technologies, even more so as they face strong pressure from both professional lobbies and public opinion that has a high trust in technological solutions to medical problems (Mechanic and Rochefort 1996). The varying ability of governments to regulate medical technology (including new drugs) is a distinctive feature of health care systems (Moran 1995), a factor that can be correlated with welfare state and political system variables, but also with the presence of medical technology and drug companies in individual countries.

Maternity care has been at the core of health care systems in the twentieth century. Maternal and infant health care were among the first services covered in all health care systems and are a focal point of intervention in developing countries today. The rise of Western health care systems has played a strong role in the medicalisation of childbirth. Although doctors' claims for childbirth started long before the development of universal health care systems, the coverage of maternity care has played a decisive role in the practice of childbirth (Benoit *et al.* 2005).

One major aim of this book is to evaluate similarities and differences across maternity regimes and to determine to what extent they match existing welfare and health care arrangements.

Maternity care is a paradigmatic example for the comparative analysis of health care because: (1) it is characterised by a high degree of state support; (2) professional dominance and conflicts are at the core of its history; and (3) technological developments have shaped and changed maternity care and birth practices. Compared with other fields of welfare provision, ill people are seen as a category with very high levels of deservingness. This is even more so for mothers and children. Thus support for the coverage of maternity and infant care is high. Co-payments for these groups are often lower for maternity than for other health care services (Sandier *et al.* 2004). Nevertheless, maternity care systems vary in their level of support for less privileged women. In a comparative analysis of maternity care provision in Canada, Finland and Iceland, Wrede *et al.* (2008) demonstrated different barriers in accessing primary care services across the childbearing period for lower income women in these three countries, as well as the factors that create poor working conditions for the predominantly female maternity care labour force. They argue that the pressure from governments to create more efficient and effective health care systems has had visible negative effects with regard to equitable health services for lower income populations and dignified working conditions for health providers.

Maternal and infant health is identified as a national goal in many countries and empirical indicators are routinely collected and reported. This strong support for maternity care should lead us to expect a high degree of similarity and convergence among different countries. However, the high importance attached to maternity care must not coincide with a strong consensus on what it should entail. Varying professional groups, and also consumers, argue for the availability of a variety of birth practices in similar situations.

The professional conflicts that we find in many areas of health care between hospitals and ambulatory settings and between general practitioners and specialists are extended by the importance of a unique profession: *midwifery*. In a comparative study of maternity services in the UK, Finland, the Netherlands and Canada, Benoit *et al.* (2005) used the profession of midwifery to illustrate why these countries have distinct maternity care systems, even though they share publicly funded universal health care and favourable health outcomes. Their analysis shows a marked variation in how these countries: (1) approached legalising midwifery and negotiating the role of the midwife in the division of labour; (2) how professional boundaries in the maternity care domain are organised; and (3) how consumer mobilisation plays a role in the support of midwifery and maternity issues

The role midwives play in the birth process has therefore been a matter of sociological analysis of maternity care systems. Technological developments also shape birth practices. Whether these procedures are medically indicated or whether they should be controlled by the women in labour is highly contested and varies significantly across countries. Thus we attempt to leverage both a welfare state and a health care perspective on different aspects of maternity care.

Rights and maternal and infant health

Citizenship is central to debates in social policy. Decommodification – one's ability to survive outside the labour market – has received much attention in welfare regime scholarship. The degree to which social rights are stratified in different societies has implications for citizens. This is useful for deconstructing maternal and infant health care systems, which is one of the goals of this book. Basically, it allows for the investigation of the rights and responsibilities associated with belonging to a particular group. Therefore it is concerned with exclusion and inclusion and with equality of status. This is important for maternity. Citizens have differential rights as service users and as professionals. Such rights can entail responsibilities. For example, when women have a right to attend antenatal care, are they obliged to attend for antenatal care and education? Do women have a right to a home birth? Do midwives and obstetricians have equal rights to practise and what responsibilities go along with such rights?

Risk and maternal and infant care

Risk is associated with potential harm, danger and adversity. Social policy is a collective response to risk. Kemshall (2002) explores the relationship between social policy and risk and argues that risk is replacing need as the key principle of social policy formation and delivery. This could be said to apply to maternity policy. Although childbirth has always been associated with risk, there are now new risks associated with the use of technology, lifestyles and deferred maternity. Giddens (1999) refers to 'the runaway world', characterised by internally produced or manufactured risks in contrast with the external risks of the natural world. Technology expands the range of personal choice and also expands uncertainties and risk.

This results in unintended side-effects and consequences, the expansion of choice and the reduction of traditional norms, trust and social bonds: 'as customary ways of doing things become problematic, people must choose in many areas which used to be governed by taken-for-granted norms' (Giddens 1998: 5). In this context, personal anxiety stakes rise, traditional bonds such as those between family and community are eroded and individuals are increasingly exposed to risk. Risks have their source in social change, economic forces, scientific developments and technological developments. Social risks have been identified as a result of the economic and social changes associated with the transition to what some social scientists call 'a postindustrial society'. As a consequence, risk management has now become a well-established domain in research and practice and one of the dominant organising concepts worldwide (Adam *et al.* 2000; Collingridge 1996; Power 2004; Rasmussen 1997; Rothstein *et al.* 2006). Managing risks is central to maternity provision. Mackenzie Bryers and van Teijlingen (2010: 494) state:

> Firstly, perceptions of risk in maternity care can be interpreted at three levels: theoretical/societal, institutional and professional – the way health boards/management groups decipher risk policy affects how risk is managed within that organisation and this, in turn, can influence professional and individual practice.

Risk is associated with clinical governance and how this operates in different societies is worthy of comparison.

We have argued that this limited epidemiological and clinical focus on risk can, in fact, create more risk – the risk of an imbalance in perspective that is connected with the loss of childbirth as a holistic, natural event in society and in the lives of women and families. On the other hand, the focus on risk can support the implementation of midwife-led care and birthing as it gives assurance and confidence to midwives, obstetricians and women whose care is being managed within an evidence-based framework.

Mackenzie Bryers and van Teijlingen (2010) differentiate between, first, 'absolute risk', which they relate to the collection and analysis of maternity outcome data and the importance that this has in the way maternity services are managed and, second, cultural influences, i.e. the way risk is perceived. To understand the relevance of risk to maternal and infant health, and the different trajectories taken by each country, it is necessary to understand the medical and social models of childbirth.

Social and medical models of maternal and infant health

There are two principal schools of thought underlying maternal health care provision. These are closely related to risk assessment and management in maternity care. Wagner argues that behind the social and medical approaches to childbirth there lies 'a set of assumptions, ideas and thinking' (Wagner 1994: 27). He stresses that he is not concerned with labelling one model as right and another as wrong, but rather 'to explore how to combine them by identifying the elements in each that might be effective in addressing specific health issues'. Wagner (1994) explains how the conflict between the two models dates from ancient Greek philosophy, but has become deeply ingrained in Western thought. The models relate to the dichotomised world that views on one side art and all that is subjective as feminine, based on intuition and quality; on the other side there exists science, objectivity, masculinity, logic and quantity. He claims that, before the modern era, health and birth were related to the artistic side, the social model, whereas

> About a hundred years ago, the profession of medicine aligned itself with science and classical, mechanical physics, applying them to the body, its functions and its disease processes: this was the basis for the medical model of health. As pregnancy and birth were brought into the medical domain this view was applied to birth and birth technology.
>
> (Wagner 1994: 27–28)

Murphy-Lawless (1998) suggests that:

> Obstetric science has organised itself as a rational practice. It argues that its beliefs about how to manage women in childbirth are the sum of its cumulative experiences and are provable in scientific terms ... so like other sciences, it presents itself to the larger non-scientific community as a superior model of rationality when compared with alternative non-scientific or pre-scientific accounts of childbirth
>
> (17)

The medical model of childbirth according to Wagner views life as a problem associated with danger and risk, which, he argues, is 'an

assumption easily accepted if one's professional career is spent sur-
rounded by pathology, suffering and death' (Wagner 1994: 28). Furthermore, Wagner suggests that in the medical model:

> The body is seen as imperfect or even corrupt and health is obtained
> only with help from the outside. Health is the success of external
> agents (treatments) over nature in temporarily eliminating disease
> or other pathological conditions from the body.... The best weapons
> in the struggle against disease and death, according to the medical
> model result from the use of the power of science to create the
> necessary interventions and to determine when and on whom to use
> them.
>
> (Wagner 1994: 28)

The social model of childbirth adheres to a 'holistic' view of women,
encompassing women as social, emotional and physical entities. It views a
woman in biographical terms, a person with a past and a future and as
part of a larger social structure. This model is synonymous with the
'natural childbirth' philosophy, associated with Dick-Read (1942), Leboyer
(1975, 1991), Kitzinger (1978, 1983, 1988) and Odent (1984). According
to Wagner (1994), the social model views life as a solution rather than a
problem, which is based on a belief that people can heal themselves and
that 'medical care should help them in this task, respecting their integrity
and supporting them with the least intervention necessary' (Wagner 1994:
29). With the social model,

> The person is seen as a kind of ecological system that is not yet well
> understood. This system includes the body, mind and spirit, each of
> which is involved in health and disease. Psychological and social
> factors (such as love and social support or lack of them) are emphas-
> ised in curing as well as producing illness.
>
> (Wagner 1994: 29)

The social model is associated with home births and domiciliary midwifery
throughout the Western world (Ehrenreich and English 1973; Donnison
1977, 1988; Murphy-Lawless 1998).

Maternity services and policy reforms: convergence or divergence?

This book explores whether there is convergence or divergence, or both, in
maternity services and policy across advanced industrial economies. As previously noted, health accounts for one of the largest proportions of public
spending in every advanced industrial economy. Moreover, health care
systems often share the fundamental collective values and solidarity upon

which the welfare state was constructed (Alber 1982; Esping-Andersen 1990; Rothstein 1998; Saltman *et al.* 2004; Skocpol and Ikenberry 1983; Meulen *et al.* 2001). There is a constant tension between the much-needed innovation in health services on the one hand and a reluctance to carry out any radical changes on the other. These difficult choices and inertia within formal institutions are the main reasons for the immobilism (i.e. an antipathy to change) of health reforms. However, exogenous factors (e.g. demographics and adverse events) exert a significant impact on the system

Changes in population have crucial impacts on a government's policy direction in many areas, ranging from economics, the labour market, education and social protection to health policy. Needless to say, maternity services are directly influenced by this.

Figure 1.1 shows the changing fertility rates in the last three decades in the eleven countries discussed in this book. Fertility rates in New Zealand, Ireland and the USA have been steadily high, around 2.0, whereas Sweden and Australia have trailed behind, although they have recently reached almost 2.0. The Netherlands, Scotland and Canada showed upward trends from 2000–2009. Fertility rates in Italy, Germany and Japan have been below 1.5 since 1995.

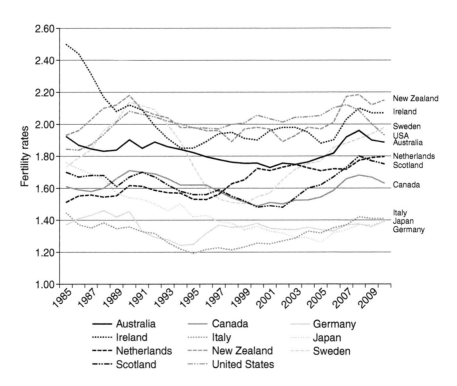

Figure 1.1 Total fertility rates (1985–2010), selected eleven countries (source: OECD 2012. Adapted by the authors).

   The book investigates maternity services in countries selected on the basis of welfare state typologies (six examples from English-speaking welfare states, two from Continental European states, and one each from Nordic, Mediterranean and East Asian states) (Table 1.1). The six English-speaking welfare states share common features in terms of low levels of spending on social protection, although health care provision and financing in these countries varies greatly. It is worth looking more closely at the differences among these six countries.

   Just as with other types of exogenous events such as wars and economic recessions, unexpected events can mark a 'critical juncture' where a new path emerges in maternity care services and policy (Kennedy and Einasto 2010; Kennedy 2012). In addition, the responsiveness or non-responsiveness of central government to public concerns is another key element in understanding changes in maternity services and the reform strategy chosen for a country's maternity services. For example, scandals and crises highlighted by some adverse events often instigate a public outcry for clearer accountability, resulting in policy changes (Butler and Drakeford 2005; Cantelli *et al.* 2011; Kodate 2012). As discussed later in this book, social risks and uncertainty cause anxiety, thus mobilising power and attracting wider public attention to decisions made at the micro-, meso- and macro-levels by various actors involved in dealing with potential harm. Maternity care is no exception and risk and uncertainty have become one of the strong features of this policy domain (Kenyon 2009). Risk management and the standardisation of clinical practice have brought some convergence in maternity services across different countries. However, remarkable differences still exist, which this book will highlight.

Understanding maternity services and policy in an international context

This chapter has introduced the literature on welfare regimes and how it has been expanded to address health policy and services. It has

Table 1.1 Total fertility rates and welfare state regimes in the eleven countries selected for study in this book

Welfare regime	*Total fertility rates (1985–2010)*		
	Low (below 1.5)	*Medium (1.5–2.0)*	*High (approx. 2.0)*
English-speaking	–	Australia, Canada, Scotland	Ireland, New Zealand, USA
East Asia	Japan	–	–
Mediterranean	Italy	–	–
Continental	Germany	The Netherlands	–
Nordic	–	Sweden	–

introduced two important concepts, rights and risk, which are central to the debates on social policy and maternal and infant health. It has discussed the medical and social models of maternity. It is clear that unearthing the nature of maternity policy is a complex task. We argue that, aside from the empirical differences in countries' attachments to certain groups or regimes, there are a number of theoretical arguments about why health care systems can be detached from their general welfare regimes.

1   How maternal and infant health are perceived in a given society. Are the recipients perceived as deserving/undeserving and do they have rights? How is the risk associated with childbirth perceived at the macro-, micro- and meso-level?
2   How is the role of the professions played out in relation to maternity care and services? In a given society, who defines risk? Does one profession have superior rights to practise to another?
3   How does the development of technology in a given society relate to maternal services and policy? What rights and risks are associated with this?

By answering these questions, this book will explore the similarities and differences in maternity services and policy across eleven advanced industrialised economies and will shed light on the factors that are bringing convergence and divergence.

References

Adam, B., Beck, U. and Loon, J. van (2000) *The Risk Society and Beyond: Critical Issues for Social Theory*. London: Sage.
Alber, J. (1982) *Vom Armenhaus zum Wohlfahrtsstaat: Analysen zur Entwicklung der Sozialversicherung in Westeuropa* (From the Workhouse to the Welfare State: Analysis of the Development of Social Security in Western Europe) [in German]. Frankfurt: Campus.
Alber, J. (1995) 'A framework for the comparative study of social services', *Journal of European Social Policy*, 5 (2): 131–149.
Arts, W.A. and Gelissen, J. (2010) 'Models of the welfare state'. In: F.G. Castles, S. Leibfried, J. Lewis, H. Obinger and C. Pierson (eds), *The Oxford Handbook of the Welfare State*. Oxford: Oxford University Press, pp. 569–583.
Bambra, C. (2005) 'Worlds of welfare and the health care discrepancy', *Social Policy and Society*, 4 (1): 31–41.
Benoit, C., Wrede, S., Bourgeault, I., Sandall, J., De Vries, R. and Teijlingen, E.R. van (2005) 'Understanding the social organisation of maternity care systems: midwifery as a touchstone', *Sociology of Health & Illness*, 27 (6): 722–737.
Blekesaune, M. and Quadagno, J. (2003) 'Public attitudes toward welfare state policies: a comparative analysis of 24 nations', *European Sociological Review*, 19 (5): 415–427.

Burau, V. and Blank, R.H. (2006) 'Comparing health policy: an assessment of typologies of health systems', *Journal of Comparative Policy Analysis: Research and Practice*, 8 (1): 63–76.

Butler, I. and Drakeford, M. (2005) *Scandal, Social Policy and Social Welfare*. Bristol: Policy Press.

Cantelli, F., Kodate, N. and Krieger, K. (2011) 'Towards democratic governance of uncertainty? Contesting notions of participation, control and accountability', *Journal of Risk Research*, 14 (8): 919–932.

Castles, F.G. and Mitchell, D. (1991) *Three Worlds of Welfare Capitalism or Four?* Discussion Paper No. 21, Public Policy Program. Canberra: ANU.

Collingridge, D. (1996) 'Resilience, flexibility, and diversity in managing the risks of technologies'. In: C. Hood and D.K.C. Jones (eds), *Accident and Design. Contemporary Debates in Risk Management*. London: UCL Press, pp. 40–45.

Conrad, P. (1992) 'Medicalization and social control', *Annual Review of Sociology*, 18: 209–232.

De Vries, R., Wrede, S., Teijlingen, E. van and Benoit, C. (eds) (2001) *Birth by Design: Pregnancy, Maternity Care and Midwifery in North America and Europe*. New York: Routledge.

Dick-Read. G. (1942) *Revelation of Childbirth: The Principles and Practice of Natural Birth*. London: William Heinemann Medical Books.

Donnison, J. (1977) *Midwives and Medicine Men*. New York: Schocken.

Donnison, J. (1988) *Midwives and Medicine Men: a History of the Struggle for the Control of Childbirth*. London: Historical Publications.

Ehrenreich, B. and English, D. (1973) *Witches, Midwives, and Nurses: a History of Women Healers*. New York: The Feminist Press.

Esping-Andersen, G. (1990) *The Three Worlds of Welfare Capitalism*. Cambridge: Cambridge University Press.

Esping-Andersen, G. (1999) *Social Foundations of Postindustrial Economies*. Oxford: Oxford University Press.

Ferrera, M. (1996) 'The "Southern model" of welfare in Social Europe', *Journal of European Social Policy*, 6 (1): 17–37.

Giddens, A. (1998) 'Risk and responsibility', *Modern Law Review*, 62 (1): 1–10.

Giddens, A. (1999) *Runaway World*. London: Profile Books.

Hacker, J.S. (1998) 'The historical logic of national health insurance: structure and sequence in the development of British, Canadian, and U.S. medical policy', *Studies in American Political Development*, 12 (1): 57–130.

Hassenteufel, P. and Palier, B. (2007) 'Towards neo-Bismarckian health care states? Comparing health insurance reforms in Bismarckian welfare systems', *Social Policy & Administration*, 41 (6): 574–596.

Huber, E. and Bogliaccini, J. (2010) 'Latin America'. In: F.G. Castles, S. Leibfried, J. Lewis, H. Obinger and C. Pierson (eds), *The Oxford Handbook of the Welfare State*. Oxford: Oxford University Press, pp. 644–655.

Immergut, E.M. 1992. *Health Politics: Interests and Institutions in Western Europe*, Cambridge Studies in Comparative Politics. Cambridge: Cambridge University Press.

Jensen, C. (2008) 'Worlds of welfare services and transfers', *Journal of European Social Policy*, 18 (2): 151–162.

Kautto, M. (2002) 'Investing in services in West European welfare states', *Journal of European Social Policy*, 12 (1): 53–65.

Kemshall, H. (2002) *Risk, Social Policy and Welfare*. Buckingham: Open University Press.

Kennedy, P. (2012) 'Change in maternity provision in Ireland: "elephants on the move"', *The Economic and Social Review*, 43 (3): 377–395.

Kennedy, P. and Einasto, H. (2010) 'Changes and continuities in maternity policies: comparison of maternity legislation in Estonia and Ireland', *European Societies*, 12 (2): 187–207.

Kenyon, C. (2009) 'Risk management standards in midwifery are no substitute for personal knowledge and accountability', *Complementary Therapies in Clinical Practice*, 15 (4): 209–211.

Kitzinger, S. (1978) 'Pain in childbirth', *Journal of Medical Ethics*, 4 (3): 119–121.

Kitzinger, S. (1983) *The New Good Birth Guide*. Harmondsworth: Penguin.

Kitzinger, S. (1988) *Freedom and Choice in Childbirth*. London: Penguin Health Books.

Kodate, N. (2010) 'Events, public discourses and responsive government: quality assurance in health care in England, Sweden and Japan', *Journal of Public Policy*, 30 (3): 263–289.

Kodate, N. (2012) 'Events, politics and patterns of policy-making: impact of major incidents on health sector regulatory reforms in the UK and Japan', *Social Policy and Administration*, 46 (3): 280–301.

Kornai, J. (1992) *The Socialist System: the Political Economy of Communism*. Oxford: Oxford University Press.

Kuhlmann, E., Allsop, J. and Saks, M. (2009) 'Professional governance and public control: a comparison of healthcare in the United Kingdom and Germany', *Current Sociology*, 57 (4): 511–528.

Leboyer F. (1975) *Birth Without Violence*. London: Wildwood House.

Leboyer F. (1991) *Birth Without Violence*, 2nd edn. London: Mandarin.

McIntyre, M., Francis, K. and Chapman, Y. (2012) 'Primary maternity care reform: whose influence is driving chamge?' *Midwifery*, 28 (5): e705–e711.

Mackenzie Bryers, H. and Teijlingen, E. van (2010) 'Risk, theory, social and medical models: a critical analysis of the concept of risk in maternity care', *Midwifery*, 26 (5): 488–496.

Mechanic, D. and Rochefort, D.A. (1996) 'Comparative medical systems', *Annual Review of Sociology*, 22 (1): 239–270.

Meulen, R.H.J. ter, Arts, W.A. and Muffels, R.J.A. (2001) *Solidarity in Health and Social Care in Europe*. Dordrecht and London: Kluwer Academic.

Moran, M. (1995) 'Three faces of the health care state', *Journal of Health Politics, Policy and Law*, 20 (3): 767–785.

Murphy-Lawless, J. (1998) *Reading Birth and Death: a History of Obstetric Thinking*. Cork: Cork University Press.

Odent, M. (1984) *Birth Reborn*. New York: Pantheon.

OECD (2012) *Family Database*. Paris: OECD.

Oorschot, W. van (2007) 'Culture and social policy: a developing field of study', *International Journal of Social Welfare*, 16 (2): 129–139.

Orloff, A.S. (1993) 'Gender and the social rights of citizenship: the comparative analysis of state policies and gender relations', *American Sociological Review*, 58 (3): 303–328.

Peng, I. and Wong, J. (2010) 'East Asia'. In: F.G. Castles, S. Leibfried, J. Lewis, H. Obinger and C. Pierson (eds), *The Oxford Handbook of the Welfare State*. Oxford: Oxford University Press, pp. 656–670.

Pierson, C. (2011) *The Modern State*. London: Routledge.

Power, M. (2004) *The Risk Management of Everything*. London: Demos.

Rasmussen, J. (1997) 'Risk management in a dynamic society: a modelling problem', *Safety Science*, 27: 183–213.

Reibling, N. (2010) 'Healthcare systems in Europe: towards an incorporation of patient access', *Journal of European Social Policy*, 20 (1): 5–18.

Rosenthal, M.B. (2008) 'Beyond pay for performance – emerging models of pro-vider–payment reform', *New England Journal of Medicine*, 359 (12): 1197–1200.

Rothstein, B. (1998) *Just Institutions Matter: the Moral and Political Logic of the Universal Welfare State*. Cambridge: Cambridge University Press.

Rothstein, H., Huber, M. and Gaskell, G. (2006) 'A theory of risk colonization: the spiraling regulatory logics of societal and institutional risk', *Economy and Society*, 35: 91–112.

Saltman, R.B., Busse, R. and Figueras, J. (2004) *Social Health Insurance Systems in Western Europe*. Maidenhead: Open University Press.

Sandier, S., Paris, V. and Polton, D. (2004) 'France: health system review', *Health Systems in Transition*, 6 (2): 1–145.

Skocpol, T. and Ikenberry, G.J. (1983) 'The political formation of the American welfare state in historical and comparative perspective', *Comparative Social Research*, 6: 87–148.

Taylor-Gooby, P. (2004) *New Risks, New Welfare: the Transformation of the European Welfare State*. Oxford: Oxford University Press.

Tuohy C.J. (1999) *Accidental Logics: the Dynamics of Change in the Health Care Arena in the United States, Britain, and Canada*. Oxford: Oxford University Press.

Wagner M. (1994) *Pursuing the Birth Machine: the Search for Appropriate Birth Technology*. Sevenoaks: ACE Graphics.

Wendt, C. (2009) 'Mapping European healthcare systems: a comparative analysis of financing, service provision and access to healthcare', *Journal of European Social Policy*, 19 (5): 432–445.

Wilsford, D. (1994) 'Path dependency, or why history makes it difficult but not impossible to reform health care systems in a big way', *Journal of Public Policy*, 14: 251–283.

Wrede, S., Benoit, C. and Einarsdottir, T. (2008) Equity and dignity in maternity care provision in Canada, Finland and Iceland. *Canadian Journal of Public Health*, 99 (2): s16–s21.

2 New Zealand

*Riz Firestone, Anna Matheson, Barry Borman,
Laura D. Howe and Lis Ellison-Loschmann*

Background

Aotearoa (literally defined as *ao* = cloud, *tea* = white/pale, *roa* = long, i.e. 'long white cloud') (Maori Language Information 2014), or New Zealand, has a land area of 269,652 km², comparable with the size of the UK. Located in the southern hemisphere, sitting on the Pacific Rim, the country consists of North Island (*Te Ika-a-Māui*), South Island (*Te Waipounamu*) and many small islands. *Māori*, the Indigenous people of New Zealand, are believed to have arrived from Hawaiki, East Polynesia (Smith 2012). The British navigator, Lieutenant James Cook, was the first explorer to chart New Zealand on the world map from the late 1760s and this paved the way for British colonisation. Today, New Zealand is a multicultural nation in the Pacific Ocean. It is a constitutional monarchy with a unitary parliamentary democracy.

Māori have a special place and status in New Zealand that are enshrined in the Treaty of Waitangi, which has become the cornerstone for *Māori* rights through strenuous *Māori* political and civil action since the 1970s (Ministry for Culture and Heritage 2014). It is a powerful founding document that offers opportunities for both the *Māori* people and the Crown to work towards a common purpose: equality within one nation (Hill 2009; Smith 2012). Thus the *Māori* people have a priority status in terms of the ownership and use of land and natural resources; they have equal rights to employment and are a health priority group when addressing issues of health and social inequalities, particularly in improving access to, and passage through, health services.

In 2002, over 85 per cent of the population lived in a main urban area, thus New Zealand had become one of the most urbanised countries in the world (Bayley and Goodyear 2004). In New Zealand, the main urban areas are defined as being very large and centred on a city or main urban centre with populations of a minimum of 30,000. Rural centres are defined as having a population of 300–999 people in a small defined area that services the surrounding area (district territory) (Statistics New Zealand 2013a). European and *Māori* people largely reside in highly rural and remote areas; they account for one in three people, particularly in the Eastern Bay of Plenty regions (Bayley and Goodyear 2004).

New Zealand as a welfare regime

New Zealand's post-colonisation system of welfare has had a relatively short history, beginning when British settlers arrived in the late eighteenth century. A targeted pension (to deserving recipients, i.e. those of 'good moral standing') was introduced in 1898 and was regarded as the first instance of welfare in the newly colonised nation.

A dramatic expansion of entitlements occurred following World War I through the creation of many more 'deserving' individuals for whom the state needed to provide both medical and rehabilitation support and disability pensions. Much of the infrastructure for the post-1938 New Zealand welfare state was developed from this time. The Great Depression impacted substantially on the notion of deserving and undeserving individuals. The Labour Party came into power in 1935 on a platform of active management of the economy and a welfare system built on this example of the influence of the international environment.

The Social Security Act 1938 is frequently identified as setting the founding structure of New Zealand's welfare system. Following the austerity required of governments during the Great Depression in the 1930s, the Labour government, elected in 1935 on a platform of every New Zealander having the right to a decent standard of living, introduced and passed the 1938 Act. The Act, often viewed as one of the most important pieces of legislation in New Zealand's history, introduced a universal pension and an array of other welfare benefits, including an unemployment benefit. The Act also marked the introduction of a comprehensive free universal health system (French *et al.* 2001) and can therefore be regarded as a critical juncture in the development of New Zealand's welfare system.

During the post-war period, Labour policies were aimed at maintaining full employment at whatever cost, increasing birth rates and supporting men in the labour force. During the period from 1949 to 1972 and a barely interrupted reign of the National Party – there was little change or public appetite for reform of the welfare system.

This trend towards an inclusive view of citizenship was reinforced through the Social Security Act 1964 and further articulated and promoted with the establishment of the Royal Commission on Social Security in 1972. The Commission advanced and supported the vision for a compassionate and citizen-based view of those in need of welfare from the state, effectively doing away with notions of deserving and undeserving individuals.

From the mid-1980s, New Zealand's welfare regime was uniquely bold in its adoption of neoliberal ideals and their application to health and welfare. However, even the National Party government began to pull back from wholehearted market approaches in the mid-1990s. In 1996 the National Party–coalition government re-introduced the universal provision for doctors' visits for children under six years of age, discarded outpatient charges and reinstated universal superannuation. This pull back was extended when Labour came into power again in 1999.

Through the 2000s Labour expanded the public sector and the welfare state, but there was a growing public disillusionment with the 'nanny state' approach. The National Party was subsequently returned to power in 2008 and again began to dismantle public services. Both the political left and right have maintained the replacement of 'full citizenship' with indicators of labour market participation and a strong focus on work (O'Brien 2013).

To categorise New Zealand's welfare regime, Barnett and Barnett (2005) proposed a useful typology developed by Ware and Goodin (1990). The classification identifies residualist (needs-based), insurance (contributions-based) and social citizenship (rights-based) models of welfare. In Esping-Andersen's typology, New Zealand is classified as liberal, as are Canada and the UK, for its low decommodification index (Esping-Andersen 1990). However, Castles (1985) identified a radical Antipodian welfare state variant in New Zealand (together with Australia), with minimum wage legislation, compulsory arbitration and a protectionist consensus. Comparing the reforms of New Zealand's 'radical' or 'wage-earners' welfare state with those in Austria, Denmark and Switzerland, Obinger *et al.* (2010) found that New Zealand assumed the characteristics of a 'liberal' and 'residual' welfare state. However, in health care, Bambra (2005) underlined the high decommodification scores in New Zealand, Canada and the UK.

Health care system

New Zealand's health system is tax-based, universal in intended reach and has developed within and alongside the welfare system. An analysis of eleven high-income countries found that countries with tax-based health systems tend towards certain priorities (Tenbensel *et al.* 2012). For example, social insurance regimes tend to focus the system on efficiency and risk, whereas tax-based systems are more likely to consider population health outcomes in their health agendas. Moreover, centre-left governments are more likely to have the reduction of inequalities as a goal; systems that are tax-based are more likely to go beyond the health sector to address health outcomes. As described in the preceding section, New Zealand has oscillated between centre-left and centre-right governments, with reform to the health system reflecting these shifts in ideology.

In terms of health care expenditure, there is no defined right amount of what should be spent on health and, in making comparisons with other OECD countries, caution should be exercised given the different contexts and health needs of the population. Over a forty-year period, New Zealand's expenditure has fluctuated compared with other OECD countries. Total health care expenditure as a percentage of GDP was at an all-time low (5.2 per cent) in 1970 (French *et al.* 2001). It then increased to 7.1 per cent in the late 1970s and steadily returned to 5 per cent in the late 1980s. This reflected a depression in the economy. Through the next decade (the 1990s) there was a steady increase to 8.2 per cent on health expenditure, despite efforts to contain costs, and this was lower than the European Union average (French *et al.* 2001). By 2000, New Zealand ranked sixteenth in the OECD for health expenditure as a percentage of GDP and nineteenth for per capita health expenditure (French *et al.* 2001). This was an indicator that health expenditure in New Zealand was expected, given the state of its economy at the time. In 2011, the total expenditure on health was 8.5 per cent (OECD 2013).

Table 2.1 gives data for the human resources in primary health care and public health services in New Zealand. The most common physicians in New Zealand are general practitioners (GPs). Approximately 27 per cent of GPs work in sole private practices and 6 per cent in other organisations (French *et al.* 2001). More than 80 per cent of the total population had visited a GP in the last 12 months, as they hold the gate-keeping role to access public secondary and tertiary level services (French *et al.* 2001). With regard to maternity services, births were previously managed and supervised by a physician until the Nurses Amendment Act (1990), which permitted midwives to operate solely as an independent provider of pregnancy and childbirth services (French *et al.* 2001). The Health and Disability Services Act (1993), Notice under Section 51 (1996) introduced the concept of a Lead Maternity Carer (LMC), who retains overall clinical responsibility for a woman's maternity care; this notice mandated midwifery services at the time of birth. The biggest effect of this Amendment to the Act was evident in the change from a previously physician-dominated service to a midwifery maternity care system. In other primary care services, more than 3000 nurses work alongside GPs in private practices or in community-based or district health care services (French *et al.* 2001).

Table 2.1 Human and physical resources in health care in New Zealand

Physicians per 1,000 population	2.6
Nurses per 1,000 population	10
Medical graduates per 100,000 population	7.9
Nursing graduates per 100,000 population	36.7
Total hospital beds per 1,000 population	2.8
Curative (acute) care beds per 1,000 population	2.6
Obstetricians and gynaecologists per 100,000 women	14.5
Midwives per 100,000 women	112.8

Source: OECD (2013).

During the nineteenth century, public health administration was either non-existent or practised, often ineffectively, by local authorities with little or no central guidance. At the end of the century, fear of the introduction of plague led to the establishment of a professionally staffed Department of Health with a primary focus on public health, such as clean water, safe food, effective waste disposal and decent housing. Beyond public health, the early health services had little, other than compassion and comfort, to offer individuals for the treatment of established diseases (Martin and Salmond 2001).

This changed with the introduction of penicillin and other antibiotics in the 1940s. Following the surge in effective medical treatments, the focus of medical activity shifted strongly towards hospitals. Coinciding with a period of relative affluence and steady growth in the New Zealand economy, resources began flowing into the hospital system through the 1950s and up to the end of the 1970s (Martin and Salmond 2001). One outcome of these changes was the dominance of the medical profession in policy-making for health services.

Structural changes were introduced into the public sector from 1983 to 1991. For the health system, this meant decentralisation and the establishment of fourteen Area Health Boards as well as a move towards more autonomy for managers and purchase-of-services contracting (French *et al.* 2001). The year 1991 heralded the most severe market reforms in both health and welfare, with both Green and White papers outlining the changes to come and the 1993 Health and Disability Services Act shaping the implementation of the health reforms. The changes included the establishment of purchasing agencies in the form of four Regional Health Authorities charged with purchasing health services from both public and private providers, the targeting of primary health care resources and the introduction of a 'budget-holding' programme for GPs. This period also saw the emergence of alternative providers, especially non-profit community mental health services, services for the *Māori* population and primary care trusts. By 1996 the promises of these reforms were not being achieved and public tolerance was waning, with the notion of hospitals as businesses becoming increasingly unpopular (French *et al.* 2001). By 1997 the four Regional Health Authorities were collapsed into one Health Funding Authority and there was a move to less competition and greater collaboration.

With the election of a Labour-led coalition government in 1999 the reforms of the 1990s were almost completely overturned, including re-integrating the functions of purchasing and providing within one organisation. Hospitals were thus re-incorporated into regional agencies and twenty-one District Health Boards (DHBs) were established. The DHBs were designed to democratise (through elected boards) and decentralise planning and decision-making, as well as to coordinate and integrate regional health services. This change was essentially a return to the role hospitals held prior to the 1993 reforms (Toth 2010). From 2002 the government governed the creation of eighty Primary Healthcare Organisations designed to work across disciplines and to better manage complex conditions and reach population health goals (Gauld 2012). The New Zealand Health Strategy 2000 and the Primary Health Care Strategy 2001 were two important documents providing broad guidance to the health sector.

The implementation and operation of these new organisations did not entirely live up to their design intentions and, even before the election that led to a National Party government in 2008, their structure was revisited. For a small country of 4.3 million people, twenty District Health Boards and eighty Primary Healthcare Organisations were considered excessive, with high transaction costs and considerable duplication of planning, purchasing and administration. Whereas the Labour-led reforms had focused on community involvement in governance, local decision-making, public health strategies and reducing inequalities, the 2008 centre-right government prioritised clinical engagement, productivity, quality improvement and service access, particularly to elective surgery and cancer treatment (Gauld 2012).

Demographic profile

Overall, New Zealanders are generally well-educated, healthy and have a good standard of living (Statistics New Zealand 2013b). Table 2.1 shows the profile of New Zealand's demographics. Recent national health survey results indicated that nine out of ten adults rated their health as good, very good or excellent and nearly all parents (98 per cent) consider their children to be in good health (Ministry of Health 2013). A good proportion of adults (79 per cent) and children (75 per cent) had visited a GP in the past year and this was comparable with previous findings in national surveys (Ministry of Health 2013). The single most reported barrier to addressing health needs was cost. This continues to be a major issue, particularly for people residing in the most deprived areas (Ministry of Health 2013).

Recorded in mid-year 2013, approximately 50 per cent of the population of New Zealand was older than 37.1 years of age, compared with 32.0 years in June 2003. The ageing population is primarily due to low fertility and increasing life expectancy. On average, life expectancy for women is 83.0 years, compared with 79.4 years for men (Statistics New Zealand 2013c).

A total of 64,485 completed pregnancies were recorded during the calendar year 2010. The total birth rate was 7.0 completed pregnancies per 100 women of reproductive age (15–44 years). Asian women had the lowest birth rate (5.3 pregnancies per 100 women) and Pacific women had the highest birth rate (11.4 pregnancies per 100 women) (Ministry of Health 2012a).

The median age of New Zealand mothers giving birth is thirty years, compared with twenty-six years in the 1960s (Statistics New Zealand 2013c). There are large discrepancies between ethnic groups in New Zealand. The median maternal age for *Māori* women is twenty-five years, for Pacific women twenty-eight years, for Asian women thirty years and for other women thirty-one years (Ministry of Health 2012a). Pacific women have a much wider age range (20–33 years) of giving birth, whereas *Māori* women are much younger in age than other women (Ministry of Health 2012a). In terms of socio-economic deprivation, the median maternal age of women ranges from young (twenty-seven years) for the most deprived, to older (thirty-two years) for the least-deprived women (Ministry of Health 2012a).

As the population in New Zealand is progressively ageing, the number of deaths is expected to gradually increase as a result of the population growing older; this is partially explained by a longer life expectancy. Overall, deaths are largely concentrated in the older age group, with the median age at death in 2012 being seventy-eight years for men and eighty-three years for women. In comparison, a decade earlier, the median ages at death for men and women were seventy-two and seventy-nine years, respectively (Statistics New Zealand 2013c).

There is reasonable cultural diversity in New Zealand (Table 2.2). In 2013, the percentage of people who self-identified as belonging to the

Table 2.2 Demographic profile of New Zealand

Population[b]	*4,242,048*
Percentage of population women[b]	51.3
Percentage of population aged 0–14 years[b]	20.1
No. of women of childbearing age (15–44 years)[a]	919,720
Percentage of population aged 65 years and older[b]	14.3
Percentage annual growth of population[b]	0.7
Population density per square kilometre[c]	16.6[c]
Total fertility rate (births per woman)[a]	2.05
Crude birth rate (per 100 women)[a]	2.0
Infant mortality rate (per 1,000 live births)	4.4
Percentage population in urban areas[c]	37.0
Ethnic groups (%):	
European	74.0
Māori	14.9
Asian	11.8
Pacific peoples	7.4
Other	2.9

Notes
People who identify with more than one ethnic group are included in each ethnic population, so the percentages add up to more than 100.
a Ministry of Health (2012b).
b Statistics New Zealand (2013d).
c Measured in 2010 (New Zealand Economic Indicators 2014).

Māori population was 14.9 per cent (598,605 people). Pacific people made up 7.4 per cent of the population; this group comprises people from independent countries around the wider South Pacific region, such as Samoa, the Cook Islands, Tonga, Fiji, Niue and Tokelau – each of these countries has large communities residing in New Zealand and have identified a unique position in New Zealand society. People of European ethnicity make up 74 per cent, the largest proportion of the total population. Interestingly, Asian ethnic groups (mostly Chinese) make up 11.8 per cent of the total population and this group has almost doubled in size since 2001. English is the most common language in which people could hold a conversation about everyday things. The next most common languages are *Māori*, Samoan and Hindi (Statistics New Zealand 2013d).

Maternity provision

New Zealand's current maternity system has been characterised as woman-centred and community-based with continuity of care (between home and hospital, labour and postnatal care, and primary and secondary care) as a core tenet (Grigg and Tracy 2013). Midwives are currently autonomous practitioners and are the primary care-givers for most women (Lawton *et al.* 2013). Midwives have their own regulatory body (the Medical Council of New Zealand) and professional organisation (New Zealand College of Midwives). In line with welfare and health provision in New Zealand, maternity care is funded through taxation and is universal.

However, during the 1920s through to the 1980s, New Zealand was in plentiful company with other Western countries in its perspective and delivery of maternity care. This perspective saw the increasing hospitalisation and medicalisation of maternity care, shaped by regulatory and legislative changes giving greater control to the obstetric and nursing professions (Grigg and Tracy 2013).

An important factor in the blurring of the boundaries between nursing and midwifery was the shift of birthing from home to hospital. This shift took place between the 1920s and 1930s. As Tully and Mortlock indicate: 'As childbirth came to be understood as a pathological event most safely managed in hospitals by doctors, the role of midwives as independent birthing practitioners both in hospital and in the community was diminished' (2005: 135).

Reconstituting midwifery as a specialist nursing practice was formalised legally in the Nurses Act 1971, essentially removing the right of midwives to practice independently of doctors. The period following World War II also marked a time of relative affluence, aspirational welfare and health policy directions which saw resources flowing into hospitals and the medical profession generally having unparalleled authority and influence in health policy matters. The reach of globalisation, including an influx of new technologies and effective medicines and treatments during this time, also helped to further shape and strengthen a medicalised approach to childbirth in New Zealand.

The early 1970s saw the medical profession at the height of its authority and the third Labour government (elected in 1972) was forced to fight a hard battle over social security in health. A number of related pieces of legislation impacted on the shift to a midwifery-led maternity service. These included: the Public Health and Disability Act (2000), which enshrines the notion that pregnancy and childbirth are a 'normal' life stage; the Accident Compensation Corporation Act (2001), which protects health professionals from civil action and personal law suits; and the Health Practitioners Competence and Assurance Act (2003), which requires all health professions to have a regulatory body.

Maternity entitlements

Women in New Zealand are entitled to employment rights and maternity leave by way of a paid parental leave scheme. Women must have worked for the same employer for a minimum of ten hours per week for six to twelve months prior to their due date; however, the exact entitlement varies with each employer and it may depend on the length of time employed. Women and their respective partners can claim up to fourteen weeks of paid parental leave after the baby is born. Payment under this scheme replaces a woman's salary up to a weekly maximum amount and it ends if the woman resigns from her job or returns to work within the fourteen-week payment period. In comparison with Australia, New Zealand's paid parental leave system is at the lower end of international comparisons, falling well short of international best practice in terms of time offered, generosity of payment and gender equity provision. Financial support for Australian parents is more generous than that offered in New Zealand and takes better account of the realities of a flexible labour market (St John and Familton 2011).

Childbirth in New Zealand

In New Zealand, maternity care is free to women who: (i) are citizens or have permanent residency; (ii) have a work permit and stay for two years; or (iii) are eligible for other reasons (e.g. the woman's partner may be eligible for publicly funded maternity-related services). Babies born in New Zealand are also eligible for free health care until the age of six years if their mother is eligible for free maternity care. The nature of maternity services in New Zealand is collaborative and complex; however, there are two predominant maternity care providers: (i) community-based LMCs; and (ii) DHB-funded primary care providers. Maternity providers are defined as any organisation or individual that provides primary maternity services and holds a current annual certificate to practice.

Antenatal care

Expectant mothers are encouraged to register with an LMC or a primary care provider during their first trimester as this will provide free early care and advice during the first critical period of embryonic development. Registration involves the expectant mother selecting an appropriate LMC (usually personalised to the woman's needs and preferences) and registering with the maternal facility affiliated with the LMC or primary provider. Previously, under Section 88 of the Maternity Notice, community-based LMCs and DHB-funded providers were able to claim the costs related to maternal care during antenatal, labour and postnatal care. This is no longer the case. There is also variability in practice across the country and this makes it difficult to locate and compare information for specific regions where routine data are not available. However, from the data available in New Zealand, it is clear that midwives provide the most common form of maternity care for pregnant women.

The LMC or primary provider ensure there is continued maternal care, characterised by periodic engagement between the mother and the LMC or provider during the antenatal phase, labour, birth and through the four to six weeks of the postnatal period. Thus the nature of maternal care is continual and consistent for the mother and her baby throughout the entire care period. In 2010, 85.7 per cent (55,254) of women registered with an LMC at some point during the maternal care process and the remaining 14.3 per cent received care through other sources (e.g. DHB-funded services) or no care at all (Ministry of Health 2012a).

Women attend a maternity facility that is defined as a primary, secondary or tertiary service depending on the specialist services available. Women also have the option of choosing the place to give birth – whether this is at a maternity facility with a birthing unit or at home. The differences in facility use by women depend on a number of factors, including clinical need, bed availability, personal choice and geographical access (Ministry of Health 2012a). LMCs are responsible for all the care and provide necessary information during the antenatal screening phase. This includes the first antenatal blood screen to identify conditions that may affect the foetus and the mother (e.g. HIV screening, blood group and rhesus factor). Diagnostic testing occurs around 15–20 weeks of pregnancy and includes amniocentesis or chorionic villous sampling to detect genetic chromosomal conditions. As a result of the high risk of miscarriage (1 in 200 women) during diagnostic testing, women have the choice not to have these tests (Ministry of Health 2012a). Other antenatal tests can be offered to 'at-risk' women around 26–28 weeks of pregnancy to screen for gestational diabetes. Receiving care from a specialist or specialist services, such as ultrasound scans (charged fees) or laboratory tests (often free of charge), may become necessary should complications arise during pregnancy or labour. The LMC discusses the reasons for the use of these options and conducts the referral or transfers the responsibility of care to a specialist, if necessary (Ministry of Health 2012a). Antenatal education classes are optional and, unless pregnant women attend government-funded classes, a fee is charged for their services. Although there is a range of services and options available for women during this phase of pregnancy, the LMC is responsible for her overall care. Visits with the LMC usually occur once every six weeks in the first trimester, once a month in the second trimester and then fortnightly in the early stage of the third trimester and weekly from thirty-four weeks of pregnancy until delivery. However, women are free to contact their LMC at any stage to seek advice, or should they wish to be seen by the LMC.

Information on maternal smoking is routinely collected at the time of registration and two weeks postpartum. The prevalence (18.1 per cent) of smoking among all adults in New Zealand is low compared with other OECD countries such as Greece, which has the highest rate of 39.7 per cent (Ministry of Social Development 2010). *Māori* (55.9 per cent) and Pacific (26.3 per cent) women are demonstrably the groups with the highest percentage of smokers and maternal smoking rates almost mirror those of the general population (Ministry of Health 2013). Of all women registered in 2010, 16.2 per cent of women smoked at the time of registration and the rate of smoking was higher in younger women (37.0 per cent) and among *Māori* women (38.4 per cent). Researchers have reported that women who smoke during pregnancy have a two-fold risk of having maternal asthma, a low birthweight baby and a baby that dies from sudden infant death syndrome.

Intrapartum care

In New Zealand, a large proportion (65 per cent) of women give birth by spontaneous vaginal delivery (including home births) and 23.6 per cent of women give birth by caesarean section (Ministry of Health 2012a) (Table 2.3). Caesarean sections are classified in two ways: (i) an elective caesarean, where the date of the procedure is planned before the onset of labour, regardless of whether it is performed before or following the onset of labour; and (ii) an emergency caesarean carried out due to an emergency situation (e.g. foetal distress) (Ministry of Health 2012a). *Māori* and Pacific women are more likely to have a spontaneous vaginal birth (74.9 and 71.5 per cent, respectively) than Asian women and women in other ethnic groups (57.4 and 60.4 per cent, respectively). Approximately 28 per cent of the women who give birth by caesarean section are more likely to be in the least-deprived socio-economic group, which is the opposite trend to that for women who experience a spontaneous vaginal birth (Ministry of Health 2012a).

Spontaneous vaginal births are more common (74 per cent) in women aged less than twenty years compared with women aged 40+ years. The proportion of women who underwent caesarean sections increases with maternal age, ranging from 14.2 per cent of women less than twenty years old to 38.5 per cent of women aged forty and over (Ministry of Health 2012).

The percentage of women who opt to give birth at home and not in a maternity facility or birthing unit is small. Only 3.2 per cent of women actually gave birth at home in 2010 and 3.6 per cent of women intended to have a home birth, but ended up giving birth at a maternity facility (Ministry of Health 2012).

New Zealand's infant mortality rate is historically low and continues to be stable compared with that in other developed countries (Ministry of Health 2012b). The main cause of death for 62.7 per cent of all foetal and infant deaths was classified as conditions originating in the perinatal period (ICD Code P969, Condition originating in the perinatal period, unspecified) and 72.8 per cent of these deaths were foetal deaths (National Centre for Classification in Health 2008). This includes data aggregated for 2008 and 2009 due to a small number of deaths from some causes. Maternal death is the:

> death of a woman while pregnant or within 42 days of termination of pregnancy, irrespective of the duration and site of the pregnancy, from any cause related to or aggravated by the pregnancy or its man-agement, but not from accidental or incidental causes.
> (National Centre for Classification in Health 2008)

In 2007, of 65,602 pregnant women there were eleven recorded maternal deaths, resulting in a maternal mortality ratio of 16.8 per 100,000 maternities. Five of these deaths were directly related to pregnancy (maternal mortality ratio 7.6 per 100,000 maternities) and were related to the suboptimum management of hypertension, reduced care in women with complex medical problems and barriers in accessing care (Perinatal and Maternal Mortality Review Committee 2007). Regardless of the small number of maternal deaths, recommendations to improve services to address hyper-tension in pregnancy and access to services have been strongly endorsed. Table 2.3 provides an overview of the available data of selected birth inter-ventions and outcomes from 1970 to 2010.

Postnatal care

LMCs provide up to six to eight weeks of postnatal care for the new mother and her baby. During this time, the baby is screened for many health conditions or problems while in hospital and at home – the LMC visits the mother and baby at home up to ten times. Babies are offered a screening test for hearing within forty-eight hours of birth and, if neces-sary, are referred to an audiologist for further diagnostic testing.

Table 2.3 Birth interventions and outcomes for selected years in New Zealand

	1970s	1980s	1990s	2000s	2010
Maternal mortality ratio	0.32	1.4	18.0	12.0	15.0
Perinatal deaths per 1,000 total live births	19.6[a]	12.2[b]	7.4[c]	9.5	10.2
Perinatal deaths per 1,000 total still births	–	7.2[b]	8.2	3.1	3.0
Neonatal deaths per 1,000 live births	10.3[a]	6.0	4.2[c]	3.8	3.6
Infant mortality per 1,000 live births (approx.)	16.7	13.0	8.4[c]	6.3	5.5
Induction rate per 100 deliveries	–	–	27.2	20.4	19.8
Forceps-only delivery per 100 deliveries	–	–	5.3	0.1	3.3
Vacuum extraction only delivery per 100 deliveries	–	–	4.8	6.0	5.8
Caesarean section (per 100 live births)	–	–	27.5	20.8	24.0
Episiotomy rate per vaginal delivery (%)	–	–	12.1	13.0	12.5

Notes
a National Health Statistics Centre (1972).
b National Health Statistics Centre (1982).
c Ministry of Health (1994).

There is a strong culture of encouraging mothers to breastfeed their newborn babies to provide the best start in life, as well as to develop a maternal bond between mother and child. Breastfeeding is more than a physiological process. It is a learned activity that involves a dynamic interaction within a complex set of social, cultural and experiential factors (National Breastfeeding Advisory Committee of New Zealand 2009). Over 91 per cent of babies were recorded to be breastfed at discharge either exclusively (70.4 per cent), fully (including breast milk stored in bottles) (9.4 per cent) or partially (12.1 per cent) (Glover *et al.* 2007). According to Plunket Society data for 2006, the overall rate of breastfeeding at six weeks was 66 per cent and 55 per cent at three months, with lower rates in the *Māori* and Pacific populations; Asian mothers have similar breastfeeding rates to *Māori* and Pacific women at six weeks (Thornley *et al.* 2007). In 2007 the Ministry of Health adopted a breastfeeding target to 'increase the proportion of infants exclusively and fully breastfed at six weeks to 74 per cent or greater, three months to 57 per cent or greater, and six months to 27 per cent or greater'. There is also a large amount of knowledge generated from groups who have found that, in general, women want to breastfeed their babies and understand that it is the best nutritional form for their baby, although a range of barriers may inhibit their capability and capacity to do so. Therefore breastfeeding promotional campaigns are used to support women in a range of contexts, including the health system, home, community settings and workplaces (Thornley *et al.* 2007).

Section 88 of the Primary Maternity Services Notice legally requires the LMC to record the transfer of the woman and her baby to a primary care provider such as a GP and/or another national service that supports growing families (e.g. the Plunket Society). For New Zealand, the majority of women and their babies are referred to their GP at discharge (91.5 per cent) and, at the same time, referrals are also made to other services (the Plunket Society, 92.5 per cent). Infants begin their schedule of immunisation for protection against a variety of diseases at six weeks and this continues at three months, five months, fifteen months and four years after birth. The vaccinations are freely available and completely optional, although strongly endorsed. In 2010, the national uptake of vaccinations for infants up to two years of age was 88.3 per cent (Ministry of Health 2011).

Consumer involvement

By the 1980s, relationships between doctors and patients were becoming more problematic and the supremacy of the professions was being challenged on a number of fronts. A number of researchers attribute the strong move in New Zealand to the reclaiming of maternity services by the midwifery profession to the growing strength of consumer groups and to the politically active role women have played historically (Belgrave 2004; Tully and Mortlock 2005; Grigg and Tracy 2013). In particular, the role of the Royal New Zealand Plunket Society (founded in 1907), which grew into a large and powerful consumer-led organisation, is viewed as critical (Bryder 2003). The Plunket Society provides nurses to go into the homes of newborn babies and provide health monitoring and advice, offers clinics for older babies and provides antenatal care. Plunket Society services have been, and continue to be, free services to all women, with funding to the organisation coming through voluntary donations and from the government. In 1940 the Director General of Health argued that infant health should be integral to the work of the Health Department and not the responsibility of a voluntary organisation. Thus a series of decisions and policy arrangements began that were aimed at excluding, or at least controlling, the Plunket Society's role in infant health. Despite these attempts, the Plunket Society retained its role in infant care. It is argued that they had huge public support and were politically astute as an organisation, which gave them a significant voice in the direction taken by maternity care (Bryder 2003).

A further major event that eroded public confidence in the medical profession was a series of controversial experiments in the treatment of abnormal Pap smears at National Women's Hospital in Auckland (Beere and Brabyn 2006). The ensuing Cartwright Enquiry (1987–1988) exposed questionable practices, including a lack of consent from women, with the fallout from these experiments resulting in the setting up of national ethical standards and processes in health research (New Zealand Committee of Inquiry into Allegations Concerning the Treatment of Cervical Cancer at National Women's Hospital, & into Other Related Matters 1988).

Consumer groups with strong voices and a withering of confidence in the medical profession influenced the trajectory of maternity services, leading to the current midwifery-led services provided in New Zealand. A pivotal event was the passing of the 1990 Nurses Amendment Act. The Act resulted in midwifery again being recognised as a separate profession from nursing and gave autonomy to the status of midwifery as a nursing specialty. The then Minister of Health, Helen Clark, in her preamble to the Act stated that: 'The majority of women have been socialised to perceive birth as an illness. The challenge of this legislation is to change that perception' (Grigg and Tracy 2013: e59).

Risk and rights

Perceived risks and adverse outcomes have been identified as being linked to communication challenges between health professionals and to different opinions about when referral from primary to secondary care is necessary (Rowland *et al.* 2012). For New Zealand, three high-level strategies have been developed to guide the planning, funding, provision and monitoring of maternity services (Ministry of Health 2011): These are: (i) to provide safe, high-quality services that are consistent across the country and achieve optimal health outcomes for mothers and babies; (ii) to ensure a woman-centred approach that acknowledges pregnancy and childbirth as a normal life stage; and (iii) to ensure all women have access to a nationally consistent, comprehensive range of maternity services that are funded and to remove financial barriers to access for eligible women.

The National Maternity Monitoring Group (NMMG) was established in 2012 to oversee the maternity system and the implementation of these standards to ensure best practice was achieved. The NMMG analysed DHB and National Maternity Collection 2012 data to ascertain how the level of, and access to, LMC registration could be improved. Once the data had been reviewed, the NMMG wrote to each DHB requesting information about how they engaged women to register with an LMC, encouraged women to engage with primary maternity services in the first trimester and facilitated service links with GPs to support referrals between GPs and LMCs (NMMG 2013).

The NMMG reported the following themes, which serve to protect the rights and reduce the risks to pregnant women. DHBs should: (i) develop governance structures that include LMC and consumer representation at governance level; (ii) use dedicated resources to coordinate a specific programme; (iii) have good consumer engagement at different levels of the programme and learn how to communicate with consumers and consumer groups (e.g. newsletters, web sites, focus groups); (iv) review how they collate and use data; (v) integrate information to improve or establish programmes; (vi) establish communication networks to improve information-sharing between community and hospital-level clinicians, and between women and families; and (vii) carry out local audits against the New Zealand maternity standards to improve quality and safety.

Advances in technology and improved maternity systems have reduced the incidence of maternal and infant deaths in New Zealand compared with those in the 1970s. The Perinatal and Maternal Mortality Review Committee (established in 2006) in New Zealand conducts a national audit, reviewing each death and morbidity (e.g. preterm birth) as an indicator for improving the quality of care. The review committee also evaluates overall care from the consumer's point of view and the results are that mothers are generally satisfied with the maternity care they have received (Rowland *et al.* 2012).

With regard to the health professionals overseeing maternity care, as noted earlier, a 1996 Notice was issued under Section 51 of the Health and Disability Services Act (1993), which gave rise to the concept of an LMC who would provide overall responsibility for maternity care. Although the New Zealand College of Midwives accepted the Notice, the New Zealand Medical Association rejected it outright, resulting in an amendment in 1998 to separate out the fee for doctor LMCs when using hospital-based midwifery support services. In addition, doctor LMCs were not required to formalise subcontracts with midwives. In 1999 the National Health Committee reviewed the system and highlighted areas for improvement; however, this did not result in any substantive changes to the framework.

Since the New Zealand Public Health and Disability Act (2000) (previous Sections and the current Section 88), the issue of a Notice, the Primary Maternity Services Notice (2007), and, subsequently, an Amendment Notice (2012), have attempted to reduce any tension between professionals by defining the specifications, roles and responsibilities of:

- **Maternity objectives:** the main objective is to empower service users with knowledge, support and skills to: (i) access pregnancy and parenting advice, support and services; (ii) make informed choices relating to pregnancy, childbirth and early parenting; (iii) develop positive and responsible early parenting skills; (iv) build self-esteem and confidence to improve their experience of pregnancy, childbirth and early parenting, and (v) the service is expected to contribute to the reduction in health inequalities by tailoring the intensity of service provided depending on the needs of different service users.
- **Services:** to provide a layered service offering pregnancy and parenting education and information and support, as necessitated by the service user;
- **Service users:** defined as pregnant women, expectant fathers/partners, parents of new babies and their families.
- **Access:** to the service is self-referral or referral from the following:
  - general practitioner, LMC or other maternity care provider;

- other non-governmental organisations/*Māori* health service providers;
- primary and secondary mental health services;
- *whānau* (family), *marae*-based services (marae means a traditional *Māori* tribal meeting place);
- teachers, school nurses and social workers; and
- other social agencies, e.g. Child Youth and Family.
- **Other general service components:** e.g. service linkages, exclusions, quality requirements and service purchasing units are also defined within this Notice.

Conclusion

New Zealand's maternity care system fulfils a crucial component within public health services. It is considered to be a unique maternity system in which the relationship between the carer and the woman is viewed as a partnership. Midwives dominate the provision of these services and provide a high level of independent professional care, often working collaboratively with specialists and specialist services. The welfare system has been underpinned by a mix of needs- and rights-based approaches, with the current balance seeing a greater emphasis on 'needs' rather than 'rights' and with greater links between welfare and work incentives. New Zealand's health system is tax-based, universal in intended reach and has developed within and alongside the welfare system. Health care, including maternity care, is mostly free for citizens and permanent residents of New Zealand up to the age of six years; thereafter health care is partly subsidised by the government. Public and government investments in the relevant maternity entitlements, particularly in postnatal care, paid parental leave, breastfeeding and smoking cessation campaigns, are encouraging. Reducing social health inequalities for high priority groups such as *Māori* and Pacific women and their babies will be an ongoing challenge, yet many public health efforts that aim to improve overall care and accessibility and to reduce barriers are being addressed.

References

Bambra, C. (2005) 'Worlds of welfare and the health care discrepancy', *Social Policy & Society*, 4 (1): 31–41.

Barnett, P. and Barnett, R. (2005) 'Reform and change in health service provision'. In: K. Dew and P. Davis (eds), *Health and Society in Aoteroa New Zealand.* Melbourne: Oxford University Press, pp. 178–193.

Bayley, A. and Goodyear, R. (2004) *New Zealand: an Urban/Rural Profile. Developing the Classifications.* Wellington: Statistics New Zealand Tatauranga Aotearoa.

Beere, P. and Brabyn, L. (2006) 'Providing the evidence: geographic accessibility of maternity units in New Zealand', *New Zealand Geographer*, 62: 135–143.

Belgrave, M. (2004) 'Needs and the state: evolving social policy in New Zealand'. In: B. Dalley and M. Tennant (eds), *In Past Judgement: Social Policy in New Zealand History.* Dunedin: Otago University Press, pp. 23–38.

Bryder, L. (2003) 'Two models of infant welfare in the first half of the twentieth century: New Zealand and the USA', *Women's History Review,* 12: 547–558.

Castles, F.G. (1985) *The Working Class and Welfare. Reflections on the Political Development of the Welfare State in Australia and New Zealand 1890–1980.* Wellington: Allen & Unwin.

Esping-Andersen, G. (1990) *The Three Worlds of Welfare Capitalism.* Cambridge: Cambridge University Press.

French, S., Old, A. and Healy, J. (2001) *Health Care Systems in Transitions: New Zealand.* Copenhagan: The European Observatory on Health Care Systems.

Gauld, R. (2012) 'New Zealand's post-2008 health system reforms: toward re-centralization of organisational arrangements', *Health Policy,* 106: 110–113.

Glover, M., Manaen-Biddle, H and Waldon, J. (2007) 'Influences that affect Maori women breastfeeding', *Maori Breastfeeding Review,* 15 (2): 5–14.

Grigg, C. and Tracy, S. (2013) 'New Zealand's unique maternity system', *Women and Birth,* 26: e59–e64.

Hill, R.S. (2009) 'Maori and State'. In: G. Byrnes (ed.), *The New Oxford History of New Zealand.* Melbourne: Oxford University Press, pp. 33–54.

Lawton, B., Koch, A., Stanley, J. and Geller, S. (2013) 'The effect of midwifery care on rates of cesarean delivery', *International Journal of Gynecology & Obstetrics,* 123: 213–216.

Maori Language Information (2014) *Maori Language Information* [online]. Available from: www.maorilanguage.info/index.html. Accessed January 2014.

Martin, J. and Salmond, G. (2001) 'Policy making: the "messy reality"', In: P. Davis, and T. Ashton (eds), *Health and Public Policy in New Zealand.* Auckland: Oxford University Press, pp. 44–61.

Ministry for Culture and Heritage (2014) *NZ History Online* [online]. Available from: www.mch.govt.nz/research-publications. Accessed 18 January 2014.

Ministry of Health (1994) *Fetal and Infant Deaths. Wellington: New Zealand Health Information Service.* Wellington: Ministry of Health.

Ministry of Health (2011) *Immunisation Handbook 2011.* Wellington: Ministry of Health.

Ministry of Health (2012a) *Fetal and Infant Deaths 2008 and 2009.* Wellington: Ministry of Health.

Ministry of Health (2012b) *Report on Maternity, 2010.* Wellington: Ministry of Health.

Ministry of Health (2013) *Health, New Zealand Health Survey: Annual Update of Key Findings 2012/2013.* Wellington: Ministry of Health.

Ministry of Social Development (2010) *The Social Report.* Wellington: Ministry of Social Development.

National Breastfeeding Advisory Committee of New Zealand (2009) *National Strategic Plan of Action for Breastfeeding 2008–2012: National Breastfeeding Advisory Committee of New Zealand's advice to the Director-General of Health.* Wellington: Ministry of Health.

National Centre for Classification in Health (2008) *The International Statistical Classification of Diseases and Related Health Problems,* 6th edn (ICD-10-AM). Sydney: National Centre for Classification in Health.

National Health Statistics Centre (1972) *National Health Statistics 1972.* Wellington: Department of Health.

National Health Statistics Centre (1982) *National Health Statistics 1982.* Wellington: Department of Health.

National Maternity Monitoring Group (2013) *Annual Report 2013* [online]. Available from: www.health.govt.nz/publication/national-maternity-monitoring-group-annual-report-2013. Accessed 30 June 2014.

New Zealand Committee of Inquiry into Allegations Concerning the Treatment of Cervical Cancer at National Women's Hospital, & into Other Related Matters (1988) *The Report of the Committee of Inquiry into Allegations Concerning the Treatment of Cervical Cancer at National Women's Hospital and into Other Related Matters* [online]. Available from: www.moh.govt.nz/notebook/nbbooks.nsf/0/64D0EE1 9BA628E4FCC256E450001CC21/$file/The%20Cartwright%20Inquiry%201988. pdf. Accessed 30 June 2014.

New Zealand Economic Indicators (2014) *Trading Economics* [online]. Available from: www.tradingeconomics.com/new-zealand/indicators. Accessed May 2014.

O'Brien, M. (2013) 'Welfare reform in Aotearoa/New Zealand: from citizen to managed worker', *Social Policy and Administration*, 47: 729–748.

Obinger, H., Starke, P., Moser, J., Bogedan, C., Gindulis, E. and Leibfried, S. (2010) *Transformations of the Welfare State: Small States, Big Lessons.* Oxford: Oxford University Press, 334 pp.

OECD (2013) 'Country statististical profiles: New Zealand' [online]. Available from: www.oecd-ilibrary.org/economics/country-statistical-profile-new-zealand_ 20752288-table-nzl. Accessed 30 June 2014.

Perinatal and Maternal Mortality Review Committee (2007) *Perinatal and Maternal Mortality in New Zealand 2007: Third Report to the Minister of Health July 2008 to June 2009.* Wellington: Ministry of Health.

Rowland, T., McLeod, D. and Froese-Burns, N. (2012) *Comparative Study of Maternity Systems.* Wellington: Malatest International Consulting and Advisory Services.

St John, S. and Familton, A. (2011) *Paid Parental Leave in New Zealand: Catching Up with Australia.* Auckland: Child Poverty Action Group.

Smith, A. (1986) *The Ethnic Origins of Nations.* Oxford: Blackwell.

Smith, P.M. (2012) *A Concise History of New Zealand*, 2nd edn. Melbourne: Cambridge University Press.

Statistics New Zealand (2013a) *New Zealand in Profile 2013: an Overview of New Zealand's People, Economy, and Environment.* Wellington: Statistics New Zealand Tatauranga Aotearoa.

Statistics New Zealand (2013b) *Births and Deaths Year Ending December 2012.* Wellington: Statistics New Zealand Tatauranga Aotearoa.

Statistics New Zealand (2013c) *National Population Estimates: at 30 June 2013.* Wellington: Statistics New Zealand Tatauranga Aotearoa.

Statistics New Zealand (2013d) *2013 Census Quick Stats About National Highlights.* Wellington: Statistics New Zealand Tatauranga Aotearoa.

Tenbensel, T., Eagle, S. and Ashton, T. (2012) 'Comparing health policy agendas across eleven high income countries: islands of difference in a sea of similarity', *Health Policy*, 106: 29–36.

Thornley, L., Waa, A. and Ball, J. (2007) *Comprehensive Plan to Inform the Design of a National Breastfeeding Promotion Campaign.* Wellington: Quigley and Watts/Ministry of Health.

Toth, F. (2010) 'Healthcare policies over the last 20 years: reforms and counter-reforms', *Health Policy*, 95: 82–89.

Tully, E. and Mortlock, B. (2005) 'Professionals and practices'. In: K. Dew and P. Davis (eds), *Health and Society in Aotearoa New Zealand*. Melbourne: Oxford University Press, pp. 130–145.

Ware, A. and Goodin, R.E. (1990) *Needs and Welfare*, Vol. 26. London: Sage.

WHO (2012) *Obesity and Overweight*. Available from: www.who.int/mediacentre/factsheets/fs311/en/. Accessed 30 June 2014.

World Bank (2014) *Birth Rate, Crude (per 1,000 People)* [online]. Available from: http://data.worldbank.org/indicator/SP.DYN.CBRT.IN/countries/NZ–XS?display=graph. Accessed 30 June 2014.

3 Ireland

Patricia Kennedy

Background

Ireland is an island on the periphery of Europe. It has been a republic since it achieved independence from Britain in 1922. Ireland joined the European Economic Community (now the European Union) in 1973. The population of Ireland is 4.6 million (Central Statistics Office 2011). Ireland was predominantly monocultural until it experienced unprecedented immigration at the end of the 1990s; since then it has quickly become a multicultural society. The number of Irish residents who were born outside Ireland continues to increase and was 766,770 in 2011, an increase of 25 per cent from 2006 and representing 17 per cent of the population. Ireland experienced strong economic growth between the late 1990s and 2007, earning it the name 'Celtic Tiger'. Between 1994 and 2007 there was an annual average growth of 7.3 per cent in the GDP and 6.6 per cent the GNP. Since 2007 Ireland has experienced severe economic recession. In 2010 the level of the GDP was 11 per cent below the level of the GNP and both measures were, in real terms, about 15 per cent below their respective levels in 2007. The unemployment rate rose from 4.6 per cent in 2007 to 13.8 per cent in 2010 (Central Statistics Office 2011). The gap between government receipts and spending was almost €19 billion in 2010 (National Recovery Plan 2010). Since the recession, Ireland's policies have been strongly influenced by the troika of the European Central Bank, the International Monetary Fund and the European Commission. This has had implications for the provision of both social services and health services.

Ireland as a welfare regime

During the Celtic Tiger period there was much interest in Ireland from scholars of welfare regimes because of its strong and strident economic growth. Payne and McCashin referred to 'the persistent problem of placing Ireland in regime terms' (2005: 16). In 1990 Esping-Andersen located Ireland in the liberal category of welfare states on the basis of its low decommodification score. He described Ireland as having low scores on socialist regime attributes, low scores on liberal attributes and medium scores on conservatism (Esping-Andersen 1990). Lewis (1992) described Ireland as a 'strong male breadwinner state', characterised by a strong influence from the church, Catholic social teaching, a traditional role for the family, the under-representation of women in full-time employment and under-developed childcare services. Cochrane and Clarke (1993) described Ireland as Catholic–corporatist. A decade later, Millar and Adshead (2004; cited in Payne and McCashin 2005) concluded that Catholic–corporatism is still useful in categorising the Irish welfare state. Daly and Yeates (2003: 94) point to the strong British influence in the emergence and later development of the Irish social security system and identify a 'new corporatism' as an important factor in the development of social security policy. Bonoli (1997) presents a 'two-dimensional' analysis of the scale of state social spending and the source of revenue (whether taxation or social insurance); Ireland is categorised as liberal associated with a low level of state spending and a low share of social insurance in the overall social spending. The National Economic and Social Council (NESC 2005) described Ireland as a hybrid welfare regime, a mix of liberal and corporatist welfare.

Health care system

The Irish health care system has been described as an 'extraordinary symbiosis of public and private medicine' (Barrington 1987: 285). Ireland is unique among Western European countries because universal coverage for primary care only applies to low income groups. In 2012, 45.8 per cent of the population was covered by private health insurance (Health Insurance Authority 2012). The Irish health care system has been classified by the OECD as a 'duplicate' system – that is, one in which insurance complements, supplements, but also duplicates the health care offered by the public system (OECD 2004). In duplicate systems, private health insurance usually guarantees a level of care, choice and speed of access superior to that of the public system. Entitlement to public health services in Ireland is primarily based on residency and means-testing, rather than on the payment of tax or pay-related social insurance or medical need. Any person, regardless of nationality, who is ordinarily resident in Ireland is entitled to either full eligibility (category 1 or medical card holders) or limited eligibility (category 2) for health services. By the end of 2012, 40 per cent of the population had a medical card compared with 28 per cent in 2005.

In category 1 eligibility, the medical card holder and their dependent spouse or partner and children are covered for the same range of health services and can receive certain health services free of charge. To qualify for a medical card, a person's cash income, savings, investments and property (except for the family home) are taken into account in the means-testing. In category 2 eligibilty, those who do not have a medical card are entitled to free public hospital services and subsidised prescribed drugs and medicines, but may have to pay inpatient and outpatient hospital charges. Since 2005 some people who do not hold a medical card may be entitled to a general practitioner (GP) visit card, which guarantees free GP visits to those over the maximum income for medical cards. In 2012, 131,102 people (2.9 per cent of the population) had GP visit cards. A range of services is provided free of charge for children, even if their parents do not have a medical card. These services are generally provided as part of the Maternity and Infant Care Scheme, health services for pre-school children and school health services, including free vaccination and immunisation services. In the 2014 budget it was announced that free GP care will be introduced during 2014 for all children aged five years and under. This is a critical juncture as it is only the second time that universal health services will be provided to a cohort of the population. In 2001, entitlement to medical cards was extended to all those aged seventy years and older, but this was rescinded in 2009 when means-testing was re-introduced.

Overall responsibility for the health care system lies with the Department of Health under the direction of the Minister of Health. In 2005, the eight Health Boards that had been responsible for the provision of health care and personal social services were abolished and replaced by the Heath Services Executive (HSE), a single body that manages all the public health services in Ireland. The HSE has three key divisions responsible for (i) population health, (ii) hospitals and (iii) primary, community and continuing care. The hospital sector incorporates both voluntary and HSE-owned hospitals. Voluntary hospitals are primarily financed by the state, but may be owned and operated by religious or lay boards of governors. Beds within these hospitals may be designated for either public or private use. There is also a small number of private hospitals. Hospital consultants have contracts with the public sector, but also supplement their income through private activity.

The government has promised to reform the health system completely, as outlined in the report Future Health: a Strategic Framework for Reform of the Health Service 2012–2015 (Department of Health 2012). It plans to introduce a single-tier health service, supported by a universal health insurance designed in accordance with the principles of social solidarity. This will shift the emphasis and entitlement from income to medical need and everyone will be insured for a standard package of health services. This is another critical juncture for the Irish health services, as it is a move away from a two-tiered general taxation and privately funded system towards a more continental model based on social insurance.

There is ample evidence that the Irish health care system is in crisis (Wren 2003; O'Connor 2007; Burke 2009). Considine and Dukelow (2009) outlined how the HSE 'has been subjected to a barrage of criticism' in relation to the adequacy of the health budget, the appropriateness of budgetary decisions, accountability, and administrative and other failures all 'highlighted by a number of high-profile cases involving misdiagnosis and inappropriate care' (Considine and Dukelow 2009: 265). This is particularly pertinent to maternity care as two high-profile cases have recently come to public attention: the death of Savita Halappanavar (Health Information and Quality Authority 2013) from septicaemia in 2012 and the death of an unprecedented number of newborn babies in the Midlands Hospital (Holohan 2014) over several years. Prior to these, malpractice by Dr Michael Neary, who performed an excessive number of peripartum hysterectomies, was investigated in 2006 (Harding Clarke 2006). In 2007 a statutory, government-funded agency, the Health Information and Quality Authority (HIQA) was established to monitor the safety and quality of health and social care in Ireland. A year later there was an inquiry into the death of Mrs Tania McCabe and her infant son Zach at Our Lady of Lourdes Hospital, Drogheda in March 2007 (Tania McCabe Inquiry 2008).

A number of professional associations and statutory bodies play a role in regulating health care professionals in Ireland. The Clinical Indemnity Scheme is managed by the State Claims Agency, which deals with clinical negligence claims and associated risks of hospitals and other health agencies. Under the Scheme, the government is fully responsible for the indemnification and management of all clinical negligence claims, which include birth-related claims. Since 2008, the Clinical Indemnity Scheme has covered medical malpractice indemnity in respect of self-employed community midwives (SECMs).

An Bord Altranais agus Cnáimhseachais na hÉireann, the Nursing and Midwifery Board of Ireland (NMBI) is the regulatory body for the nursing profession. Since the Nurses Act 1985, midwifery has been subsumed under nursing; in 2012 An Bord Altranais (the Nursing Board) was replaced by the NMBI to reflect the recognition of midwifery as a separate and distinct profession to that of nursing. In 2011 the Nurses and Midwives Act was signed into law. This Act updated the provisions relating to the regulation of nurses and midwives. One of the functions of the Board is to inquire into the conduct of a registered nurse on the grounds of alleged professional misconduct or alleged unfitness to engage in such practice by reason of physical or mental disability. In 2013 there were 94,715 nurses registered and, of this total, 87,295 were women and 7420 men, of whom 66,419 were active. This included 18,344 midwives (18,316 women and twenty-eight men). In total, 11,525 midwives were active. There were, in total, four advanced midwives, all women and all active (Register Statistics 2012). In Ireland, to qualify as a midwife, general nurse training has to be completed for three years before two years of additional training. Since 2006, a direct-entry to midwifery programme (a four-year honours degree) has also been offered.

The Institute of Obstetricians and Gynaecologists is the professional and training body for obstetrics and gynaecology in Ireland. Its functions include advising government, statutory bodies and other expert groups on all matters of obstetrics and gynaecology, and representing members' interests at a national and international level on professional, legislative and regulatory matters. The Medical Council (Comhairle na nDochtúirí Leighis) regulates medical doctors in the Republic of Ireland. The Council's purpose is to protect the public by promoting and ensuring high standards of professional conduct and professional education, training and competence among doctors. The Medical Council can look into complaints about individual doctors. Anyone can make a complaint to the Medical Council about a doctor, including members of the public, employers and other health care staff. The Medical Council itself may also make a complaint about a doctor.

Health spending in Ireland represents 8.9 per cent of the GDP, lower than the OECD average of 9.3 per cent (OECD 2013). The number of physicians in Ireland is 2.7 per 1,000 population, below the OECD average of 3.1 per 1,000 population (OECD 2013). The number of practising nurses in Ireland is 12.2 per 1,000 population, above the OECD average of 8.4. Table 3.1 shows the ratios of health care practitioners and hospital beds to the population in Ireland.

Demographic profile

Ireland is experiencing an unprecedented demand for maternity services, with in excess of 76,023 births in 2009, the highest since the 1970s when Ireland last experienced a 'baby boom' (Table 3.2). There has been a decrease since 2009, with 75,600 births in 2010, 74,377 births in 2011 and 71,986 births in 2012 (Department of Health 2014). This is due, in part, to a slight reduction in fertility rates and to the declining number of women of childbearing age. At 15.8 per 1,000 live births, Ireland has the highest birth rate of the 27 European Union countries. The average is 10.4 per 1,000 population. After Ireland, the countries with the next highest birth

Table 3.1 Human and physical resources in Ireland

Total number of physicians per 1,000 population	2.7
Total number of nurses per 1,000 population	12.2
Medical graduates per 100,000 population	16.1
Nursing graduates per 100,000 population	37.6
Total hospital beds per 1,000 population	3
Curative (acute) care beds per 1,000 population	2.2
Total number of obstetricians and gynaecologists	126
Total number of midwives	11,529 active 2013
Total expenditure as percentage of GDP	8.9

Source: OECD (2013).

Table 3.2 Demographic profile of Ireland, 2013

Total population	4,593,125
Women	2,319,279
Men	2,273,846
Population aged 0–14 years	1,007
Women of childbearing age (15–44 years)	980,930
Population aged 65 years and older	568,103
Annual population growth (%)	0.2
Population density per square kilometre	67 (2011)
Fertility rate (total births per woman)	2.01
Crude birth rate per 1,000 people	15.8 (2012)
Crude death rate per 1,000 people	6.41
Dependency ratio	50.8 (0–14 years, 32.7; 65+ years, 15.1)
Urban population (%)	62 (1.736 people per square kilometre)

Source: Compiled by author from: *Health in Ireland Key Trends* for selected years. Available from: http://health.gov.ie/publications-research/statistics/statistics-publications/.

rates are the UK (12.9), France (12.7), Belgium (11.9) and Sweden (11.8). In 2011, Germany (8.1) had the lowest birth rate, with Hungary (8.8) the next lowest.

In 2012 almost a quarter of births were to mothers born outside Ireland, with births to mothers from the EU-15 to EU-27 countries at 11.6 per cent, followed by mothers from Asia at 4.0 per cent. The highest peri-natal mortality rate was recorded for babies born to mothers from Africa (13.9 per 1,000 live births and stillbirths). The total period fertility rate for 2011 was 2.01, the highest of the EU-27 countries; the average rate for the EU-27 countries was 1.57. The total period fertility rates for Sweden and Finland were 1.90 and 1.83, respectively, while Hungary (1.23) and Romania (1.25) recorded the lowest total period fertility rate for in 2011.

Maternity provision

The classification of Ireland as Catholic–corporatist is understandable when the historical development of maternity policy and services is exam-ined. The Catholic Hierarchy intervened in 1951 when there was a polit-ical move towards introducing universal medical care for mothers and children. This had long-term implications (Kennedy 2002, 2012). The Catholic Hierarchy focused on the principle of subsidiarity, arguing that such a scheme would undermine the privacy of the family. This was coupled with a fear of non-Catholic doctors educating Irish women about such issues as sex, chastity and marriage, and a fear of socialism. Resist-ance from the medical profession was financially motivated, as doctors made between 70 and 80 per cent of their income from looking after young children and a free service would lead to an increase in salaried doctors (Barrington 1987). GPs in Ireland are self-employed. The rejection of what became known as the Mother and Child Scheme, associated with the then Minister for Health Dr Noël Browne, and the introduction of the Maternity and Infant Care Scheme under the 1953 Health Act shaped maternity policy for the subsequent sixty years. This was a critical juncture and an example of institutional lock-in that limited the scope for future policy variation (Kennedy 2012).

Under the 1954 Maternity and Infant Care Scheme, all women in Ireland are entitled to free maternity care during pregnancy and for six weeks postnatally. Interestingly, the Maternity and Infant Care Scheme only covers maternity-related illnesses, while care for other illnesses which the woman may experience during pregnancy is not covered. Postnatally, the GP will examine the baby (not the mother) at two weeks postpartum and both mother and baby at six weeks. GPs have agreements with the HSE to provide services. Mothers are entitled to free inpatient and out-patient public hospital services in respect of pregnancy and birth and are not liable for any of the standard inpatient hospital charges. Despite the availability of free maternity care, an important feature of maternity services in Ireland is the coexistence of private maternity care.

The duplicate system of health care, as identified by the OECD (2004), is visible when maternity provision is examined. In Ireland, obstetrics is a profession which guarantees a high income. O'Connor (2006) highlights the great divide in the Irish maternity service:

> The market for private obstetrics is worth at least 49 million annually; this is divided among the country's 104 obstetricians. Dublin doctors can earn an estimated €503,000 on average from private maternity fees. Outside Dublin, where births are less centralised, revenues tend to be slightly lower, averaging €447,000 per head annually.... These incomes are further boosted by public salaries (ranging from €125 to €150,000) and private gynaecological fees.
>
> (O'Connor 2006: 10)

To put this in perspective, it is worth noting that the average annual earnings in Ireland in 2012 were €33,327 per year. There has recently been an investigation into top-up payments made to the Masters of the three Dublin maternity hospitals, where in excess of 40 per cent of all births in Ireland occur. The term 'Master', used in the three Dublin maternity hospitals, describes the combined role of chief executive officer and clinical director of the maternity hospital.

There is a dearth of analysis of maternity provision in Ireland, with some notable exceptions (Murphy-Lawless 1998, 2011a, 2011b, 2011c; Kennedy 2002, 2004, 2008, 2010, 2012; Begley and Devane 2006; Devane *et al.* 2007; Mander and Murphy-Lawless 2013). There is no national audit of maternity hospitals in Ireland. The Lourdes Hospital Inquiry into peripartum hysterectomy in 2006 recommended that annual clinical reports of activity and clinical outcomes should be prepared and published within nine months of the previous year-end (Harding Clarke 2006). A welcome development was the establishment of the National Perinatal Epidemiology Centre (NPEC) in 2007, with the overall objective of translating outcome data from Irish maternity hospitals and evidence-based best practice into improved clinical services for Irish patients. The NPEC is funded by the HSE and aims to provide Irish maternity providers with a facility to undertake in-depth reviews of their own medical practices through monitoring outcomes and regular audit. All nineteen maternity hospitals/units are participating in the voluntary audit. There is no agreed national data set for the collection of quality and safety measures for maternity services in Ireland.

In 2011, the Obstetrics and Gynaecology Clinical Care Programme within the HSE provided maternity units for the first time with individual perinatal reports produced by the Economic and Social Research Institute and sent the rates of caesarean section back to individual units for local review. The three Dublin maternity hospitals have collected the same key activity data for decades, allowing for comparison and bench-marking of performance between the three hospitals (Kennedy 2002). However, only eight of the remaining hospitals/units in Ireland complete reports and these vary significantly in style, format and degree of detail (HIQA 2013). HIQA (2013: 59) recommends that the HSE must develop, publish and implement a suite of national performance measures for maternity services with a clear focus on patient outcomes; these would form the basis of a national maternity 'dashboard', which should be collected and analysed. Appropriate action should be taken where local variance exists. They should be published and reported nationally on a regular basis.

Despite the current awareness of the need for tighter regulation, particularly monitoring the quality of maternity services, a picture of inadequate and flawed services had already been presented back in 2006 by the review of maternity provision conducted by the Institute of Obstetricians and Gynaecologists in the light of health policy reform (Institute of Obstetricians and Gynaecologists 2006). KMPG (2008) suggests that this 2006 report 'uncovers much which is undesirable', including poor infrastructure, overcrowding, lack of privacy, long waiting times, operational difficulties and, sometimes, problems with accessing emergency caesarean sections:

> The dominance of a medically led, hospital-centred model of care provides effective services for women with non-routine clinical conditions. However, approximately 60 per cent of women experience a normal pregnancy and birth. It does therefore limit the choice for women whose routine clinical needs could be provided for in a wider range of settings.
>
> (KPMG 2008)

This 2006 review by the Institute of Obstetricians and Gynaecologists reported that maternity provision in Ireland continues to be obstetric-led and is synonymous with the 'active management of labour', ensuring a highly medicalised model of care. This is due, in part, to the way in which the Maternity and Infant Care Scheme has been delivered by GPs and hospitals and also the two-tiered system of medical care, in which private health insurance offers a lucrative income to obstetricians. Women in Ireland have been denied choice in relation to the place of birth and type of care provided. This is despite recognition in other jurisdictions that woman-centred care involves informed choice and a variety of options for women.

Maternity services in Ireland have consistently become more medicalised and hospital-based over the past fifty years. There has been a trend in Ireland since the 1970s towards larger maternity units (Kennedy 2002). This has implications for the type of service provided. Women in Ireland are more likely to undergo a caesarean section than previously. The caesarean rate for 2012 was 29 per cent. The number of women giving birth at home has declined from about one-third in 1950 to less than 1 per cent today.

A public outcry in 2012, when Savita Halappanavar died in an Irish maternity unit from septicaemia, led to a demand for transparency in relation to maternity services. The subsequent report (HIQA 2013) was the first comprehensive exploration of maternity services in Ireland ever undertaken and also the first time that basic as well as sensitive information was made available to the public online. HIQA identified a wide variation in the local clinical and corporate governance arrangements in place in the nineteen maternity hospitals/units around the country and a lack of accessible, consistent and reproducible data relating to the quality of maternity services. HIQA claimed it was impossible to assess the performance and quality of maternity service nationally as no national review or national population-based needs assessment has been undertaken to demonstrate the appropriate allocation of resources, including multidisciplinary workforce arrangements, for the provision of maternity services in Ireland.

HIQA found that there are variations in models of maternity care, with the predominance of consultant-led care and a wide variation in the availability of obstetric beds in relation to the number of births within hospitals. The average birth to inpatient bed ratio is 69:1. There is no recommended birth to inpatient bed ratio for the model of maternity care provided in Ireland. The number of births by maternity hospital/unit ranged from 1,179 births in South Tipperary General Hospital to 9,109 in the National Maternity Hospital, Dublin. The number of births per inpatient bed ranged from 45:1 in South Tipperary General Hospital to 94:1 at Wexford General Hospital, a difference of almost 109 per cent. HIQA noted that there were many areas where maternity service needs were not being fully met and expressed concern in relation to the inconsistency in the provision of maternity services. HIQA recognised a need to ensure that all pregnant women have appropriate access to the right level of care and support at any given time.

Governance structures and arrangements vary in the nineteen maternity hospitals/units throughout the country. At a national level, the HSE's Director of Integrated Services is responsible for the delivery of maternity services and reports directly to the Director General of the HSE. The HSE Office of the Director of Integrated Services reports quality and safety concerns directly to the Director of the Quality Patient Safety Directorate, which has responsibility for investigating patient quality and safety events. There are three stand-alone maternity hospitals in Dublin, each headed by a Master, who is both the senior clinician and chief executive officer. These hospitals are funded through the HSE and are linked to acute general hospitals for gynaecology services and act as local tertiary and national subspecialty referral centres for other obstetric units. These hospitals are managed through service level arrangements with the Integrated Service Area managers for their respective HSE region. Until 2014 there was one independent hospital, Mount Carmel Hospital, providing private maternity services in Dublin, but it was closed due to financial difficulties.

Outside Dublin, maternity services are provided through statutory HSE hospitals, mostly within the structure of an acute hospital. Some are provided in stand-alone hospitals on the campus of the main general hospital (e.g. the Cork University Hospital Group) or located off-site (e.g. the Mid-Western Regional Hospital Group, Limerick) and the governance arrangement for the majority of these maternity hospitals/units is through the hospital general manager and respective Integrated Service Area manager to the Regional Director of Operations or the chief executive officer, up to the National Director for Integrated Services. The Mid-Western Regional Hospital Group and the Galway and Roscommon University Hospitals Group have different governance and reporting structures. They both have a chief executive, a hospital group board chairperson and a group board. The Group chief executive reports to the HSE through the National Director for Integrated Services and to the National Director for Quality and Patient Safety in relation to patient safety issues. The establishment of hospital groups in Ireland, as a step to creating independent hospital trusts, proposes a reorganisation of maternity services in the context of the integration of services and the supporting governance arrangements.

In Ireland, the Report of the National Task Force on Medical Staffing (Hanly Report 2003) concluded that there was a clinical need for a consultant obstetrician and gynaecologist to be present on-site in each regional obstetric unit on a twenty-four hour basis. To achieve this, they recommended that 191 consultant posts in obstetrics and gynaecology would be needed by 2013. At the end of 2012, the HSE reported that there were in total 126 consultant obstetricians and gynaecologists. In 2006, the Institute of Obstetricians and Gynaecologists produced a report entitled The Future of Maternity and Gynaecology Services in Ireland 2006–2016, in which it found clear variations in the quantum and mix of midwifery/nursing staff across maternity hospitals/units and no national reference for setting staffing level standards. This report included a series of recommendations and standards for Irish maternity services. In relation to consultant staffing of labour wards, it recommended that there should be twenty-four hour on-site, on-call consultant obstetric cover on the labour ward of units handling 6,000 deliveries per annum or more – or a dedicated consultant presence on the labour ward. It recommended that, by 2016, there should be at least one consultant per 350 births to allow maternity units with between 3,000 and 4,500 births to provide dedicated consultant cover on the labour ward for forty hours per week.

HIQA reviewed a paper produced by the HSE's Obstetrics and Gynaecology Clinical Care Programme on consultant workforce planning for obstetrics and gynaecology in the Republic of Ireland 2012–2022 (HIQA 2013: 51). It reported that there are a relatively low number of consultant obstetricians and gynaecologists in Ireland and that action should be taken to increase the numbers of trainees in the national system. It highlighted that a failure to address this issue could potentially lead to serious adverse consequences for the provision of health care services in the medium and long term, which could be associated with poorer outcomes for women and children. HIQA reviewed a 2009 national review of the skill-mix in maternity services (HIQA 2013: 55). This review found that the number of health care assistants employed by many of the nineteen maternity hospitals/units was low and there was an under-utilisation of health care assistants in maternity services in general. It concluded that the role of the health care assistant should be part of any workforce planning or reconfiguration of the maternity services to enable midwives to realise their full potential in clinical practice. HIQA (2013: 56) reported that a 2012 review of the midwifery service workforce indicated that the total number of midwife whole-time equivalents in post on 30 November 2011 was 2,249.84 and the national number of vacant posts on this date was 123.88. The review concluded that a more in-depth analysis of the skill-mix needed to be undertaken to more accurately determine the requirements for all staff who work in maternity services in the future and that this analysis needs to take place after models of care for maternity services are agreed for implementation by the HSE. HIQA recommended that the HSE must, as a priority, conduct a review of national maternity services and agree and implement standard, consistent models for the delivery of a national maternity service to ensure that all pregnant women have appropriate choice, access to the right level of safe care and support on a twenty-four hour basis.

Maternity entitlements

Women in Ireland are entitled to twenty-six weeks maternity leave; two weeks must be taken before the expected date of delivery. It is possible to take an additional sixteen weeks of unpaid leave. This has gradually been extended since it was first introduced under the 1981 Maternity Protection of Employees Act. Health and Safety Leave for pregnant and breastfeeding women was introduced under the 1994 Maternity Protection (Health and Safety) Act. Parental leave was introduced under the 1998 Parental Leave Act as amended by the Parental Leave (Amendment) Act 2006. It can be taken by either parent, but as it is unpaid it cannot be used by all of the population. There is no paid paternity leave in Ireland, although some employers allow fathers to take paid leave at the time of the birth. *Force majeure* leave allows for three days in any twelve month period or five days in a thirty-six-month period with full pay. It arises when, for urgent family reasons, the immediate presence of the employee is indispensable owing to injury or illness of a close family member.

Maternity benefit is paid to employed/self-employed mothers who meet certain criteria. The payment has been gradually eroded during the current economic downturn and, since 2013, is taxable for the first time. A small one-off means-tested maternity grant of €10.16 is available to women who have medical cards. Women on low incomes can apply for an exceptional needs payment to help meet the costs of maternity and baby clothes, a cot and a pram.

Childbirth in Ireland

Antenatal

The medical model of childbirth dominates maternity provision in Ireland. Childbirth is universally associated with risk and obstetrics emphasises this risk. The medical model is based on the assumption that something can go wrong and that mothers and babies are at risk of potential harm. Women are assessed for risk when they attend for antenatal care. Risk in childbirth is associated with age, parity, social class, obstetric history, coexisting disease, hypertension, diabetes and obesity, among other factors. A woman's risk status is assessed and she is viewed in that context throughout her pregnancy and labour. Maternity care in Ireland begins with a visit to a GP. Combined care refers to the system in Ireland where women attend both their GP and maternity unit for maternity care. In 2012, 77.3 per cent of all live births involved combined antenatal care and 22.4 per cent of live births were attended by a hospital/obstetrician only. Only 0.2 per cent of live births were attended by only a GP and 0.1 per cent were attended by none. This is a limited use of 'care' as it is more like surveillance and supervision. A schedule of antenatal care is recommended in Ireland. The GP provides an initial examination, if possible before twelve weeks, and a further six examinations during pregnancy, which are alternated with visits to the hospital maternity unit. The schedule of visits may be changed by the GP or the hospital obstetrician, or both, depending on medical need. A woman with a significant illness, e.g. diabetes or hypertension, may have up to five additional visits to the GP. A woman availing of domiciliary care or midwifery-led care will have continuity of care with a specific midwife or team of midwives. Traditionally, antenatal care involved touch, conversation and weighing. Nowadays women are more likely to experience a number of ultrasound scans; other interventions include chorionic villous sampling and amniocentesis.

Intrapartum

HIQA (2013) found there are many areas where maternity service needs were not being fully met in Ireland. There is an inconsistency in the provision of maternity services and the need to ensure that all pregnant women have appropriate choice, access to the right level of care and support at the right time. There are differences in the model of maternity care provided to pregnant women in different parts of the country. In the HSE Dublin Mid Leinster region, the model of care has a stronger focus on midwifery-led care than in other regions, with the availability of a midwifery-led Domiciliary Care In and Out of Hospital (DOMINO) scheme. There are midwifery-led units based in the HSE Dublin North East region. These came about as a result of the closure of maternity units there, the Report of the Maternity Services Review Group to the North Eastern Health Board (Kinder 2001) and the establishment of the NEHSE Maternity Services Task Force, which oversaw the implementation of the recommendations of the Kinder Review (Kennedy 2010). In contrast, many other maternity hospitals/units in the country are predominantly consultant-led.

Some hospitals operate a limited home birth service, the largest being that run by the National Maternity Hospital in Dublin. Home birth services provided by a hospital or HSE scheme are provided free of charge as the woman is regarded as a public patient. There are currently schemes in the counties of Cork, Kerry, Waterford and Wexford. Most of the home births in Ireland are attended by SECMs, registered with the HSE and practising independently. Although individual SECMs attend all the women who engage their services, hospital-employed midwives work as a team with a shared caseload. Midwives employed by the hospitals are under the supervision of hospital obstetricians. SECMs are professionals in their own right and are qualified to practice independently in providing all the services associated with a home birth. The SECM provides full antenatal care, attends the labour and delivery, and provides postnatal care up to and including a six-week check-up, regular paediatric newborn checks and the PKU (heel-prick test) on the baby. The services of an SECM are partially covered by a direct payment of €2,400 from the HSE for attending each woman. This covers a minimum of eleven visits (including both antenatal and postnatal care) and attendance at the birth. This amount is exclusive of travelling expenses and any additional services. Thus the SECM may charge extra. Private health insurers give grants towards the costs of a home birth.

Maternity services have come under increasing pressure in Ireland as a result of the general rise in the number of births, alongside an older population of mothers. Increased maternal age can lead to higher rates of complications in pregnancy. In addition, the increased use of human-assisted reproduction has led to a higher rate of multiple births and there are now also higher rates of comorbid diseases (HIQA 2013: 44). The number of babies born to women who themselves were born outside Ireland has risen and these mothers may experience communication difficulties and other social and clinical challenges in accessing and receiving maternity care. The Confidential Maternal Death Enquiry Ireland report for 2009 to 2011 identified that 40 per cent of all maternal deaths occurred in women who were not born in Ireland (five of six direct deaths, four of thirteen indirect deaths and one of six coincidental deaths) (HIQA 2013: 45). This was also reflected in the NPEC's Severe Maternal Morbidity Audit 2011, which reported that the incidence of severe maternal morbidity was disproportionately higher among non-Irish national ethnic minorities (HIQA 2013: 45).

In 2012 there were 71,986 births, a 16.1 per cent increase since 2003. Just over 44 per cent of the total births took place in fifteen maternity units accommodating between 1,000 and 3,999 births each annually. Four maternity units each accommodated 8,000 or more births, accounting for almost 49 per cent of the total births. The mothers' average length of stay was four days in 2003 and 3.4 days in 2012. For 22.8 per cent of mothers, the length of hospital stay was recorded as 0–1 day. There were 176 home births attended by independent domiciliary midwives in 2012.

Primiparous mothers accounted for 39.9 per cent of all maternities, with 60.1 per cent of maternities having one or more previous live births or stillbirths. Of mothers aged younger than 20 years, 89.2 per cent gave birth for the first time, with only 9.6 per cent delivering for the second time and 1.2 per cent delivering for a third time or more. For women aged 30–34 years, 38.4 per cent gave birth for the first time and 37.2 per cent delivered for the second time. The average age of mothers giving birth was 31.9 years compared with 30.6 in 2003. Two per cent of those giving birth were younger than twenty years and 30 per cent of women giving birth were thirty-five years or older. A total of 39 per cent of women gave birth for the first time and the average age was 30.0 years. The number of those women under thirty years of age giving birth for the first time fell and those aged over thirty years increased. The average parity (number of live and stillbirths) has remained stable at 1.0 over the decade.

Spontaneous vaginal deliveries fell from 61.2 per cent in 2003 to 55.6 per cent in 2012. The percentage of babies delivered by spontaneous vaginal delivery declined with age and was reported at 65.5 per cent for mothers aged less than twenty years compared with 45.9 per cent to mothers aged forty years and older. Just over 16 per cent of the total live births were assisted by instrumental delivery (breech/forceps, forceps or vacuum extraction) with higher percentages for live singleton births (16.2 per cent) compared with live multiple births (12.7 per cent). The caesarean section rate was 28.9 in 2012, up from 24.2 in 2003. However, there is major variation in the caesarean section rate between hospitals, with a rate of 38 per cent in St Luke's Hospital, Kilkenny and 19.1 per cent in Sligo General Hospital (Association for the Improvement of Maternity Services 2014). The caesarean section rates ranged from 15.1 per cent for mothers aged less than twenty years to 43.6 per cent for mothers aged forty years and older (Table 3.3).

Postnatal

The perinatal mortality rate is 5.9 per 1,000 births and stillbirths, a reduction of 3.1 per cent since 2003, when the perinatal mortality rate was 8.6 per 1,000 live births and stillbirths. The national morbidity rate reported by the NPEC was 3.8 cases per 1,000 maternities, or 1 in 263 maternities. This morbidity rate is reported in terms of births rather than maternities.

The 2012 report Infant Feeding Policy for Maternity and Neonatal Services (Health Services Executive 2012) recommends that all hospital staff should encourage and enable mothers to breastfeed exclusively for the first six months and continue thereafter as part of a wider diet until two years of age or beyond. It states that all parents have the right to receive

Table 3.3 Birth interventions and outcomes for selected years in Ireland

	2012
Total number of live births	71,986
Stillbirths	3.9
Early neonatal death	2.0
Perinatal mortality	5.9
Adjusted perinatal mortality	4.3
Spontaneous vaginal delivery	55.6
Caesarean section rate	28.8
Vacuum extraction	11.2

Source: Economic and Social Research Institute (2013).

Notes
Rates are calculated per 1,000 births. For stillbirths, perinatal deaths and adjusted perinatal deaths, the rates are calculated on the total live births and stillbirths. For early neonatal deaths, the rates are calculated on total live births.

clear evidence-based information to enable them to make fully informed decisions about how their babies are fed and cared for. It recommends that staff should support women in their chosen method of infant feeding, regardless of method chosen. Fifty-five per cent of mothers recorded any breastfeeding in 2012, compared with 51 per cent in 2007 and 44 per cent in 2002. Forty-seven per cent of mothers in 2012 exclusively breastfed, compared with 45 per cent in 2007 and 41 per cent in 2002 (Economic and Social Research Institute 2012). The Baby-Friendly Hospital Initiative (BFHI) began in Ireland in 1998, when the prevalence of any breastfeeding on discharge was 31 per cent. Research published online in February 2013 indicated that the initiation of breastfeeding in Ireland is more likely in a Baby-Friendly Hospital (BFHI 2013). The name of the Initiative was later amended to use 'Health' rather than 'Hospital' Initiative to reflect the potential activity that extends further than hospitals. All of the Irish maternity units participated in the BFHI in 2013. Forty-two per cent of births occurred in a Baby-Friendly designated hospital. This is higher than Germany, England, Finland, the USA, Italy, France and Spain, among others.

Consumer involvement

The United Nations Millennium Development Goals in 2000 placed maternal health on the international agenda. Jentsch *et al.* (2007) refer to the UK, where there has developed, during the last decade, a strategy which involves consumers in health service planning to '…ensure that services are tailored to meet local needs and that consumer involvement may act as a catalyst for change thereby overcoming some of the inequalities in healthcare provision' (Jentsch *et al.* 2007: 129). McGregor (2003) suggests that '…a benefit of public involvement is that public confidence in decision-making and information-sharing is increased as citizens most affected by a health issue contribute to its possible solutions early in the policy planning and review process' (McGregor 2003: 169). WHO defines community participation as: '…going beyond consultation to enable citizens to become an integral part of the decision making and action process' (WHO 2002: 1). Such issues are emerging in Ireland.

In his speech to the *Dáil* (Irish parliament) on the launch of the Health Reform Programme (27 June 2003), the then Minister for Health Mícheál Martin referred to '…the most important voice to be heard in planning the delivery of services is the patients, clients and their families'. This reflected one of the goals of the Health Strategy *Quality and Fairness: a Health System for You*, which stated that '…Provision will be made for the participation of the community in decisions about the delivery of health and personal services. Deliverables; regional advisory panels/co-ordinating committees established by mid 2002' (Department of Health and Children 2001: 4). The Strategy Document outlined its principles as '…equity, people-centredness, quality and accountability. They are aimed at achieving the goals of better health for everyone, fair access, appropriate and responsive care delivery and high performance' (Department of Health and Children 2001: 130) and, again, '...the central contribution of staff, users, communities and voluntary organisations in shaping this'.

Despite this aspiration, maternity units do not have structured maternity liaison committees. In recent years the first maternity liaison groups have been established as part of a major restructuring of maternity services in the north-east of the country. The North East Health Services Executive developed two initiatives in the north-east following on from the Kinder Review, which recommended the establishment of maternity liaison committees:

> We consider that a region-wide Consumer Committee for Maternity and Childcare Services should be put in place. Representatives of Consumer organisations would have the opportunity to be involved in consultation about present operations and future developments and should be able to assess the quality of the services being provided.
>
> (Health Services Executive 2011: 35)

Consumer involvement in maternity services in Ireland has, for the most part, been initiated by community activists and represented by a number of voluntary organisations, including *Cuidiú* – The Irish Childbirth Trust, the Association for the Improvement of Maternity Services (AIMS) and the Home Birth Association.

Cuidiú, the Irish Childbirth Trust was established in 1983 and is based on the UK's National Childbirth Trust. With branches throughout Ireland, it provides information for parents in relation to pregnancy, childbirth and breastfeeding. It publishes a Consumer Guide to Maternity Services in Ireland, organises antenatal classes, postnatal and parenting support groups and 'bump, baby and toddler groups'.

AIMS Ireland is a consumer-led campaign and pressure group, founded in 2007 (previously there were two similar groups: the Association for the Improvement of Maternity Services and Irish AIMS, which disbanded) by mothers dissatisfied with the maternity care system and eager to campaign for change. AIMS is committed to highlighting and supporting normal birth and mother-friendly birth practices in Ireland.

The Home Birth Association of Ireland was founded in 1982 to give information and support to those considering and opting for a home birth. It runs open meetings for those interested in planning a home birth to meet with those who have experienced home births. It organises workshops and conferences, and lobbies the relevant authorities, urging them to provide more information on home births, to reintroduce practical domiciliary midwifery and to integrate nationwide domiciliary care into maternity services.

Risk and rights

Ireland is perceived as a hybrid welfare regime, a mix of liberal, Catholic, conservative–corporatist and continental regimes. Looking at maternity services shows the complexity of classifying welfare regimes. There is universal maternity and infant care in Ireland, available free of charge to all women and babies. Mothers and babies are the only cohort in the Irish population (prior to the proposed introduction of free health care for all children under five years of age in 2014) who have universal rights to free health care. Risk pooling is the norm when it comes to maternity provision, paid for out of general taxation, and this guarantees solidarity during this time in a woman's life. Thus women have extensive social rights where maternity care is concerned. Social citizenship rights guarantee inclusion and access to services, thus the risk of denial of care is obliterated. However, this inclusionary access to a large extent guarantees inclusion in a very specific type of maternity service where risk is emphasised.

Maternity services have increasingly become more medicalised, with fewer spontaneous vaginal deliveries and 29 per cent of births by caesarean section. This is linked directly to the discourse on risk that has come to dominate maternity services in Ireland, as in other Western societies. Personal responsibility is emphasised and women in Ireland are encouraged to attend antenatal care and education to prepare them for childbirth. Childbirth in Ireland has always been perceived as involving risk for the mother and child as maternal and neonatal mortality have always been a part of life. Now childbirth is perceived as an event that is risky, but that risk can be managed and the obstetric profession is judged as being in the best position to do so. Although the majority of women do participate in antenatal care and education, it is necessary to ask to what extent the subsequent choices they make are truly informed. Two recent high-profile cases in Ireland highlighted the powerlessness often experienced in maternity units where the obstetric profession dictates the course of events. Many women exercise active citizenship by joining maternity pressure groups such as the Irish Childbirth Trust, AIMS and the Home Birth Association to campaign and lobby for improved services.

In Ireland, while maternal and infant health is an entitlement enjoyed by all women and children under the 1954 Maternity and Infant Care Scheme, in practice there is a two-tiered 'duplicate' system, where some women enjoy private health care that ensures continuity of care, obstetric care and more luxurious accommodation in hospital. Maternity is an insurable risk and women can enjoy private care if they have paid private health insurance.

At a macro-level, maternity services are provided and regulated by the Department of Health. HIQA has a part to play in monitoring the safety and quality of health care and social care in Ireland. Since 2008 the Clinical Indemnity Scheme managed by the State Claims Agency has dealt with clinical negligence claims and the associated risks of hospitals and other health agencies. An Bord Altranais agus Cnáimhseachais na hÉireann, the NMBI, is the regulatory body for the nursing profession. The Institute of Obstetricians and Gynaecologists is the professional and training body for obstetrics and gynaecology in Ireland. The Medical Council regulates medical doctors in the Republic of Ireland.

At a meso-level, practice in maternity units has come under scrutiny, resulting in recent inquiries, such as the Lourdes Hospital Inquiry (Harding Clarke 2006) the Tanya McCabe Inquiry (2008) and the HIQA report on the treatment of Savita Halappanavar (HIQA 2013) The most recent crisis to emerge is in relation to intrapartum deaths in the Midlands Hospital (Holohan 2014). All of these cases have unearthed evidence about practices at the meso-level in maternity units as well as how risks have not been captured by the regulatory system in Ireland. Risk is associated with clinical governance and how this operates in different societies is worthy of comparison. It is necessary to understand the medical and social models of childbirth to understand the relevance of risk to maternal and infant health. These are closely related to risk assessment and management in maternity care.

At a micro-level, women in Ireland are continuing to have babies, with the birth rate remaining the highest in Europe. Although childbirth has always been associated with risk, there are now new risks associated with the use of technology, lifestyles and deferred maternity. Risk management is central to maternity provision. Perceptions of risk in maternity care are interpreted by individuals and managed accordingly. Maternity care in Ireland is very closely linked to GP services. Through the system of combined care, the GP is the first point of contact with the health services for a pregnant woman. This is how she is guided through the system, which for the majority of women involves combined care, shared between the GP and maternity unit/hospital. In Ireland in general there is very little challenge to the status quo and very little demand for a more varied range of birth practices sought from professional groups and consumers in relation to the availability of a variety of birth practices in similar situations. Women who avail of private health insurance have a greater choice when it comes to the type of hospital accommodation, antenatal and postnatal appointments and their choice of obstetrician.

Conclusion

Locating maternity services in Ireland within the welfare regime literature reveals an anomaly that is a feature of many welfare regimes. This is that the rights of women and infants to maternity services differ from their rights to other health and social services. Using risk and citizenship as the conceptual/theoretical framework, we see that maternity services within countries may diverge from the national health policy. We see the centrality of the social and medical models of health to understanding maternity policy. Risk and rights are two important concepts that straddle the combined literature on welfare regimes, health regimes and scholarship on maternity policy and practice. Reibling's model of analysis of health regimes enhances our understanding of the complexities of maternity policy (Reibling 2010). Maternity care is a paradigmatic example of the comparative analysis of health care: (i) it is characterised by a high degree of support; (ii) professional conflicts are at the core of its history; and (iii) technological developments have shaped and changed maternity care and birth practices. Compared with other fields of welfare provision, people who are ill are seen as a category with very high levels of deservingness. This is even more so for mothers and children. Thus support for the coverage of maternity and infant care is high. The case of Ireland shows that, when it comes to maternity services, users are perceived as deserving with associated rights. Service providers have the right to practise, but obstetrics has a higher status than midwifery and a more established place in maternity provision. Risk is defined by the medical profession with which the woman engages from the beginning of her pregnancy. Childbirth in Ireland has become dominated by obstetrics. GPs in Ireland also have a dominant and protected role under the Maternity and Infant Care Scheme.

Recent events in maternity units in Ireland have highlighted the inadequacies of the Irish maternity system and there is evidence of serious system failures. The HIQA enquiry (HIQA 2013) and the Holohan report (2014) have unearthed some serious problems with maternity services in Ireland and have made important recommendations pertaining to the future of maternity services in this country.

Useful websites

AIMS Ireland	www.aimsireland.com
Home Birth Association of Ireland	www.homebirth.ie
Institute of Obstetricians and Gynaecologists	www.rcpi.ie
Irish Childbirth Trust	www.cuidiu-ict.ie
Medical Council of Ireland	www.medicalcouncil.ie
National Perinatal Epidemiology Centre	www.ucc.ie/en/npec
Nursing Board of Ireland	www.nursingboard.ie

References

Association for the Improvement of Maternity Services (AIMS) (2014) *Detailed Statistics on Ireland's 19 Public Maternity Units Published for the First Time* [online]. Available from: http://aimsireland.ie/detailed-statistics-on-irelands-19-public-maternity-units-published-for-the-first-time/. Accessed 9 September 2014.

60   *P. Kennedy*

Baby-Friendly Health Initiative (BFHI) (2013) *Baby-Friendly Health Initiative Annual Report 2013* [online]. Available from: www.ihph.ie/babyfriendlyinitiative/images/BFHI%20Ireland%20Annual%20Report%202013%20public.pdf. Accessed 10 April 2014.

Barrington, R. (1987) *Health, Medicine and Politics in Ireland 1900–1970.* Dublin: Institute of Public Administration.

Begley, C. and Devane, D. (2006) *Research Progress Report: Fifteenth Research Progress Status Report to the Maternity Services Taskforce and HSE-Dublin North East 1st September 2006–31st December 2006.* Dublin: School of Nursing and Midwifery, Trinity College Dublin.

Bonoli, G. (1997) 'Classifying welfare states: a two-dimensional analysis', *Journal of Social Policy*, 26 (3): 351–372.

Burke, S. (2009) *Irish Apartheid: Healthcare Inequality in Ireland.* Dublin: New Island.

Central Statistics Office (2004) *Population and Labour 2004.* Dublin: Stationery Office.

Cochrane, A. and Clarke, J. (1993) *Comparing Welfare States.* London: Sage.

Considine M. and Dukelow, F. (2009) *Irish Social Policy, a Critical Introduction.* Dublin: Gill and Macmillan.

Daly, M. and Yeates, N. (2003) 'Common origins, different paths: adaptation and change in social security in Britain and Ireland', *Policy and Politics*, 31 (1): 85–97.

Department of Health (2012) *Future Health. A Strategic Framework for Reform of the Health Service 2012–2015.* Dublin: Department of Health. Available from: www.drugsandalcohol.ie/18790/. Accessed 9 September 2014.

Department of Health and Children (2001) *Quality and Fairness – a Health System for You – Health Strategy.* Dublin: Department of Health and Children.

Devane, D., Murphy-Lawless, J. and Begley, C. (2007) 'The invisible woman: maternity care in Ireland', *Midwifery*, 23 (1): 92–101.

Economic and Social Research Institute (ESRI) (2013) *Perinatal Statistics 2012.* Dublin: ESRI.

Esping-Andersen, G. (1990) *The Three Worlds of Welfare Capitalism.* Cambridge: Polity Press.

Hanly Report (2003) *Report of the National Task Force on Medical Staffing* [online]. Available from: http://health.gov.ie/blog/publications/report-of-the-national-task-force-on-medical-staffing-hanly-report-2/. Accessed 9 September 2014.

Harding Clarke, M. (2006) *The Lourdes Hospital Enquiry: an Inquiry into Peripartum Hysterectomy at Our Lady of Lourdes Hospital Drogheda.* Dublin: Stationery Office.

Health Information and Quality Authority (HIQA) (2013) *Patient Safety Investigation Report into Services at University Hospital Galway (UHG) and as Reflected in the Care Provided to Savita Halappanavar* [online]. Available from: www.hiqa.ie/healthcare/focus-quality-safety/investigations/galway. Accessed 10 April 2014.

Health Insurance Authority (2012) *Annual Report and Accounts.* Dublin: Health Insurance Authority.

Health Services Executive/National Breastfeeding Strategic Implementation Monitoring Committee (2012) *Infant Feeding Policy for Maternity and Neonatal Services* [online]. Available from: www.breastfeeding.ie/policy_strategy. Accessed 10 April 2014.

Holohan, T. (2014) *HSE Midland Regional Hospital, Portlaoise Perinatal Deaths (2006–date) Report to the Minister for Health Dr James Reilly TD from Dr Tony Holohan Chief*

Medical Officer, 24 February 2014 [online]. Available from: http://health.gov.ie/wp-content/uploads/2014/.../portlaoise_perinatal_deaths.pdf. Accessed 9 September 2014.

Institute of Obstetricians and Gynaecologists (2006) *The Future of Maternity and Gynaecology Services in Ireland 2006–2016.* Report from Institute Sub-Group. Dublin: Institute of Obstetricians and Gynaecologists.

Jentsch, B., Durham, R., Hundley, V. and Hussein, J. (2007) 'Creating consumer satisfaction in maternity care: the neglected needs of migrants, asylum seekers and refugees', *International Journal of Consumer Studies*, 31: 18–134.

Kennedy, P. (2002) *Maternity in Ireland: a Woman Centered Perspective.* Dublin: The Liffey Press.

Kennedy, P. (ed.) (2004) *Motherhood in Ireland; Creation and Context.* Cork: Mercier Press.

Kennedy, P. (2008) 'A woman centred maternity service for the North Eastern Health Board', *International Journal of Consumer Studies*, 32: 27–33.

Kennedy, P. (2010) 'Healthcare reform: maternity service provision in Ireland', *Health Policy*, 97: 145–151.

Kennedy, P. (2012) 'Change in maternity provision in Ireland: elephants on the move', *Economic and Social Review*, 43 (3), 377–399.

Kinder, P. (2001) *Report of the Maternity Services Review Group to the North Eastern Health Board.* Kells: North Eastern Health Board.

KPMG (2008) *Independent Review of Maternity and Gynaecology Services in the Greater Dublin Area.* Dublin: KPMG.

Lewis, J. (1992) 'Gender and the development of welfare regimes', *Journal of European Social Policy*, 2 (3): 159–173.

Mander, R. and Murphy-Lawless, J. (2013) *The Politics of Maternity.* Oxford: Routledge.

McGregor, S (2003) 'Government transparency: the citizen perspective and experience with food and health products policy', *International Journal of Consumer Studies*, 27 (2): 168–175.

Millar, M. and Adshead, M. (2004) 'Health care in Ireland: applying Esping-Andersen's typology of welfare to the Irish case', paper presented at the Political Studies Association Conference, University of Lincoln.

Murphy-Lawless, J. (1998) *Reading Birth and Death: a History of Obstetric Thinking.* Cork: Cork University Press.

Murphy-Lawless, J. (2011a) 'Stop press; news on Ireland's midwifery unit closures', *AIMS Journal*, 23: 4–7.

Murphy-Lawless, J. (2011b) 'Childbirth adrift in Ireland', *AIMS Journal*, 23 (3): 22–24.

Murphy-Lawless, J. (2011c) '"Ceiling caves in": the current state of maternity services in Ireland', *MIDIRS Midwifery Digest*, 21 (4): 446–451.

National Economic and Social Council (NESC) (2005) *The Developmental Welfare State.* Dublin: Government Publications Office.

National Recovery Plan (2010) National Recovery Plan 2010–2014 [online] Dublin: Stationery Office. Available from: www.budget.gov.ie/The%20National%20 Recovery%20Plan%202011-20. Accesssed 9 September 2014.

O'Connor, M. (2006) 'Conjuring choice while subverting autonomy: medical technocracy and home birth in Ireland'. In: A. Symon (ed.), *Risk and Choice in Maternity Care: an International Perspective.* London: Churchill Livingstone/Elsevier.

O'Connor, M. (2007) *Emergency: Irish Hospitals in Chaos.* Dublin: Gill & Macmillan.

OECD (2004) *Private Health Insurance in OECD Countries: the OECD Health Project.* Paris: OECD.

OECD (2013) *Country Statistical Profile: Ireland* [online]. Available from: www.oecd-ilibrary.org/economics/country-statistical-profile-ireland_20752288-table-irl. Accessed 30 June 2014.

Payne, D. and McCashin, A. (2005) *Welfare State Legitimacy: the Republic of Ireland in Comparative Perspective.* Series UCD Geary Institute Discussion Paper Series No. WP2005/10. Dublin: University College Dublin, Geary Institute. Available from: www.ucd.ie/geary/publications/2005/Geary.

Register Statistics (2012) [online]. Available from: http:// www.nursingboard.ie/en/homepage.aspx. Accessed 9 September 2014.

Reibling, N. (2010) 'Healthcare systems in Europe: towards an incorporation of patient access', *Journal of European Social Policy,* 20 (1): 5–18.

Tanya McCabe Inquiry (2008) *Report into the Circumstances Pertaining to the Death of Mrs Tania McCabe and her Infant Son Zach at Our Lady of Lourdes Hospital, Drogheda on Friday 9 March, 2007* [online]. Available from: www.hse.ie/eng/services/Publications/services/Hospitals/Report_into_maternaland child death at Our Lady of Lourdes Hospital.pdf. Accessed 10 April 2014.

WHO (2002) *European Sustainable Development and Health Series,* Vol. 4. Geneva: WHO.

Wren, M.A. (2003) *Unhealthy States: Anatomy of a Sick Society.* Dublin: New Island.

4   United States of America

Christine H. Morton and Megan M. Henley

Background

The USA is a republic consisting of fifty states and a federal district. It is located on the North American continent between neighbouring Canada to the north and Mexico to the south. At 3.79 million square miles, stretching from the Pacific to the Atlantic coasts, the USA is the fourth largest country in the world by total area (World Atlas Website 2014). It is a geographically diverse nation with mountain, desert, plain and coastal climates.

The modern USA began as a collection of colonies founded by European settlers in the 1500s. Delegates from these colonies issued the Declaration of Independence in 1776, declaring their independence from the Kingdom of Great Britain. The Founders ratified the Constitution and the Bill of Rights in 1791, guaranteeing many civil rights and freedoms to its citizens, such as freedom of religion, freedom of speech and freedom of the press. The USA has a federal system of government with three branches of government (executive, legislative and judicial) that serve to balance and check one another.

The USA has a capitalist economy based ostensibly on free markets, but, in practice, the system has grown increasingly monopolistic. The private sector accounts for the vast majority of the economy. It is largely a consumer society, with low levels of unionisation (12 per cent) and no national policy of paid leave for workers (Ray *et al.* 2013).

With a population close to 317.6 million, the USA is the third most populous country in the world (US Census Bureau 2014). Most Americans live in urban areas and urban living has increased in recent decades. About 80.7 per cent of Americans live in cities and urban areas, whereas only 19.3 per cent live in rural areas (US Census Bureau 2010).

The USA as a welfare regime

According to Esping-Andersen's typology of welfare regimes, the USA is a liberal welfare regime (Esping-Andersen 1990). This means that markets, rather than the state, largely dictate family and maternity care policy. In liberal welfare regimes the state only intervenes to ameliorate poverty, which has specific and malleable measures. Market and private provisions cover the health needs of the majority of Americans; the government provides health care only in cases of substantial poverty where families cannot meet basic needs.

The majority of Americans (54 per cent) therefore receive coverage of health care costs from private health insurance, another 30 per cent are covered by the public financing system (Medicaid for low income individuals who qualify, or Medicare for adults over sixty-five years of age) and the remainder pay out-of-pocket for their health care. Some individuals may receive both private and publicly funded health care. However, one of every six Americans does not have health insurance; this is likely to change with the adoption of the Affordable Care Act (Rice *et al.* 2013).

The USA is the most market-based regime in the world and there is no universal system for pricing or providing health care. As a result, those with private health insurance are dependent on their insurer to determine which health care costs they will pay; this varies widely by insurance provider and the price of the insurance policy (Kaiser Family Foundation 2013b). Insurance companies directly negotiate prices for health care services (e.g. physicians, hospitalisation and pharmaceutical drugs). This means that, in the USA, health care services vary in cost according to the type of insurance policy. Those with private employee-based coverage will pay the lowest out-of-pocket expenses for most of their care, but others can expect to pay whatever their insurance company decides they will not cover. Those without insurance rely on doctors to dictate their prices. Many people without health insurance simply do not receive medical care except in emergencies.

Health care system

The American health care system relies primarily on markets and private insurers. Health care is decentralised in the USA. Public health structures vary significantly from state to state and sometimes defer to individual counties. Federal, state and local public health services are consistently under-funded and focused more on immediate public health concerns (such as a sudden flu outbreak or a bioterrorist threat) than long-term, comprehensive health care and coverage (Rice *et al.* 2013). The public sector also covers low-income and elderly citizens and those with emergencies.

Insured Americans enter the health care system either through a primary care provider or through a specialist. Uninsured individuals often do not have a primary care provider and instead visit community health centres and hospital emergency rooms for their care. Emergency rooms in the USA are required to treat individuals who need emergency care until they are stable. However, this over reliance on emergency rooms results in a lack of continuity of care and a lack of regular health care maintenance for the uninsured population.

Vulnerable populations in the USA suffer from limited access to health care and limited resources for paying out-of-pocket costs. These populations include those with low incomes, the uninsured, the disabled, the homeless, women, children, racial and ethnic minorities, those with HIV/ AIDS, the mentally ill, the elderly, and those living in rural areas. Federal, state and local governments have programmes for reducing disparities in health care for these populations. Although there are special programmes for certain vulnerable groups (including American Indians and Alaskan Natives, military personnel, veterans and those who are institutionalised, such as prisoners), many other vulnerable populations fall through the cracks or do not qualify for government programmes. This results in a disproportionate distribution of health care services across the country.

Table 4.1 details the human and physical resources in the USA. Overall, there are a greater number of nurses (8.54 per 1,000) than physicians (2.5 per 1,000) (American Congress of Obstetricians and Gynecologists 2013). Physicians, nurses and certified nurse-midwives receive their training from public or private universities and, after graduating from their programme, they must pass a comprehensive test to obtain their medical or nursing licence. States regulate physician and nurse licensing and most states recognise licences between states.

The USA suffers from a poor distribution of health care professionals. There are more specialists than primary care physicians and specialists are not evenly distributed by region across the country. There are also shortages of physicians by racial and ethnic representation. Current predictions on the future supply of medical professionals are mixed regarding physicians, but suggest an increasing shortage of nurses overall. Because the USA expects an increase in the ageing population to be unmatched by the number of nurses, an important goal of the Affordable Care Act is expanding the health care workforce, particularly nurses (Rice *et al.* 2013).

Currently, there are 3.1 hospital beds per 1,000 people in the USA and 2.6 curative beds per 1,000 (OECD 2013). Since 1970 the number of hospital beds and the length of hospital stay have steadily decreased (OECD 2013). Total expenditure on health increased between 1970 and 2010 (OECD 2013). Some of this increase is a result of increased life expectancy. Other variables include transportation accidents, which are among the world's highest, a higher incidence of low birthweight babies and higher infant mortality rates than other OECD countries. In addition, the USA has one of the highest rates of both type 1 and type 2 diabetes, accounting for a large share of health expenditures. Finally, at 32 per cent, the USA has one of the highest rates of obesity in the world (OECD 2013). Obesity rates are higher among poorer and non-white populations.

Table 4.1 Human and physical resources in the USA

Physicians per 1,000 population	2.5[a]
Nurses per 1,000 population	8.54[b]
Medical graduates per 100,000 population	6.6[a]
Registered nurses* per 100,000 population	874[c]
Total hospital beds per 1000 population	3.1[a]
Curative (acute) care beds per 1,000 population	2.6[a]
Obstetricians per 100,000 population	27.3[a]
Gynaecologists	20,880[d]
Certified Nurse Midwives	13,071[e]
Certified Midwives	84[e]
Certified Professional Midwives	~2000[f]

Sources: a OECD (2013); b US Department of Health and Human Services & Health Resources and Services Administration (2010); c Kaiser Family Foundation (2014); d US Department of Labor & Bureau of Labor Statistics (2014); e American College of Nurse-Midwives membership, www.midwifery.org; f North American Registry of Midwives (2014).

Note
* Registered nurses include advanced practice nurses such as nurse practitioners, clinical nurse specialists, certified nurse midwives and certified registered nurse anaesthetists.

Demographic profile

Table 4.2 gives demographic information for the USA population. Of approximately 313.9 million Americans, about 159 million are women. The number of births in the USA was 3,952,937 in 2012 (Martin *et al.* 2013a). The total fertility rate has remained fairly steady at 1.9 since 2010 and the crude birth rate is thirteen births per 1,000 women (World Bank 2013). The sex ratio at birth has remained consistently balanced, with an average of 50.8 per cent of babies born being female.

The life expectancy at birth has consistently risen for both men and women over the past forty years (Rice *et al.* 2013). The latest research reports an overall life expectancy of 78.7 years. Women can expect to live to eighty-one years of age, whereas men can expect to live to 76.3 years (Miniño 2013). Accordingly, age-adjusted death rates are higher for men than for women. Overall the crude death rate is 740.6 per 100,000. For men the rate is 874.5 and for women it is 631.9 (Miniño 2013).

Since its inception, the USA has been home to an ethnically diverse population, the result of immigration from many different countries. Most immigrants live in the largest cities. The latest national census shows that 63.7 per cent of Americans identify themselves as white, 16.3 per cent identify as Hispanic or Latino, 12.6 per cent identify as African American and 4.8 per cent identify as Asian American. American Indians and Alaskan Natives make up 0.9 per cent of the population, Native Hawaiians and Pacific Islanders make up 0.2 per cent of the population, 6.2 per cent identity with some other race and 2.9 per cent of Americans identify with two or more races (US Census Bureau 2012a).

Non-white and immigrant populations are over-represented among the uninsured and those on Medicaid. Specifically, non-citizens do not receive any health care coverage except in emergency situations. Medicaid recipients must earn a low income household threshold, which is set by each state. This threshold tends to be lower than the poverty line in many states. As a result, many people are exempt because they have too high an income to qualify for state health care, but too low an income to purchase private health insurance (Amnesty International 2010). Those who do receive Medicaid have very low incomes and are disproportionately African American and Hispanic women.

Similarly, ethnic minorities are over-represented in terms of health morbidity. Premature death from stroke and coronary heart disease are significantly higher in the non-Hispanic black population than in the white population. Both life expectancy and years of life free from chronic health conditions are consistently higher for the white population than for ethnic minorities (Centers of Disease Control Office of Minority Health and Health Equity 2013).

Maternity provision

Maternity care in the USA is provided through the private insurance system and through state Medicaid programmes. Like the provision of

Table 4.2 Demographic profile of the USA

Population	313.9 million[a]
Women	159.4 million[a]
Population aged 0–14 years	61.1 million[a]
Women of childbearing age (15–44 years)	62.7 million[a]
Population aged 65 years and older	43.1 million[a]
Population annual growth (%)	0.9[a]
Population density per square kilometre	32.3[a]
Total fertility rate (births per woman)	1.88[b]
Crude birth rate per 1,000 people	12.6[b]
Crude death rate per 1,000 people	8[c]
Urban population (%)	80.7[c]
Ethnic groups (%)[d]	
White	63.7
Hispanic or Latino	16.3
African American	12.6
Asian American	4.8
American Indian/Alaska Native	0.9
Native Hawaiian/Pacific Islander	0.2
Other	6.2
Multiracial	2.9

Sources: a US Census Bureau (2012c); b Martin *et al.* (2013b); c World Bank (2013); d US Census Bureau (2012a).

health services, maternity care is decentralised and varies by payer. National investment in maternal–child health began with creation of Title V as part of the Social Security Act of 1935, which authorised the creation of the Maternal and Child Health programmes. Medicaid, a state-federal programme, is the primary payer of maternity care among low income women and covers approximately 48 per cent of all births nationally (Kaiser Family Foundation 2013a). The Title V Block Grant served 2,345,543 pregnant women in the financial year 2012 (US Department of Health and Human Services Health Resources and Services Administration and Maternal and Child Health Bureau 2014). Women of colour are disproportionately represented among those whose maternity care is covered by Medicaid (Kaiser Family Foundation 2013a). States currently have wide discretion in setting priorities for maternal health needs as well as varying Medicaid eligibility levels based on income thresholds.

The Patient Protection and Affordable Care Act (or 'Obamacare') offers major opportunities to improve the health of women in the USA by expanding access to clinical preventive services for women, assuring no cost-sharing for more than forty-seven million women. Among the most important opportunities for prevention are those linked to the content, quality and utilisation of well-woman visits, preconception care, prenatal care, inter-conception care for women with a prior adverse pregnancy outcome and the postpartum visit. The Health and Human Services Secretary's Advisory Committee on Infant Mortality (SACIM) has also given priority to 'improving the health of women before, during, and after pregnancy', as one of its six recommended strategic directions for national action to reduce infant mortality (SACIM 2013).

The expansion of Medicaid is part of the foundation of the Affordable Care Act coverage expansion and anticipated reduction in numbers of uninsured people, including pregnant women (Kaiser Family Foundation 2013a). However, at the time of writing, nineteen states have rejected Medicaid expansion and another five are still debating whether to accept the programme as a result of opposition to the Affordable Care Act. Another twenty-four states have delayed implementation, leaving some 4.8 million Americans without health insurance, representing 1.4 per cent of the population.

There are approximately 27.3 obstetricians/gynaecologists per 100,000 Americans. There are 2.65 obstetricians/gynaecologists per 10,000 women and 5.39 obstetricians/gynaecologists per 10,000 women of reproductive age (Rayburn 2011). Obstetricians/gynaecologists are more likely to be practising in metropolitan areas; approximately half (1,550, 49 per cent) of all US counties lack an obstetrician/gynaecologist. States with the highest proportion of counties without an obstetrician/gynaecologist are located in the central and mountain western states (Rayburn 2011).

Family medicine physicians are important providers of care for women of reproductive age and the breadth of the specialty includes care before, during and after pregnancy. Family physicians provided 12 per cent of prenatal visits in 1995–1996, but only 6 per cent in 2003–2004 (Cohen and Coco 2009). The proportion of family physicians that provides maternity care has declined over time, from 23.3 per cent in 2000 to 9.7 per cent in 2010 (Tong *et al.* 2012). A national survey found that a family physician attended the delivery of 7 per cent of women in 2006 and 9 per cent of women in 2012 (Declercq *et al.* 2013).

There are three types of certified midwife in the USA: Certified Nurse-Midwives (CNMs), Certified Midwives (CMs), and Certified Professional Midwives (CPMs). There are an estimated 13,071 CNMs, eighty-four CMs, and approximately 2,000 CPMs (Table 4.1). CNMs are educated in two disciplines: midwifery and nursing. They earn graduate degrees, complete a midwifery education programme accredited by the Accreditation Commission for Midwifery Education and pass a national certification examination administered by the American Midwifery Certification Board to receive the professional designation of CNM. CMs are educated in the discipline of midwifery. They earn graduate degrees, meet health and science education requirements, complete a midwifery education programme accredited by the Accreditation Commission for Midwifery Education and pass the same national certification examination as CNMs to receive the professional designation of CM (American College of Nurse-Midwives 2014).

The vast majority of direct-entry midwives in the USA are CPMs who have met the standards for certification set by the North American Registry of Midwives (National Association of Certified Professional Midwives 2014). CPMs may have a variety of training routes, from the completion of an accredited midwifery programme to apprenticeship.

State laws restrict midwifery practice as well as the type of midwife that can attend births. CPMs are legally permitted to practice in twenty-eight states. CNMs are licensed to practice in every state; Medicaid reimbursement for CNM/CM care is mandatory in all states and is 100 per cent of the physician fee schedule under the Medicare fee schedule. The majority of states also mandate private insurance reimbursement for midwifery services (American College of Nurse-Midwives 2014).

The Core Data Survey conducted in 2010 of 1998 members of the American College of Nurse-Midwives found that most CNMs were employed by hospitals (31.6 per cent) and physician-owned practices (24.1 per cent). Of the respondents, nearly 70 per cent reported attending births, the majority of which were in hospitals (American College of Nurse-Midwives 2012).

According to the US Department Bureau of Labor Statistics, in May 2012 27,000 health professionals reported they were actively providing maternity care services (5,710 CNMs and 20,880 obstetricians/gynaecologists) (US Department of Labor and Bureau of Labor Statistics 2014). The expected shortages of maternity care providers has prompted legislation to be introduced to the US Congress (Improving Access to Maternity Care

Act HR 4385) that would establish a health professional shortage area designation of maternity care under the Public Health Service Act, similar to that for primary care and dental and mental health.

The structure of the US health care system contributes to the lack of availability of maternal health care providers. High malpractice insurance premiums as well as low reimbursements for women covered by Medicaid create disincentives for providers to treat low income women. According to Amnesty International's report Deadly Delivery, 'Maternal care in the USA all too often fails to meet women's need for comprehensive care' (Amnesty International 2010). Structural gaps include a lack of or inadequate services for things such as counselling and education on nutrition, domestic violence, mental health and smoking cessation. In addition, access to sexual and reproductive health care for many low income women is severely limited.

Maternity entitlements

After Australia passed its parental leave law in 2010, the USA became the only industrialised nation not to offer paid maternity leave (OECD 2014). New parents are entitled to twelve weeks of federally protected time off work through the Family and Medical Leave Act enacted in 1993. However, the Family and Medical Leave Act guarantees job security only for those who have been employed for at least one year and who work for an organisation with fifty or more employees. The Family and Medical Leave Act is available to fewer than 50 per cent of workers and many cannot afford to take it (National Partnership for Women and Families 2012).

Although some employers offer maternity leave benefits, only 11 per cent of US workers have access to paid family leave through their employers (National Partnership for Women and Families 2012). Those employees with paid sick leave can use this benefit, but often state or municipal laws restrict this leave to three to nine days, depending on the size of the business.

States may have additional programmes or policies. For example, since 2004 in California and 2009 in New Jersey, workers can take paid leave to care for an ill family member or bond with a new child (through birth or adoption). New mothers in California are covered by Temporary Disability Insurance, which provides 60 per cent of their salaries with a maximum limit of US$840 per week for six weeks. Temporary Disability Insurance programmes for personal medical leave are also in place in Hawaii, New York, Rhode Island and Puerto Rico (National Partnership for Women and Families 2012). However, fewer than 40 per cent of workers in the USA have access to these programmes.

There are currently three federal initiatives in support of paid family and medical leave. These are: (i) proposed national paid family leave insurance legislation, which would create a federal system to provide up to sixty 'care-giving' days of partially paid leave for reasons covered by the Family and Medical Leave Act; (ii) a proposed US$5 million State Paid Leave Fund in the Federal Department of Labor's 2013 financial year budget that would help states conduct the research, planning and analysis necessary to adopt their own paid leave programmes; and (iii) the Federal Employees Paid Parental Leave Act (HR 616 in the 112th Congress), which would provide four weeks of paid parental leave to federal workers (National Partnership for Women and Families 2012).

Childbirth in the USA

Antenatal

Obstetricians/gynaecologists attend the majority of births and provide care for women during pregnancy and throughout their reproductive life span. Both the American College of Nurse-Midwives and the American College of Obstetrics and Gynecology recommend that women visit a maternity care provider monthly during the first three-quarters of their pregnancy and then every week or two until delivery. Approximately 71 per cent of women initiate prenatal care within the first three months. Black and Hispanic women were twice as likely as white women to receive prenatal care starting in their third trimester, or no prenatal care at all (American Congress of Obstetricians and Gynecologists 2011). According to Listening to Mothers III, a representative survey of 2,400 mothers from across the USA, 38 per cent of mothers surveyed could not receive prenatal care as soon as they had hoped due to financial restrictions, such as not having enough money to pay for the visit or not yet having access to Medicaid (Declercq *et al.* 2013).

Women usually see the same provider for their prenatal care and to attend their delivery (78 per cent). Listening to Mothers III found that 81 per cent of women in their study chose their obstetrician because he or she provided their gynaecological care (Declercq *et al.* 2013). In addition, 75 per cent of women chose their provider because he or she had delivered their babies in the past. However, the majority of women surveyed (96 per cent) reported that they chose their provider because he or she accepted their health insurance. This suggests that health insurance plays an essential role in the maternity care that women receive. Insurance therefore dictates where women give birth, who attends the birth and what tests and/or procedures the mother will receive.

During pregnancy, women usually have multiple tests to monitor their own health and that of their foetus. These tests include blood tests for diabetes, infections and general health, and blood tests and chorionic villous sampling or amniocentesis to check for Down's syndrome or other common foetal conditions. Nearly all mothers from the survey (98 per cent) reported having at least one ultrasound scan during their pregnancy; 70 per cent reported having three or more ultrasound scans and 23 per cent said that they had six or more ultrasound scans (Declercq *et al.* 2013).

In terms of prenatal education, women in the USA turn to a variety of sources for information. For first-time mothers, the survey found that 76 per cent reported that their maternity care provider was their primary source of information about pregnancy and childbirth. A total of 70 per cent of mothers indicated that childbirth education classes (whether hospital-based or from another organisation) served as their primary source of information. Women also relied on pregnancy/childbirth web sites (66 per cent), pregnancy/childbirth phone applications (56 per cent) and general health web sites (51 per cent) for information (Declercq *et al.* 2013).

Intrapartum

In 2010, 98.8 per cent of all births in the USA occurred in hospitals. The vast majority of hospital births are attended by a medical doctor (obstetrician or family physician) (86.3 per cent), followed by CNMs (7.6 per cent) and doctors of osteopathy (5.7 per cent) (Martin *et al.* 2012).

The postpartum length of stay in hospital of newborn babies in the USA has declined steadily from 1970 to the mid-1990s. In 1970 the average length of stay in hospital was 3.9 days, compared with 2.0 days in 1993 (Datar and Sood 2006). The mid- to late 1990s saw state and federal legislation to reduce very short hospital stays for newborn babies. Variations exist across states, but laws generally require insurance plans to cover postpartum hospital stays for newborn babies of at least forty-eight hours for vaginal deliveries and at least ninety-six hours for caesarean sections (Liu *et al.* 2004).

Among the 1.2 per cent of out-of-hospital births, 67.0 were in a residence (home) and 28.0 per cent were in a freestanding birthing centre (Martin *et al.* 2012). After a decline from 1990 to 2004, the percentage of births in the USA that occurred at home increased by 29 per cent, from 0.56 per cent of births in 2004 to 0.72 per cent in 2009. In that year there were 29,650 home births (representing 0.72 per cent of all births), the highest level since 1989 when data was first collected (MacDorman *et al.* 2010).

Table 4.3 shows birth interventions and outcomes from 1970 to 2012. The induction rate has steadily increased since 1970 to the point that 234 of every 1,000 births are induced, with or without medical indication (Martin *et al.* 2012). In contrast, the use of vacuum or forceps for delivery has sharply decreased over time. This is probably correlated with the consistent rise in the number of caesarean section births in this same time period. According to the US Centers for Disease Control and Prevention, fifty-five of every 1,000 births occurred by caesarean section in 1970

(National Center for Health Statistics 1995), whereas the latest figures indicate that 328 (around one-third) of babies are born by caesarean section (Martin *et al.* 2013b). The USA has one of the highest caesarean birth rates in the world, largely due to a fear of litigation, obstetric convenience and hospital protocol (American Congress of Obstetricians and Gynecologists 2011).

In 1991, WHO and UNICEF launched the Baby-Friendly Hospital Initiative, which promotes better maternity care services during pregnancy and especially promotes and supports exclusive breastfeeding immediately postpartum. In the USA, 175 hospitals and birthing centres in forty-one states and the District of Columbia hold the Baby-Friendly designation. Currently, 6.9 per cent of births in the USA occur in a Baby-Friendly facility. The Baby-Friendly Hospital Initiative aims to increase this percentage to 8.1 per cent by the year 2020 (Baby-Friendly USA 2014).

The Listening to Mothers III survey revealed that, at the end of pregnancy, 91 per cent of mothers intend to breastfeed and 50 per cent of new mothers breastfed exclusively during the first three months of their baby's life. This rate falls steadily over the first year. By the time their baby was 12 months old, only 10 per cent of mothers breastfed in conjunction with formula and/or solid foods (Declercq *et al.* 2013).

Postnatal

Maternal and infant health are often separated in the US context, with many more resources and attention historically allocated to organisations and efforts around improving infant outcomes. Maternal mortality in the USA reached a low of 7.4 per 100,000 in 1986, yet by 1990 the maternal mortality rate had begun to steadily increase, with 8.2 maternal deaths per 100,000, rising to a rate of 9.8 per 100,000 in 2000, and reaching 16.8 per 100,000 in 2010, with rates among African American women three to four times those of other racial ethnic groups, a troubling disparity that has persisted during this time frame (Bingham *et al.* 2011). Spending on health care in the USA is twice that of other developed nations, but its maternal and neonatal outcomes are among the worst. Most recently, research published in *The Lancet* on progress towards Millennium Development Goal 5 noted that the USA was one of just eight countries that saw a rise in maternal mortality between 2003 and 2013. The researchers estimated that 18.5 mothers died for every 100,000 births in the USA in 2013, a total of almost 800 deaths. The USA now ranks sixty for maternal deaths on a list of 180 countries, down markedly from its ranks of twenty-two in 1990 and fifty in 2010 (Bingham *et al.* 2011; Kassebaum *et al.* 2014).

This rise in maternal mortality has led to a renewed focus on examining the causes of and contributing factors to this critical public health indicator. Enhanced ascertainment has been estimated to account for no more than 30 per cent of the observed rise (Hoyert 2007). Other possible reasons for

Table 4.3 Birth interventions and outcomes for selected years in the USA

	1970	1980	1990	2000	2010
Maternal mortality rate[a]	21.5	9.2	8.2	9.8	16.8*
Perinatal mortality rate per 1,000 live and stillbirths[b]					
Definition 1: infant deaths under age 7 days and foetal deaths at 28 weeks or more of gestation	–	–	8.95	6.97	–
Definition 2: infant deaths under 28 days and foetal deaths at 20 weeks or more of gestation	–	–	13.12	11.19	–
Neonatal mortality rate per 1,000 live births[c] (deaths under 28 days per 1,000 live births)	15.08	8.48	5.85	4.63	4.2
Infant mortality per 1,000 live births[d]	19.9	12.7	9.4	7.1	6.3
Induction per 1,000 births[e]	Not available	Not available	95	160	234
Forceps per 1,000 births	Not available	176[f]	86[f]	40[f]	6.6[g]
Vacuum per 1,000 births	Not available	7[f]	61[f]	84[f]	29.6[h]
Caesarean per 1,000 births[i]	55	165	220.4	230.1	313.6
Episiotomy per 1,000 births	–	640[j]	556[j]	327[j]	Not available

Sources: * Bingham et al. (2011); a Hoyert (2007); b MacDorman et al. (2012); c UNICEF (2014); d UNICEF (2013); e US Census Bureau (2013); f Simpson and Atterbury (2003); g Martin et al. (2013a); h Martin et al. (2012); i Menacker and Hamilton (2010); j CDC/NCHS National Hospital Discharge Survey (2010).

the rise in maternal mortality and morbidity include increasing rates of caesarean deliveries with their associated risks and more women entering pregnancy with chronic health conditions, such as hypertension and diabetes. In
addition, there have been numerous calls to action; for example, in January
2010, the Joint Commission, which accredits and certifies more than 20,000
health care organisations and programmes in the USA, issued a Sentinel
Event Alert for maternal death, noting:

> Although the current maternal mortality rate may reflect increased
> identification of women who died during or shortly after pregnancy,
> there clearly has been no decrease in maternal mortality in recent
> years, and we are not moving toward the U.S. government's Healthy
> People 2010 target of no more than 3.3 maternal deaths per 100,000
> live births.
>
> (Joint Commission 2010)

In November 2011, the US Health Resources and Services Administration's Maternal Child Health Bureau announced the National Maternal
Health Initiative (Highsmith 2013). In addition, organisations such as the
Association for Maternal Child Health Programs and the US Centers for
Disease Control and Prevention support the expansion of maternal mortality reviews at the state level (Goodman *et al.* 2013). The National Partnership for Maternal Safety is another multi-stakeholder initiative, which
calls for every birthing facility in the USA to have a safety programme in
place for the most common preventable causes of maternal death and
severe morbidity (D'Alton *et al.* 2014).

The infant mortality rate in the USA has declined over the past several
decades, although it has plateaued in recent years. In 2010 the reported
rate was 6.15 deaths per 1,000 live births and the provisional rate for 2011
was 6.05 per 1,000 (SACIM 2013). Racial and ethnic disparities in maternal
and infant outcomes persist; in particular, the infant mortality rate for
non-Hispanic black women (13.31) was 2.4 times the rate for non-Hispanic
white women (5.63). Preterm birth (prior to 37 weeks of gestation) is a
factor driving disparities in infant mortality. In 2007, preterm birth among
non-Hispanic black women accounted for 78 per cent of the higher rates
of infant mortality for non-Hispanic black women compared with non-
Hispanic white women (SACIM 2013).

In 2010, the USA ranked twenty-seventh in infant mortality compared
with other nations in the OECD and the infant mortality rate in the USA is
higher than the industrialised country average of five per 1,000 live births
(OECD 2013). The USA has consistently dropped in ranking since 1960,
when it ranked twelfth, to 1980 when it was ranked nineteenth, to 2005 at
thirtieth, and then twenty-seventh among OECD countries in 2010. Differences in how live births are recorded are not seen as a main cause of the
low ranking (SACIM 2013).

Consumer involvement

Birth outcomes in the USA have been described as a perinatal paradox: despite spending more per capita on health, the maternal and neonatal outcomes are worse than in other industrialised countries that spend less. Efforts to ameliorate this deteriorating situation include the national initiatives described in the previous section. In addition, several organisations have been working for many years to improve birth outcomes, including reductions in non-medically indicated inductions and caesarean deliveries. These organisations have similar goals, but different foci; some, such as the National Partnership for Maternal Safety, work towards quality improvement by highlighting the risks of obstetric emergencies and the need for facility-based readiness. Others, with a focus on more normal birth, advocate for increased access to midwifery and/or low intervention care, including the availability of vaginal birth after caesarean through a focus on normal birth.

Some efforts are directed towards the development of perinatal quality metrics, which can be used to benchmark and publicly report hospital and provider-level rates. The National Quality Forum (NQF) is the organisation designated to review and endorse quality metrics. In 2008, the NQF convened a steering committee of twenty perinatal experts to develop national voluntary consensus standards for perinatal care. Thirty-three measures were considered and the NQF endorsed seventeen, nine of which relate to primarily obstetric practices. Once the NQF has endorsed measures, other organisations may adopt them for tracking quality outcomes. In February 2009, the Joint Commission convened a technical advisory panel of eight perinatal experts to review the NQF recommendations and select a subset for Joint Commission core performance measures of perinatal care. As a result, five measures were selected to apply to hospital discharges starting on 1 April 2010. As of 1 January 2014, hospitals that have more than 1,500 deliveries per year are required to report on these metrics, with public reporting commencing from 1 January 2015. Of note, the Joint Commission had not updated core performance measures for perinatal care since 1999.

The NQF sponsored the formation of the National Priorities Partnership, consisting of more than fifty organisations from across the health care spectrum, including payers, purchasers, providers and consumers, to target maternity care. The National Priorities Partnership decided to focus on two 'aspirational goals': to reduce the percentage of babies delivered electively prior to thirty-nine weeks of gestation to 5 per cent or less and to reduce caesarean births among low-risk women to 15 per cent or less.

The information available to the public regarding the hospital rates of typical childbirth procedures or quality metrics varies by state. Hospitals can select which set of Joint Commission quality measures to report and, until 2014, were under no obligation to choose the perinatal set. Even when they are collected, publicly available data are difficult to find, often highly technical, and/or not presented in user-friendly formats. Most measures typically rely on administrative data obtained from hospital patient discharge diagnoses and vital statistics, which means that the most recent data are typically three to four years old. This makes the data unsuitable for data-driven quality improvement and makes it difficult for payers, consumers, childbearing women and other interested stakeholders to make relevant, informed maternity care decisions about how much to pay for, and where to get, quality care.

Childbirth Connection, an advocacy organisation devoted since 1918 to improving the value and quality of maternity care through consumer engagement and health system transformation, has in recent years focused its energies on promoting evidence-based maternity care, policy and quality issues, and shared decision-making. Centrally engaged in the quality metric and health policy arenas, it has also partnered with the Foundation for Informed Decision Making to develop awareness and create tools for shared decision-making around maternity. Childbirth Connection also maintains a comprehensive web site with information for pregnant women, providers and policy-makers, and has sponsored three national surveys of women who have recently given birth, Listening to Mothers, from 2002 to 2012.

Advocacy for women's access to information and a full range of choices in maternity care has been a key aim of organisational and entrepreneurial efforts. At the national level, several organisations advocate the expansion of access to CPMs and out-of-hospital maternity care. These include professional organisations such as the Midwives Alliance of North America, the National Association of Certified Professional Midwives, educational and lobbying organisations such as the Midwives and Mothers in Action Campaign, the Big Push for Midwives Campaign and Citizens for Midwifery. State-based organisations work to advance legislative efforts pertaining to the legal status and scope of practice of CPMs.

Some organisations are single-issue, such as the International Caesarean Awareness Network, which provides information and local support groups for women about non-medically indicated caesarean delivery and access to vaginal birth after a prior caesarean section. Entrepreneurial efforts, possibly due to the leverages afforded by effective use of social media, have emerged in the past decade. Started as blogs by one or two individuals, they continue as entrepreneurial enterprises offering workshops, such as Jennifer Kamel's VBACFacts.org, whereas others serve as information clearing houses and shared support, such as the Unnecesarean.com blog, whose founder, Jill Arnold, published previously difficult to locate or unpublished caesarean section rates by state (and, where possible, by hospital) on CesareanRates.com.

The numerous membership organisations for doulas and childbirth educators, such as DONA International or Lamaze International, vary in their level of advocacy and engagement in maternity policy. The Coalition for Improving Maternity Services, founded in 1997, is a coalition of individuals and national organisations promoting evidence-based mother- and baby-friendly maternity care. The recent arrival of newcomers, such as ImprovingBirth.org in 2011, has mobilised grassroots Labor Day rallies since 2012 in nearly all fifty states, yet its connection with older, more established organisations is unclear. The diversity of organisations engaged in this space makes it difficult to gauge their overall size or impact. Most of these efforts operate independently, with little funding for national coordination and strategic alliances.

All advocacy efforts to improve maternity care outcomes and experiences do so in a context in which 83 per cent of women rate the quality of care in the USA as good or excellent (Declercq *et al.* 2013). Under the Affordable Healthcare Act, reimbursement rates are tied to patient satisfaction and there is considerable interest among hospitals to develop patient satisfaction surveys that capture the unique features of the maternity hospitalisation experience, as well as developing programmes and models to enhance patient satisfaction.

Risk and rights

In the USA, health care in general and maternity care in particular are organised around a biomedical framework within a neoliberal political and economic context that defines pregnancy as a risky endeavour and a matter of individual, rather than public, responsibility. Poor outcomes are attributed to the individual characteristics of women taken at the aggregate level: women giving birth are said to be older, fatter and sicker. Solutions are therefore largely seen as the responsibility of individuals. Pregnant women are encouraged to take responsibility for managing their weight at optimum levels preconception, inter-conception and during pregnancy, to refrain from potentially harmful practices, such as smoking or drinking alcohol, to seek prenatal care early, and to minimise exposure to stress and other reproductive hazards.

The USA does not consider health care to be a citizen's right; individuals desiring or in need of health care services either purchase them directly or access care through private or public insurance. Neither can the USA be said to have a 'maternity care system', in that access to care and the provision of services are governed by a variety of federal, state and local conditions; care is of varying quality and cost, and outcomes show significant racial and ethnic disparities. As noted in the 2010 Amnesty International report on maternal mortality in the USA, 'the fragmented nature of healthcare financing and delivery also leads to a fragmented and uncoordinated approach to oversight' (Amnesty International 2010). This state of affairs may be changing, with leadership from the Maternal Child Health Bureau proposing a National Maternal Health Initiative and efforts to coordinate hospital readiness and response to obstetric emergencies (Highsmith 2013; D'Alton *et al.* 2014). Furthermore, the Affordable Care Act promises to expand the coverage of preventive care for women as well as to require insurers to offer maternity and newborn care, although, as we have shown, half of all fifty states have either rejected or are considering rejecting Medicaid expansion for their poorest citizens (Rice *et al.* 2013).

There have been recent efforts to put the 'M' for maternal back in maternal–child health or maternal–foetal medicine (D'Alton *et al.* 2012). In the face of persistently poor neonatal outcomes and worsening maternal outcomes, there is a growing recognition that a concerted effort is needed to reverse these trends, as well as to reduce the widening racial and ethnic disparities seen among non-Hispanic black women and their babies. As an example of this, the Secretary's Advisory Committee on Infant Mortality of the US Health and Human Services Department identified improving women's health as the first strategic direction in the national framework to reduce infant deaths (SACIM 2013).

Maternity care clinicians (physicians, midwives and nurses) and hospitals are regulated by public agencies at the federal and state level and by national non-governmental and provider regulatory organisations (Rice *et al.* 2013). Most clinicians are accredited by the licensing boards in states in which they practice. These boards issue new licences to health care clinicians with approved educational credentials, renew licences and enforce basic standards of practice through their power to suspend or revoke licences to practice (Rice *et al.* 2013). They also review complaints and have public databases regarding licensure and discipline information.

The American Board of Obstetrics and Gynecology is an independent, not-for-profit organisation that certifies obstetricians and gynaecologists in the USA and is one of twenty-four specialty boards recognised by the American Board of Medical Specialties. The American Board of Obstetrics and Gynecology also certifies the subspecialty area of maternal and foetal medicine. Other medical specialties that provide maternity care services include family medicine, overseen by its own Board.

The National Council of State Boards of Nursing is a not-for-profit organisation that oversees and develops licensure examinations for nurses and its membership comprises boards of nursing in the fifty US states, the District of Columbia and four territories. The American Midwifery Certification Board is the national certifying body for candidates in nurse-midwifery who have received graduate level education in programmes accredited by the American Midwifery Certification Board. Certification from the American Midwifery Certification Board is recognised in all fifty states in the USA; however, state licensure (in nursing) provides the legal basis for practice. The North American Registry of Midwives is the agency that sets the standards for the nationally accredited CPM credential, which is currently recognised in twenty-eight states in the USA.

Hospitals in the USA are regulated via certification and accreditation requirements by the non-governmental Joint Commission and federal law on who must be treated at hospitals, and by eligibility for reimbursement criteria by Centers for Medicare and Medicaid Services (Rice *et al.* 2013). Founded in 1951, the Joint Commission evaluates and accredits more than 20,000 health care organisations and programmes in the USA and reaccreditation takes place every three years via an on-site survey. Joint Commission standards address a hospital's level of performance in key functional areas, such as patient rights, patient treatment, medication safety and infection control (Joint Commission 2014). Since 1997 the Joint Commission has integrated outcomes and other performance measurement data into the accreditation process. As noted earlier, the perinatal core measure set was adopted in 2009 and will be publicly reported for hospitals with more than 1,500 births annually starting in 2015. Out-of-hospital birth accounts for less than 1 per cent of all births in the USA and the Commission for the Accreditation of Birth Centers is the only accrediting body for freestanding birth centres. The Commission for the Accreditation of Birth Centers has accredited sixty-six birth centres, with six in process, out of a total of 200 birth centres. Neither the federal government nor all states require birth centre accreditation.

Pregnancy and childbirth represent the vast majority of hospitalisations (23 per cent in 2009) and caesarean section is the most common operating room procedure in the country (Childbirth Connection 2012). In 2010, 45 per cent of all maternal childbirth-related hospital stays were billed to Medicaid and 48 per cent to private insurers, with the total facility charges billed reaching a combined total of US$111 billion (Childbirth Connection 2012). About half (51 per cent) of the 6.6 million pregnancies in the USA are unintended and access to comprehensive sexual and reproductive health care varies significantly by income, race and ethnicity, and region of the country (Guttmacher Institute 2013).

Thus, overall, maternity care in the USA is highly medicalised and most women receive care from physicians, predominantly obstetrician/gynaecologists, and give birth in hospitals. In recent years, the proportion of caesarean deliveries has increased by 50 per cent, so that now one in three women have a surgical birth. Whereas vaginal birth after prior caesarean section was seen as optimum two decades ago, reaching a high point of 28 per cent of all births in 1996, it has steadily declined so that by 2005 it was less than 10 per cent. Data have not been available to track national trends since 2005 due to the inconsistent adoption of the revised (2003) birth certificate form across jurisdictions.

Medical specialties that utilise technology and surgery have been shown to have a high degree of geographical variation in utilisation and such variation cannot be attributed to differences in patient population. Obstetrics has dominated maternity care provision in the USA and analyses have shown how variation, both within one facility or across several facilities, in caesarean deliveries, particularly those for labour dystocia (failure to progress) is largely driven by factors such as providers' decision-making (Main *et al.* 2011). Given the dominant position of obstetricians in maternity care delivery, solutions to the over-use of caesarean section are being proposed largely by obstetric leaders and their organisations (Spong *et al.* 2013). CNMs currently attend just 7.6 per cent of births, a slight rise from previous years (Martin *et al.* 2012). Few Americans know what midwives are and/or how to access them and CNMs work in subordinate structures in which physicians hold more power, whether in hospitals or in physician-owned practices.

More ominously, several states have introduced, and Tennessee has recently passed, legislation that criminalises the behaviour of pregnant women if it results in (unintended) harm to the foetus. A study of 413 criminal and civil cases between 1973 and 2005 (after the Roe Supreme Court decision legalising abortion) showed that state authorities have used a number of measures, including foeticide and anti-abortion laws recognising separate rights for fertilised eggs, embryos and foetuses, as the basis for depriving pregnant women – whether they were seeking to end a pregnancy or go to term – of their physical liberty (Paltrow and Flavin 2013).

Conclusion

The maternity care system in the USA is in transition. The Affordable Care Act is in the midst of implementation and rollout and new national efforts aimed at improving maternal health, both in its own right and as a means to further improve infant health, are gaining momentum through the advocacy of maternity organisations and key individual leaders. Yet political opposition to the health care reform legislation means that a significant proportion of women will not have access to affordable health insurance for prenatal and maternity care. Maternity outcomes are highly disparate by race and ethnicity, with non-Hispanic black women having a three- to four-fold higher rate of maternal mortality than women of other races or ethnicities. This is the largest disparity in public health. Despite some gains in infant outcomes overall, racial and ethnic disparities remain a persistent and widening problem.

Although most women who give birth rate the maternity system in the USA as good or excellent, a growing number are voicing displeasure and anger about the over-use of procedures, such as induction and caesarean deliveries, which have weak clinical justification and demonstrate harm without improving overall maternal or neonatal outcomes. Their concerns are echoed by key organisational advocates, such as Childbirth Connection, which focuses on informing policy-makers on issues of maternal quality and safety, or the Big Push for Midwives, which seeks increased access to home birth through legislative action.

The neoliberal context in which maternity care services are delivered means that many of the drivers for system change come from payers and purchasers of health care. The USA is an anomaly in a comparative analysis of maternity care. Health care, even during pregnancy, is not considered a right; professional interests have outweighed those of pregnant women and their babies and the fragmentation of services and oversight means that there is little central regulation, resulting in the over-use of technology even as outcomes worsen. Recent changes have come about by broad coalitions of government agencies, including public health, professional associations and not-for-profit organisations that represent payers (public and private), purchasers and pregnant women.

Useful web sites

VBACFacts.org
Unnecesarean.com blog
CesareanRates.com.
ImprovingBirth.org

References

American College of Nurse-Midwives (2012) *Core Data Survey.* Silver Spring, MD: American College of Nurse-Midwives.

American College of Nurse-Midwives (2014) *Fact Sheet: Essential Facts About Midwives.* Silver Spring, MD: American College of Nurse-Midwives.

American Congress of Obstetricians and Gynecologists (2011) *Women's Health: Stats and Facts.* Washington, DC: American Congress of Obstetricians and Gynecologists.

American Congress of Obstetricians and Gynecologists Workforce Studies and Planning Group (2013) 'The obstetrician-gynecologist distribution atlas'. Washington, DC: American Congress of Obstetricians and Gynecologists.

Amnesty International (2010) *Deadly Delivery: the Maternal Health Care Crisis in the USA* [online]. Available from: www.amnestyusa.org/sites/default/files/pdfs/deadlydelivery.pdf. Accessed 24 June 2014.

Baby-Friendly USA (2014) *Find Facilities* [online]. Available from: www.babyfriendly-usa.org/find-facilities. Accessed 20 May 2014.

Bingham, D., Strauss, N. and Coeytaux, F. (2011) 'Maternal mortality in the United States: a human rights failure', *Contraception*, 83: 189–193.

CDC/National Hospital Discharge Survey (2010) *Number of All-listed Procedures for Discharges From Short-stay Hospitals, By Procedure Category and Sex: United States, 2010* [online]. Available from: www.cdc.gov/nchs/data/nhds/4procedures/2010pro4_numberproceduresex.pdf. Accessed 24 June 2014.

CDC Office of Minority Health and Health Equity (2013) *CDC Health Disparities and Inequalities Report–U.S. 2013.* Washington, DC: CDC Office of Minority Health and Health Equity.

Childbirth Connection (2012) *United States Maternity Care Facts and Figures.* New York, NY: Childbirth Connection.

Cohen, D. and Coco, A. (2009) 'Declining trends in the provision of prenatal care visits by family physicians', *Annals of Family Medicine*, 7 (2): 128–133.

D'Alton, M.E., Bonanno, C.A., Berkowitz, R.L., Brown, H.L., Copel, J.A., Cunningham, F.G., Garite, T.J. *et al.* (2012) 'Putting the "M" back in maternal-fetal medicine', *American Journal of Obstetrics and Gynecology*, 208 (6): 442–448.

D'Alton, M.E., Main, E.K., Menard, M.K. and Levy, B.S. (2014) 'The National Partnership for Maternal Safety', *Obstetrics and Gynecology*, 123 (5): 973–977.

Datar, A. and Sood, N. (2006) 'Impact of postpartum hospital-stay legislation on newborn length of stay, readmission, and mortality in California', *Pediatrics*, 118 (1): 63–72.

Declercq, E., Sakala, C., Corry, M.P., Applebaum, S. and Herrlich, A. (2013) *Listening to Mothers III: Pregnancy and Childbirth*. New York: Childbirth Connection.

Esping-Anderson, G. (1990) *The Three Worlds of Welfare Capitalism*. Princeton, NJ: Princeton University Press.

Goodman, D., Stampfel, C., Creanga, A.A., Callaghan, W.M., Callahan, T., Bonzon, E., Berg, C. and Grigorescu, V. (2013) 'Revival of a core public health function: state- and urban-based maternal death review processes', *Journal of Women's Health*, 22 (5): 395–398.

Guttmacher Institute (2013) *Fact Sheet: Unintended Pregnancy in the United States* [online]. Available from: www.guttmacher.org/pubs/FB-Unintended-Pregnancy-US.html. Accessed 24 June 2014.

Highsmith, K. (2013) *National Maternal Health Initiative: a Comprehensive Collaborative Strategy* [online]. Maternal and Child Health Bureau, Health Resources and Services Administration. Available from: www.hrsa.gov/advisorycommittees/mchb advisory/InfantMortality/natlmentalhlthinitiative.pdf. Accessed 24 June 2014.

Hoyert, D.L. (2007) 'Maternal mortality and related concepts', *Vital Health Statistics*, 3 (33). Hyattsville, MD: National Center for Health Statistics.

Joint Commission (2010) *Preventing Maternal Death. Sentinal Event Alert, Issue 44* [online]. Available from: www.jointcommission.org/sentinel_event_alert_issue_44_preventing_maternal_death/. Accessed 30 June 2014.

Joint Commission (2014) *Facts about the Joint Commission* [online]. Available from: www.jointcommission.org/about_us/fact_sheets.aspx. Accessed 30 June 2014.

Kaiser Family Foundation (2013a) *Issue Brief: Health Reform: Implications for Women's Access to Coverage and Care*. Menlo Park, CA: Kaiser Family Foundation.

Kaiser Family Foundation (2013b) 'Visualizing health policy: the role of Medicaid and Medicare in women's health care', *Journal of the American Medical Association*, 309 (19): 1984.

Kaiser Family Foundation (2014) *Registered Nurses per 100,000 Population. State Health Facts* [online]. Available from: http://kff.org/other/state-indicator/registered-nurses-per-100000-population/. Accessed 10 April 2014.

Kassebaum, N.J., Bertozzi-Villa, A., Coggeshall, M.S. Shackelford, K.A. Steiner, C., Heuton, K.R. *et al.* (2014) 'Global, regional, and national levels and causes of maternal mortality during 1990–2013: a systematic analysis for the Global Burden of Disease Study 2013', *The Lancet*, 2 May 2014.

Liu, Z., Dow, W.H. and Norton, E.C. (2004) 'Effect of drive-through delivery laws on postpartum length of stay and hospital charges', *Journal of Health Economics*, 23 (1): 129–155.

MacDorman, M., Kirmeyer, S.E. and Wilson, E.C. (2012) 'Fetal and perinatal mortality, United States, 2006', *National Vital Statistics Report*, 60 (8). Hyattsville, MD:

National Center for Health Statistics. Available from: www.cdc.gov/nchs/data/nvsr/nvsr60/nvsr60_08.pdf. Accessed 20 June 2014.

MacDorman, M., Menacker, F. and Declercq, E. (2010) 'Trends and characteristics of home and other out-of-hospital births in the United States, 1990–2006', *National Vital Statistics Reports*, 58 (11). Hyattsville, MD: National Center for Health Statistics. Available from: www.cdc.gov/nchs/data/nvsr/nvsr58/nvsr58_11.PDF. Accessed 20 June 2014.

Main, E.K., Morton, C.H., Hopkins, D., Giuliani, G., Melsop, K. and Gould, J.B. (2011) *Cesarean Deliveries, Outcomes, and Opportunities for Change in California: Toward a Public Agenda for Maternity Care, Safety and Quality.* CMQCC White Papers. Palo Alto, CA: California Maternal Quality Care Collaborative.

Martin, J.A., Hamilton, B.E., Ventura, S.J., Osterman, M.J., Wilson, E.C. and Mathews, T.J. (2012) 'Births: final data for 2010', *National Vital Statistics Reports*, 61 (1). Hyattsville, MD: National Center for Health Statistics. Available from: www.cdc.gov/nchs/data/nvsr/nvsr61/nvsr61_01.pdf. Accessed 20 June 2014.

Martin, J.A., Hamilton, B.E., Ventura, S.J., Osterman, M.J. and Mathews, T.J. (2013a) 'Births: final data for 2011', *National Vital Statistics Report*, 62 (1). Hyattsville, MD: National Center for Health Statistics. Available from: www.cdc.gov/nchs/data/nvsr/nvsr62/nvsr62_01.pdf. Accessed 20 June 2014.

Martin, J.A., Hamilton, B.E., Osterman, M.J., Curtin, S.C. and Mathews, T.J. (2013b) *Births: final data for 2012. National Vital Statistics Report*, 62 (9). Hyattsville, MD: National Center for Health Statistics. Available from: www.cdc.gov/nchs/data/nvsr/nvsr62/nvsr62_09.pdf. Accessed 30 June 2014.

Menacker, F. and Hamilton, B.E. (2010) 'Recent trends in cesarean delivery in the United States', *NCHS Data Brief No. 35*. Hyattsville, MD: National Center for Health Statistics.

Miniño, A.M. (2013) 'Death in the United States, 2011'. *NCHS Data Brief No. 115*. Hyattsville, MD: National Center for Health Statistics.

National Association of Certified Professional Midwives (2014) *What is a Certified Professional Midwife?* [online]. Available from: www.nacpm.org/what-is-cpm.html. Accessed 1 April 2014.

National Center for Health Statistics (1995) 'Rates of cesarean delivery – United States, 1993', *Morbidity and Mortality Weekly Report*, 44 (15): 303–307. Available from: www.cdc.gov/mmwr/preview/mmwrhtml/00036845.htm. Accessed 30 June 2014.

National Partnership for Women and Families (2012) *Fact Sheet: Paid Family and Medical Leave: an Overview* [online]. Available from: www.nationalpartnership.org/research-library/work-family/paid-leave/paid-family-and-medical-leave.pdf. Accessed 1 April 2014.

North American Registry of Midwives (2014) [online]. Available from: http://narm.org/certification/current-status/. Accessed 1 April 2014.

OECD (2013) *Health at a Glance 2013: OECD Indicators.* Paris: OECD.

OECD (2014) *OECD Family Database* [online]. Available from: www.oecd.org/social/family/database. Accessed 1 April 2014.

Paltrow, L.M. and Flavin, J. (2013) 'Arrests of and forced interventions on pregnant women in the United States, 1973–2005: implications for women's legal status and public health', *Journal of Health Politics, Policy and Law*, 38 (2): 299–343.

Ray, R., Sanes, M. and Schmitt, J. (2013) *No-vacation Nation Revisited.* Washington, DC: Center for Economic and Policy Research. Available from: www.cepr.net/documents/publications/no-vacation-update-2013-05.pdf. Accessed 30 June 2014.

Rayburn, W.F. (2011) *The Obstetrician/gynecologist Workforce in the United States: Facts, Figures, and Implications.* Washington, DC: American Congress of Obstetricians and Gynecologists.

Rice, T., Rosenau, P., Unruh, L.Y., Barnes, A.J., Saltman, R.B. and Ginneken, E. van (2013) 'United States of America: health system review', *Health Systems in Transition*, 15 (3): 1–431.

Secretary's Advisory Committee on Infant Mortality (SACIM) (2013) *Report of the Secretary's Advisory Committee on Infant Mortality: Recommendations for Department of Health and Human Services Action and Framework for a National Strategy* [online]. Health Resources and Services Administration. Available from: www.hrsa.gov/advisorycommittees/mchbadvisory/InfantMortality/Correspondence/recommendationsjan2013.pdf.

Simpson, K.R. and Atterbury, J. (2003) 'Trends and issues in labor induction in the United States: implications for clinical practice', *Journal of Obstetric, Gynecologic, and Neonatal Nursing*, 32 (6): 767–779.

Spong, C.Y., Berghella, V., Wenstrom, K.D., Mercer, B.M. and Saade, G.R. (2013) 'Preventing the first cesarean delivery: summary of a joint Eunice Kennedy Shriver National Institute of Child Health and Human Development, Society for Maternal-Fetal Medicine, and American College of Obstetricians and Gynecologists workshop' [reply]. *Obstetrics and Gynecology* 121 (3): 687.

Tong, S.T., Makaroff, L.A., Xierali, I.M., Parhat, P., Puffer, J.C., Newton, W.P. and Bazemore, A.W. (2012) 'Proportion of family physicians providing maternity care continues to decline', *Journal of the American Board of Family Medicine*, 25 (3): 270–271.

US Census Bureau (2010) *2010 Census Urban Area Facts* [online]. Available from: www.census.gov/geo/reference/ua/uafacts.html. Accessed 1 April 2014.

US Census Bureau (2012a) *2012 Statistical Abstract* [online]. Available from: www.census.gov/compendia/statab/2012edition.html. Accessed 1 April 2014.

US Census Bureau (2012b) *Percentage of Births to Teens, Unmarried Mothers, and Births with Low Birth Weight: 1990 to 2008* [online]. Available from: www.census.gov/compendia/statab/2012/tables/12s0086.pdf. Accessed 1 April 2014.

US Census Bureau (2012c) *Resident Population, by Age, Sex, Race and Hispanic Origin: United States, Selected Years 1950–2012* [online]. Available from: www.cdc.gov/nchs/data/hus/2012/001.pdf. Accessed 1 April 2014.

US Census Bureau (2014) *Monthly Population Estimates for the United States: April 1, 2010 to December 1, 2014* [online]. Available from: http://factfinder2.census.gov/faces/tableservices/jsf/pages/productview.xhtml?src=bkmk. Accessed 1 April 2014.

US Department of Health and Human Services, Health Resources and Services Administration (2010) *The Registered Nurse Population: Initial Findings from the 2008 National Sample of Registered Nurses* [online]. Available from: http://bhpr.hrsa.gov/healthworkforce/rnsurveys/rnsurveyinitial2008.pdf. Accessed 1 April 2014.

US Department of Health and Human Services, Health Resources and Services Administration, and Maternal and Child Health Bureau (2014) *Number of Individuals Served by Title V, by Class of Individuals, Title V Information System* [online]. Available from: https://mchdata.hrsa.gov/tvisreports/ProgramData/NumIndiServe.aspx. Accessed 10 April 2014.

US Department of Labor and Bureau of Labor Statistics (2014) *Occupational Employment and Wages: Obstetricans and Gynecologists* [online]. Available from: www.bls.gov/OES/current/oes291064.htm. Accessed 1 April 2014.

UNICEF (2013) 'Trends in infant mortality rates, 1960–2012'. In: *Statistics by Area: Child Survival and Health* [online]. Available from: www.childinfo.org/mortality_imrcountrydata.php. Accessed 1 April 2014.

UNICEF (2014) *Child Mortality Estimates: United States of America* [online]. Available from: www.childmortality.org/index.php?r=site/graph&ID=USA_United States of America. Accessed 1 April 2014.

World Atlas Website (2014) *United States of America* [online]. Available from: www.worldatlas.com/webimage/countrys/namerica/us.htm. Accessed 30 June 2014.

World Bank (2013) 'Fertility rate, total (births per woman)'. *Data* [online]. Available from: http://data.worldbank.org/indicator/SP.DYN.TFRT.IN. Accessed 5 February 2014.

5 Australia

Meredith McIntyre

Background

Australia is located in Oceania between the South Pacific Ocean and the Indian Ocean. Australia is a federal state with a parliamentary democracy and constitutional monarchy; it consists of six states and seven territories. Rich in natural resources, it is reported to be one of the largest capitalist economies in the world, ranked fifth in the world in terms of per capita GDP (International Monetary Fund 2014). Since the early 1990s, Australia has experienced its longest period of continuous economic growth on record as a result of the global boom in natural resources (Greenville *et al.* 2013). The nation has developed a highly diversified economy with considerable strengths, particularly in the mining and agricultural sectors, and has become increasingly integrated economically with the countries of East Asia. It has also avoided some of the more severe effects of the global financial crisis as a consequence of a highly regulated banking sector (Australian Bureau of Statistics 2010). The distribution of wealth in Australia reflects that of other OECD countries (Australian Bureau of Statistics 2013a). The average household net-adjusted disposable income per capita is US$31,197 per year, more than the OECD average of US$23,938 per year. However, there is a considerable gap between the richest and poorest – the top 20 per cent of the population earn almost six times as much as the bottom 20 per cent (OECD 2013).

Australia was claimed by Britain in 1770 after Captain James Cook charted the east coast. Britain established penal colonies in New South Wales and Tasmania from 1788, and later also in Western Australia. The great Australian gold rush, commencing in the 1850s, attracted great waves of immigrants from all over the world, quickly outnumbering the convict communities and creating the beginnings of a multicultural society. From the 1850s to the 1890s, when few other countries in the world were democratic, the Australian colonies progressively established universal male suffrage and were also among the first to give women the vote. The six colonies united in 1901 to form the federal Commonwealth of Australia (Department of Foreign Affairs and Trade 2013), although they still remained a member of the British Commonwealth. While the Aboriginal and Torres Strait Islander peoples are the traditional inhabitants of the land, immigrants from more than 200 countries also call Australia home. In the early years after World War II, the majority of migrants came from Europe. These days, Australia is the destination for migrants and refugees from Asia, Africa and the Middle East. Australia's immigration policy welcomes people from all over the world and does not discriminate on racial, cultural or religious grounds (Department of Foreign Affairs and Trade 2013). The estimated resident population of Australia on 30 June 2013 was 23,130,900 people and the annual population growth rate for the year ended 30 June 2013 was 1.8 per cent, higher than the world's average of 1.2 per cent (Australian Bureau of Statistics 2013b). Modern Australian society represents a melting pot of diverse cultures and is one of the world's most multicultural nations.

Australia as a welfare regime

Australia is usually listed within the English-speaking family of welfare regimes, which includes Canada, Ireland, New Zealand, the USA and the UK (Castles 2010). These countries are categorised as the 'residual welfare model' (Titmuss 1987) or 'liberal' welfare state (Esping-Andersen 1990). Selectivism predominates, particularly in the realm of income transfers (i.e. means-tested assistance, modest universal transfers or social insurance). Entitlement rules are strict and are often associated with stigma; decommodification effects are therefore limited. However, the welfare models that exist within this grouping vary. Castles and Mitchell (1991) identified several unique characteristics of the Australian welfare state, including the combination of high-level minimum wage policies and a strong emphasis on relatively generous means-tested welfare programmes. The 'wage-earners' welfare regime, recognised by Castles (1996) and Schwartz (1998), is a more labour market centred and work-oriented model than its American and British counterparts and shows similarities to Singapore, South Korea and Japan. However, Australia belongs to a highly selective and residual type of welfare regime and most social security schemes are non-contributory, except for the health insurance scheme. About half of all the taxes collected in Australia are directed to social spending. In 2007 Australia spent 16 per cent of GDP on cash benefits (including pensions and unemployment payments, health care and community services), compared with an OECD average of just over 19 per cent (OECD 2013). Australian citizens are eligible to receive government support payments if they are unemployed, live with a disability or are single parents to pre-school children. A pension is available for the older population, subject to age and asset restrictions. Unlike the other government support payments, this pension provides only a bare living, marginally above the poverty line. Welfare spending in Australia represented 18.8 per cent of the GDP in 2013 (OECD 2013).

Health care system

The Australian government provides high-quality, tax-funded health services, regardless of the ability to pay, through a Medicare levy system applied to all tax-payers. The health care system is complex, involving many funders and health care providers. As a federal state, responsibilities are split between different levels of government, and between the government and non-government sectors. As a generalisation, the Australian government is primarily responsible for the funding of health care through health insurance arrangements and direct payments to the States and Territories, while the States and Territories are primarily responsible for the direct provision of services. The system is a mixture of public and private sector health service providers and a range of funding and regulatory mechanisms. The Australian government has the primary role of developing broad national policies, regulation and funding. The State and Territory and local governments are primarily responsible for the delivery and management of public health services. They are also responsible for maintaining direct relationships with most of the health care providers, including the regulation of health professionals and private hospitals, private practitioners (including general practitioners, specialists and consultant physicians) and for-profit and non-profit organisations and voluntary agencies.

The Australian government's funding includes three major national subsidy schemes: Medicare, the Pharmaceutical Benefits Scheme and the 30 per cent Private Health Insurance Rebate. Medicare provides the entire population with subsidised access to medical care, free public hospital care, subsidised pharmaceutical drugs and basic dental care. The people of Australia make their contribution to the health care system through taxes and the Medicare levy based on their income, and through private financing such as private health insurance. Despite this safety net, disparities in access to health services are evident between urban and rural health services, with those living in rural areas reporting poorer health outcomes, and the continuing poor health status of Indigenous Australians.

The Pharmaceutical Benefits Scheme subsidises payments for a high proportion of prescription drugs purchased from pharmacies, with individuals contributing out-of-pocket payments for services (Australian Insitute of Health and Welfare 2012b). Under Medicare, the Australian and State governments also jointly fund public hospital services, so these are provided free of charge to people who choose to be treated as public patients.

Australians are encouraged by the government to take out private health insurance by way of the Medicare levy surcharge. This is applied to people earning over a certain amount who do not have appropriate hospital cover. Private health insurance can cover private and public hospital charges (public hospitals only charge those patients who elect to be private patients in order to be treated by the doctor of their choice) and a portion of medical fees for inpatient services. Private insurance can also cover allied health/paramedic services (such as physiotherapy and podiatry services) and some aids and appliances (such as spectacles).

Expenditure on health in Australia was 9.5 per cent of GDP in 2011–2012, up from 9.3 per cent in 2010–2011 and up from 8.4 per cent in 2001–2002 (Australian Insitute of Health and Welfare 2013a). The estimated recurrent expenditure on health was US$5,881 per person. Governments funded 69.7 per cent of the total health expenditure, a slight increase from 69.1 per cent in 2010–2011. The largest components of health spending were public hospital services (31.8 per cent of recurrent expenditure), followed by medical services (18.1 per cent) and medications (14.2 per cent). The private health insurance schemes contributed 8 per cent of funding for the health system. Less than 2 per cent of the total health budget is spent on public health (disease prevention and health promotion at the population level) (Australian Insitute of Health and Welfare 2013a). Funding for primary health care is invested in the growing general medical practice (small business) sector through Medicare payments. In recent years there has been a decline in the number of general medical practice services that do not require an out-of-pocket co-payment. This situation is exerting additional stress on the public hospital sector, as those who cannot pay choose to wait for medical care in the overcrowded local hospital emergency departments.

The cost of funding health care has increased at a greater rate than the economy as people of all ages expect to receive the best that modern medical technology and health care can provide. Health and medical research spending comprises 14 per cent of all research development funding in Australia (Australian Insitute of Health and Welfare 2012b).

Medical practitioners in Australia, as the main providers of primary health care, are funded by the government via Medicare payments. The medical practitioner workforce experienced a 10.7 per cent rise in numbers between 2007 and 2011 (Australian Insitute of Health and Welfare 2013b). The gender balance has continued to shift, with women making up 37.6 per cent of practitioners in 2011 compared with 34 per cent in 2007. Specialists-in-training in the public sector worked the longest average hours per week (47.6 hours), while general practitioners in the public sector worked the least (20.5 hours) (Australian Insitute of Health and Welfare 2013b). All doctors must be registered with the Medical Board. The Medical Board looks after complaints about doctors and issues of professional conduct. The Medical Board also ensures that only properly trained doctors are registered and administers the registration of doctors who have trained overseas. To meet the projected medical workforce demands across the nation, new enrolments into medical courses have almost doubled from 1889 in 2003 to 3686 in 2012 (Health Workforce Australia 2013).

Between 2007 and 2011, the number of nurses and midwives employed in nursing increased by 7.7 per cent (Table 5.1). The average age of the workforce increased from 43.7 to 44.5 and the proportion of nurses and midwives aged 50 or older increased from 33.0 to 38.6 per cent (Australian Insitute of Health and Welfare 2012d). In 2011, the Australian supply of full-time equivalent nurses was 1056 per 100,000 population. In 2011, four out of five registered nurses and midwives provided direct patient care (Health Workforce Australia 2013). New enrolments across the country into nursing courses have increased by 33 per cent from 10,746 in 2005 to 16,328 in 2011 (Health Workforce Australia 2013). Midwives working in Australia are either dual-qualified as a registered nurse and midwife and make up 46.2 per 100,000 or hold a midwifery-only qualification as with 6 per 100,000 (Health Workforce Australia 2013).

Medical, nursing and allied health professional education in Australia is provided by the university sector, with strong links to clinical placement partner health services. Nursing and midwifery courses were the last to move into the tertiary education sector in the 1980s. The medical, nursing and allied health workforces have grown substantially since 1996 in response to steady population growth and the projected health needs of an ageing population.

Nurses, midwives and the majority of allied health professionals are not eligible to receive Medicare funding for health service provision. This has restricted the opportunities for these groups of health professionals to provide primary care services, resulting in the majority being employed in public and private health service organisations.

The Australian Health Practitioner Regulation Agency is responsible for the regulation of fourteen health professions under the National Registration and Accreditation Scheme. The Australian Health Practitioner Regulation Agency supports fourteen National Boards that are responsible for regulating individual health professions. The primary role of the National Boards is to protect the public and they set standards and policies that all registered health practitioners must meet. The Nursing and Midwifery Board of Australia and the Medical Board Australia comprise two of the fourteen boards.

Table 5.1 Human and physical resources in Australia

Physicians per 1,000 population	3.3
Nurses per 1,000 population	10.5
Total hospital beds per 1,000 population	3.86
Curative (acute) care beds per 1,000 population	3.5
Midwives per 1,000 population	0.6

Source: Health Workforce Australia (2013).

Demographic profile

Australia is the most urbanised country in the world, with 89.1 per cent of the population living in cities or within eighty kilometres of the coast (Geohive 2014). Children aged 0–14 years make up 19 per cent of the population, while people aged sixty-five years and older account for 14 per cent of the population (Table 5.2). Two-thirds of the population are therefore aged 15–64 years (67 per cent) – the group that is traditionally treated as being of working age. The median age of the population was 38.1 years in 2013. One-quarter of the population was born overseas and many residents who were born in Australia have a parent who was born in another country. Aboriginal people and Torres Strait Islanders represent 2.5 per cent of the population. Around one-half of the population aged fifteen years and older is married. The median age at first marriage in 2011 was 29.7 years for men and twenty-eight years for women (Australian Bureau of Statistics 2014).

The life expectancy at birth of Australians continues to be among the highest in the world. The life expectancy at birth of Australians is almost eighty-two years, two years higher than the OECD average of eighty years. Life expectancy for women is eighty-four years, compared with eighty for men (Australian Insitute of Health and Welfare 2012b; OECD 2013). A boy born in 2011 can expect to live 79.9 years, whereas a girl can expect to live 84.3 years. For those approaching retirement age, say sixty-five years, men can expect to live a further nineteen years and women a further twenty-two years (Australian Bureau of Statistics 2012b). In contrast, the latest data available indicate that life expectancy for Indigenous boys born between 2005 and 2007 was estimated to be 67.2 years (compared with 78.7 years for non-Indigenous boys for the period) and for Indigenous girls 72.9 years (compared with 82.6 years) (Australian Insitute of Health and Welfare 2012c).

There were 309,582 births registered in Australia in 2012, approximately 8,000 (2.6 per cent) more than the number registered in 2011

Table 5.2 Demographic profile of Australia

Population	23,235,800
Women (%)	50.22
Population aged 0–14 years (%)	18.1
Population aged 65 years and above (%)	14.2
Population annual growth (%)	1.8
Population density per square kilometre	2.91
Fertility rate (total births per woman)	1.89
Crude birth rate per 1000 people	13.6
Crude death rate per 1000 people	6.5
Urban population (%)	89

Source: Australian Insitute of Health and Welfare (2012).

(301,617). Just over half (51 per cent) of all births registered in 2012 were male babies, resulting in a sex ratio at birth of 105.6 male births per 100 female births (Australian Bureau of Statistics 2012a). In 2012, Australia's total fertility rate was 1.93 babies per woman, an increase from the 2001 total fertility rate of 1.74 babies per woman. Since 1976, the total fertility rate for Australia has been below the replacement level of 2.1 babies per woman (Australian Bureau of Statistics 2012a). Fertility rates increased slightly for women aged 20–24 years, 30–34 years, 35–39 years and 45–49 years between 2011 and 2012 and remained stable for all other age groups. At the national level, the teenage fertility rate remained stable between 2011 and 2012, with sixteen babies per 1,000 women aged 15–19 years (Australian Bureau of Statistics 2012a). In 2012, the total fertility rate for Aboriginal and Torres Strait Islander women decreased to 2.71 babies per woman from 2.74 babies per woman in 2011. Births to women aged under 30 years contributed three-quarters (76 per cent) of the total fertility rate for Aboriginal and Torres Strait Islander women in 2012, compared with less than half of the total fertility rate for all women (45 per cent) (Australian Bureau of Statistics 2012a).

The average age of first-time Australian mothers continues to rise. The report, *Australia's Mothers and Babies 2011*, shows that, in 2011, the average age of women having their first baby was 28.3 years. Of all first-time mothers in 2011, 14.2 per cent were aged thirty-five or older (Li *et al.* 2013).

Maternity provision

Australia has a relatively short history when it comes to non-Indigenous childbirth practices. At the time of colonisation, the professionalisation of medicine was well established across Europe and the USA. The practice of midwifery at the time, an inheritance from English origins, was a vocation for working class women without formal education attending births and providing domestic support to the household during the lying-in period (Hastie 2006). This level of childbirth support was all most families expected or could afford; however, a small minority of affluent women at the time engaged a medical practitioner to attend the birth (Purcal 2008). This situation established a belief in the community, still in evidence today, that medical care in childbirth represents the best care money can buy, relegating midwifery care to being the lesser option. Since this time, competition between medicine and midwifery for a market share in uncomplicated childbirth has continued unabated. The modern iteration of the struggle between obstetrics and midwifery has been sensationalised in a recent high-profile Australian-based book *The Birth Wars* (MacColl 2009). The medical professions position themselves as the guardians of safety in childbirth in the belief that only they have the training and expertise for safe birth outcomes to be achieved (Australian and New Zealand

College of Anaesthetists 2008). This position is supported by the Secretary General of the Australian Medical Association, who warned that the introduction of non-medically led services will undermine the quality of maternity services in Australia and threaten the safety of mothers and babies (Australian Medical Association 2008).

In the 1980s, fiscally responsible health service management introduced independent arbitrators in the form of maternity service managers replacing medical directors in important decision-making appointments. This change immediately challenged a funding model that incentivised (higher payments) medical interventions during birth (McIntyre *et al.* 2012a). The first decade of the twenty-first century has seen important key stakeholders in maternity service delivery join forces in a campaign to deliver pregnant women with a choice of maternity care provider (Hastie 2008). The routine presence of obstetrics in normal birth has been challenged by advocates for normal birth, drawing health management scrutiny to the financial extravagance associated with all pregnant women being allocated the same expensive resources irrespective of clinical need (McIntyre *et al.* 2012a).

Maternity care professionals in Australia include specialist obstetricians, midwives and rural doctors. Midwives registered to work in Australia have completed a three-year undergraduate course (direct-entry), an eighteen-month post-graduate course following registration as a nurse, or a four-year undergraduate double-degree nursing and midwifery course. Midwives are employed by maternity service providers, with a small number being self-employed in private group practices. Rural doctors have completed procedural obstetric and/or anaesthetic training, for which they are registered, in addition to their medical degree and internship training. The services provided by obstetricians and rural doctors are covered by a schedule of government-funded Medicare payments; private midwifery services, however, do not receive this funding and must rely on fee-for-service payments.

Maternity services in Australia are located within the public and private acute hospital sectors. The majority of Australian women (96.9 per cent) give birth in either obstetric-led public or private hospitals (Li *et al.* 2013), reflecting a widespread acceptance that birth needs to be medically managed. Risk management is a primary driver of practice in Australian maternity care (Jordan and Murphy 2009). The assessment of medical risk in childbirth has only recently been questioned in Australia in the light of the escalation in unexplained caesarean births affecting mothers of all ages, races and across all medical conditions, with an associated rise in morbidity rates (Janssens *et al.* 2008; Roberts *et al.* 2009; Laws *et al.* 2010). The universal application of risk management in Australian maternity care was associated with 33.2 per cent of primiparous women giving birth by caesarean section in 2011 (Li *et al.* 2013), reflecting a similar international trend.

Maternity entitlements

The minimum entitlement for parental leave is twelve months of unpaid leave (Office of the Fair Work Ombudsman 2012). The Australian government has introduced a paid parental leave scheme for working parents of children born or adopted on or after 1 January 2011. The scheme gives eligible employees up to eighteen weeks of pay at the National Minimum Wage. This applies to eligible primary carers of newborn babies or adopted children. The payment is made by the government to the employer, who then pays it to the employee. To be eligible for the payment, the woman must have worked for at least ten of the thirteen months prior to the birth or adoption of the child and have worked for at least 330 hours in that ten-month period (just over one day a week), with no more than an eight-week gap between two consecutive working days. Both parents can take twelve months of unpaid leave to care for a newborn baby or adopted child. The parents have to take most of their unpaid parental leave at separate times. The total amount of leave that parents can take between them is twenty-four months. The leave cannot be taken more than two years after the baby's birth or adoption date (Office of the Fair Work Ombudsman 2012).

The Australian government has incentivised natural population growth with a tax-free Baby Bonus payment of US$5,000 paid for all children born or adopted before 1 July 2013. Eligibility for the Baby Bonus has changed for all children born or adopted after 1 July 2013. The first baby born is eligible for US$5,000 and all subsequent children receive US$3,000 (Department of Human Services 2014). The government assists with the cost of raising children through a Family Tax Benefit payment for each child aged 0–15 years. To qualify, the family needs to satisfy an income test, meet residence requirements and be caring for the child at least 35 per cent of the time. A parenting payment is also available to support unemployed single parents with a child aged less than six years (Department of Human Services 2014).

Childbirth in Australia

The escalating costs of maternity service provision have been attributed to the fact that healthy informed Australian women have come to expect access to expensive high-tech specialist resources. Inequity is a strong feature of this expectation as there are insufficient maternity care resources available for women living in regional, rural or remote communities (McIntyre *et al.* 2011a). Inequity of access to maternity care in rural and remote communities was raised as a serious deficiency in current maternity service delivery, a situation exacerbated by service closures (National Rural Health Alliance 2008). The limited availability of services requires pregnant women to travel long distances for care, with many women needing to leave their community to give birth, placing a substantial burden on the families affected (National Consensus Framework for Rural Maternity Services 2008; National Rural Health Alliance 2008). New immigrants to Australia predominantly settle in the capital cities. The metropolitan areas thus have a large 'voice'. Rural regions have often felt that they are the 'poor relation' and, over time, smaller and more remote inland centres in particular have struggled to retain their populations (Muir 2007).

Australian women have experienced substantial decreases in maternal mortality rates over the past century. The rate stabilised in the 1980s to approximately ten deaths per 100,000 live births, with the most recent status in 2010 reported as seven deaths per 100,000 live births. Australia's perinatal mortality rates have declined from 21.7 perinatal deaths per 1,000 births in 1973 to 10.3 perinatal deaths per 1,000 births in 2007 – a decline of 53 per cent. Compared with other OECD nations, Australia's maternal and perinatal mortality rates remain relatively low (Li *et al.* 2013).

Antenatal

Women in Australia routinely attend a general medical practitioner for confirmation of their pregnancy and, in this process, are referred directly to private or public obstetric services, reinforcing an obstetric monopoly and the general population's belief that medical care is essential to ensure the safety of mother and baby (McIntyre *et al.* 2011a).

Antenatal care is provided in private medical consulting rooms for women receiving private obstetric care. The antenatal histories for these women are not shared with the hospital in which they are booked to give birth, creating a gap in information transfer between antenatal care and labour care. Comprehensive health and medical histories are taken during the hospital booking process to compensate for the lack of antenatal information. Women receiving publicly funded antenatal care attend medical-led antenatal clinics in large public hospitals, supplemented by a small number of midwifery-led antenatal care services. A pregnant woman attending midwifery-led antenatal care, where available, must see an obstetrician at least twice during her pregnancy. Antenatal records for these women are located within the maternity service and are available for reference during labour care. The clinical practice guidelines for antenatal care recommend ten visits for a woman's first pregnancy without complications and seven visits for subsequent uncomplicated pregnancies (National Health and Medical Research Council 2012). Australia's mothers and babies study reported that 65.7 per cent of all pregnant women attended at least one antenatal visit in the first trimester (before fourteen weeks of gestation) and 13.8 per cent did not begin antenatal care until after twenty weeks of gestation (Li *et al.* 2013).

Intrapartum

The caesarean section rate has shown an upward trend in the last decade, increasing from 27.0 per cent nationally in 2002 to a peak of 33.3 per cent in 2011 (Table 5.3). Women giving birth in private hospitals accounted for 42.8 per cent of the total, compared with 29.4 per cent of women giving birth in public hospitals. The onset of labour was spontaneous for 54.8 per cent of all women who gave birth and there was no labour for 19.1 per cent of mothers. Labour was induced for 26.0 per cent of mothers and augmented for 17.9 per cent of all mothers, representing one-third (32.8 per cent) of mothers with a spontaneous onset of labour. In subsequent pregnancies, 12.3 per cent of mothers who had previously had a caesarean section had a non-instrumental vaginal birth and 3.5 per cent had an instrumental vaginal birth. Repeat caesarean sections occurred for 84.1 per cent of mothers with a history of caesarean section (Li *et al.* 2013). Rising rates of caesarean section are the consequence of a risk management framework where caesarean section is considered a safe, low-risk childbirth option in an environment where the risks associated with caesarean birth are downplayed and the benefits overstated (McIntyre *et al.* 2011c, 2012b).

The broadly held understanding that caesarean section births are cost-neutral when compared with uncomplicated vaginal births has misled childbirth practices due to the existence of the hidden costs associated with the rising rates of short- and long-term maternal and neonatal morbidity. The use of mortality as the index measure of quality and safety in maternity care perpetuates risk management practices in healthy populations of women due to a lack of effective official reporting and practice surveillance. Changing the index measurement to include serious morbidity and unexplained caesarean births as performance measures will enable the collection of a complete data set of information generated through official reporting processes. Complete population data sets pertaining to

Table 5.3 Birth interventions and outcomes for selected years in Australia

	1970	1980	1990	2000	2010
Maternal mortality	12.7	12.9	9.3	11.1	7
Perinatal deaths per 1,000 live and stillbirths	22.6	–	–	10.1	9.9
Neonatal deaths per 1,000 live births	–	7.1	–	3.1	2.6
Infant mortality per 1,000 live births	–	12.2	–	5.2	3.3
Induction (%)	–	–	19.5	–	32.7
Forceps (%)	–	–	12.5	5.1	4.2
Vacuum (%)	–	–	2	6.1	7.9
Caesarean section (%)	–	–	17.5	23.3	32.3
Episiotomy (%)	–	–	–	12.8	16.3

Source: Li *et al.* (2013).

morbidity statistics and unexplained caesarean births are needed to obtain a clear description of current practices and associated morbidities (McIntyre *et al.* 2012b). The neonatal death rate for babies of non-Indigenous mothers was 2.4 per 1,000 live births and 6.0 per 1,000 live births to Aboriginal and Torres Strait Islander mothers (Li *et al.* 2013).

Postnatal care

The postnatal hospital stay for mothers varies, with 17.1 per cent being discharged less than two days after giving birth and 65.2 per cent being discharged between two and four days after giving birth. The postnatal stay varies depending on whether the hospital is public or private. Women with private health insurance in a private hospital have a median postnatal length of stay of four days following a vaginal birth or seven days following a caesarean section delivery, compared with two days following a vaginal birth or four days following caesarean section delivery for those in a public hospital (Li *et al.* 2013). At least one home-based postnatal visit by a midwife is offered within 24 hours of discharge from hospital. The visit is tailored to the individual requirements of the woman. Additional home visits are provided on the basis of individual clinical and psychosocial needs (Department of Health 2012).

In 2011, 1267 women gave birth at home, representing 0.4 per cent of all women who gave birth. The mean age of mothers who gave birth at home was 31.7 years. Most women who gave birth at home were living in the major cities (70.8 per cent). Of the mothers who gave birth at home, about one-quarter had their first baby (22.3 per cent) and 77.4 per cent were multiparous. Of the babies born at home in 2011, 99.2 per cent were live-born with a mean birthweight of 3614g (Li *et al.* 2013).

The Australian College of Midwives supports the choice of midwife-attended home birth as a safe option for women with uncomplicated pregnancies (Australian College of Midwives 2014b). Pregnant women who choose to give birth at home need to engage the services of an independent midwife or meet the inclusion criteria for a small number of publicly funded home birth services. The majority of independent midwives work in group practices within the National Midwifery Guidelines for Consultation and Referral (Australian College of Midwives 2014b). The guidelines have been endorsed by State and Territory governments, are embedded in practice at every level and are used extensively, from private practising midwives through to medical consultants at tertiary hospitals (Australian College of Midwives 2014b). All midwives are able to provide midwifery continuity of care or to work in private practice. A woman may choose to give birth at home, but she must be able to pay the full private fee for this service. Medicare rebates are not available for midwives engaged in the care of women who elect to give birth at home.

The demand for home birth from a small, but vocal, number of women has led to the introduction of a small number of publicly funded home birth programmes (Catling-Paull *et al.* 2011). These programmes have operated under strict inclusion and exclusion criteria and have been variably evaluated (Catling-Paull *et al.* 2012).

The National Breastfeeding Strategy 2010–2015 aims to improve the health, nutrition and well-being of infants and young children, and the health and well-being of mothers, by protecting, promoting, supporting and monitoring breastfeeding. Australia's dietary guidelines recommend exclusive breastfeeding of infants until 6 months of age, with the introduction of solid foods at around six months and continued breastfeeding until the age of twelve months, and beyond if both mother and infant wish (Australian Insitute of Health and Welfare 2012a). The majority of maternity services have a policy of exclusive breastfeeding which ensures that all newborn babies are offered the breast within the first hour of birth, resulting in 96 per cent of babies being breastfed initially. Breastfeeding rates are reported to drop quickly, with only 39 per cent exclusively breastfed to around four months of age; only 15 per cent are breastfed to the recommended six months of age (Australian Insitute of Health and Welfare 2012a).

The Australian government funds a childhood immunisation programme that aims to increase national immunisation rates by funding free vaccination programmes, administering the Australian Childhood Immunisation Register and communicating information about immunisation to the general public and health professionals. In June 2011, 92 per cent of one-year-old and 90 per cent of five-year-old children were fully immunised (Australian Insitute of Health and Welfare 2012b).

Consumer involvement

The rise of consumer influence in maternity service policy has resulted in a changing of the guard as doctors' traditional authority is questioned by strong consumer organisations and informed consumers (Reiger 2006). This powerful consumer influence can be seen as a feature of a neoliberal approach to health management and, when applied to maternity services, promotes consumer choice and individual autonomy (Newman 2009). Consistent with these values, women are encouraged through numerous web sites hosted by the Australian government to empower themselves regarding maternity care through informed decision-making (Callister 2009). The loudest voice in the consultation process comes from supporters of consumer movements such as the Maternity Coalition and Homebirth Australia, organisations dedicated to promoting natural childbirth.

Australian women's expectations of birth are situated at opposite ends of the spectrum. They either perceive the birthing experience to be a normal, natural process that women can or should achieve themselves, or to be a pathologically hazardous event, fraught with risk and danger to be feared and surrendered to medical control (Bayes *et al.* 2008). An addiction to specialised medical advancement has changed societies' expectations regarding childbirth. It is apparent that women are becoming more fearful than ever before of the birthing process, a situation compounded by feelings of vulnerability in relationships when confronted with a constant stream of unknown maternity care professionals (Dahlen *et al.* 2010).

Risk and rights

In the past five years the Australian government has sought to curtail the financial extravagance associated with healthy pregnant women being allocated the same expensive medical resources as women who require specialist medical care to give birth safely (Commonwealth of Australia 2009). In response to the findings from the National Review of Maternity Services reported in 2009, the government has sought to address the need to supply pregnant women with a genuine choice regarding options of maternity care (McIntyre *et al.* 2011c). Implementation of the recommended changes would align Australian maternity services with developments in New Zealand, Canada and the UK. The direction of the proposed changes is a move away from a reliance on tertiary and secondary level maternity care for all pregnant women irrespective of clinical need. The reforms are expected to provide the right balance between primary level care and access to appropriate levels of medical expertise as clinically required (Australian Health Ministries'Advisory Council 2008). The recommendations have endorsed the role of midwives in the provision of non-medical-led models of primary maternity care for healthy pregnant women. The introduction of a Medicare rebate for midwifery services was introduced in preparation for the change in primary care provider from obstetric to midwifery. A new status of Eligible Midwife was identified for this primary care role. Eligible Midwives have been notated by the Nursing and Midwifery Board of Australia as meeting specified advanced practice criteria. This enables an Eligible Midwife to provide Medicare-funded care and order diagnostic tests and ultrasound scans relating to pregnancy, birth and the newborn period. In addition, Eligible Midwives may seek endorsement to prescribe medications that relate to pregnancy, birth, and postnatal and neonatal care. To provide Medicare rebateable midwifery services, an Eligible Midwife is required to: (i) have a Medicare Provider Number; (ii) be working in private practice; (iii) have professional indemnity insurance; and (iv) have collaborative arrangements in place with a specified medical practitioner. Eligible Midwives have the right to apply for visiting or admitting rights to hospital, as do private practising obstetricians. Eligible midwives can receive payment from Medicare to provide care during pregnancy and after the baby is born, wherever the woman is situated, and during labour and birth, but only if the woman is situated in a hospital or birth centre. Medicare benefits enable women to claim some of the cost of private midwifery care under the same arrangement that is in place for offsetting the cost of private obstetric fees. No midwife providing care to a woman who elects to give birth at home will receive funding for this service (Australian College of Midwives 2014a).

Australian women having babies are reminded that they are not the experts in pregnancy and birth and that the consequences of any problems that may arise can be catastrophic (Klein *et al.* 2006). These messages foster pregnant women to develop high levels of fear that are sustained by women's perception of their own birth risk being disproportionate to the actual medical risk (Fisher *et al.* 2006; Jordan and Murphy 2009). Women want to avoid regret and, in doing so, place their own well-being secondary to that of their baby (Kitzinger *et al.* 2006). Authoritative knowledge is based on scientific evidence that is communicated by care providers. Non-medical knowledge is devalued by all participants, usually including the woman herself, who comes to believe that the course charted on the basis of professional medical knowledge is best for her (Munro *et al.* 2009). Women and their partners accept medical intervention because they are afraid that something will go wrong and the perfect child is more important than the perfect birth (Klein *et al.* 2006). Consequently, they put their trust in their care providers and willingly do whatever they are led to believe might help secure a healthy baby. Any woman who does not heed this advice is labelled as an irresponsible mother (McIntyre *et al.* 2011c).

Women's right to complain or question the care they receive is subjugated in their best interest by maternity care-givers. Women report distressing experiences in which their carefully considered birth plans were dismissed by their maternity care-givers as being unimportant. These women quickly discovered that the rhetoric advocating the empowerment of women during childbirth through exercising their right to informed choice had backfired. These women find themselves labelled by the health professionals, on whom they rely, as being difficult to please or a complaining nuisance (McIntyre *et al.* 2012b).

Conclusion

Australia is one of the safest countries in which to give birth or be born when measured against international maternal and neonatal mortality rates. Medicine and obstetrics believe that high-quality medically led maternity services have contributed to this excellent safety record (Australian Medical Association 2008). United in opposition to change, they are vocal in warning the general public and government that the introduction of non-medically led services will undermine the quality of maternity services in Australia and threaten the safety of mothers and babies.

Consequently, every pregnancy and birth continues to be treated as a medical event and women continue to experience difficulty in being able to access low-risk maternity care.

Maternity care is universally available to all women, irrespective of their ability to pay, as part of the welfare regime and a government commitment to a healthy start to life for all Australians. The rights of Australian women to make informed choices regarding the type of maternity care they would like to receive is overridden by the commonly held belief that potential medical risk must be managed in the best interests of the mother and baby. Consumer groups advocating for changes to the available maternity care options continue to campaign, and midwives continue to position themselves as a safe alternative to obstetric care for healthy women.

References

Australian Bureau of Statistics (2010) *1301.0 Year Book Australia 2009–2010. The Global Financial Crisis and its Impact on Australia.* Canberra: Australian Government.

Australian Bureau of Statistics (2012a) *3301.0 – Births, Australia, 2012* [online]. Canberra: Australian Government. Available from: www.abs.gov.au/ausstats/abs@.nsf/cat/3301.0. Accessed 2 September 2014.

Australian Bureau of Statistics (2012b) *3302.0 – Deaths, Australia, 2012* [online]. Canberra: Australian Government. Available from: www.abs.gov.au/ausstats/abs@.nsf/cat/3302.0. Accessed 2 September 2014.

Australian Bureau of Statistics (2013b) *3101.0 Australian Demographic Statistics, December.* [online]. Canberra: Australian Government. Available from: www.abs.gov.au/ausstats/abs@.nsf/mf/3101.0/. Accessed 2 September 2014.

Australian Bureau of Statistics (2013a) *Household Income and Income Distribution 2011–2012.* Canberra: Australian Government.

Australian Bureau of Statistics (2014) *Census.* Canberra: Australian Government.

Australian College of Midwives (2014a) *Eligible Midwives* [online]. Canberra: Australian College of Midwives. Available from: www.midwives.org.au/scripts/cgiip.exe/WService=MIDW/ccms.r?PageId=10181. Accessed 2 September 2014.

Australian College of Midwives (2014b) *National Midwifery Guidelines. Guidelines for Consultation and Referral* [online]. Canberra: Australian College of Midwives. Available from: www.midwives.org.au/scripts/cgiip.exe/WService=MIDW/ccms.r?PageId=10194. Accessed 10 September 2014.

Australian Health Ministries'Advisory Council (2008) *Primary Maternity Services in Australia – a framework for Implementation* [online]. Available from: www.AHMAC.gov.au. Accessed 2 September 2014.

Australian Insitute of Health and Welfare (2012a) *Australia's Health 2012* [online]. Canberra: Australian Governement. Available from: www.aihw.gov.au/publication-detail/?id=10737422172&tab=3. Accessed 2 September 2014.

Australian Insitute of Health and Welfare (2012b) *Australias Health 2012* [online]. Canberra: Australian Government Available from: www.aihw.gov.au/WorkArea/DownloadAsset.aspx?id=10737422169. Accessed 2 September 2014.

Australian Insitute of Health and Welfare (2012c) *Life Expectancy* [online]. Canberra: Australian Government. Available from: www.aihw.gov.au/life-expectancy/. Accessed 2 September 2014.

Australian Insitute of Health and Welfare (2012d) *Nursing & Midwifery Workforce 2011* [online]. Canberra: Australian Government. Available from: www.aihw.gov. au/publication-detail/?id=10737422167. Accessed 2 September 2014.

Australian Insitute of Health and Welfare (2013a) *Health Expenditure Australia 2011–2012.* Canberra: Australian Government.

Australian Insitute of Health and Welfare (2013b) *Medical Workforce 2011* [online]. Canberra: Australian Government. Available from: www.aihw.gov.au/publication-detail/?id=60129542627. Accessed 2 September 2014.

Australian and New Zealand College of Anaesthetists (2008) *ANZCA: Submission to Maternity Services Review* [online]. Available from: www.anzca.edu.au/communi-cations/anzca-bulletin/bulletin-release-2008/anzca-bulletin-2008-dec.pdfpage 10. Accessed 2 September 2014.

Australian Medical Association (2008) *AMA: Submission to Maternity Services Review* [online]. Available from https://ama.com.au/ama-submission-maternity-services-review. Accessed 2 September 2014.

Bayes, S., Fenwick, J. and Hauck, Y. (2008) 'A qualitative analysis of women's short accounts of labour and birth in a Western Australian public tertiary hospital', *Journal of Midwifery & Women's Health,* 53 (1): 53–61.

Callister, L.C. (2009) 'How is evidence-based decision making promoted for child-bearing women in Australia?', *MCN: the American Journal of Maternal and Child Nursing,* 34 (2): 131–131.

Castles, F.G. (1996) 'Needs-based strategies of social protection in Australia and New Zealand'. In: G. Esping-Andersen (ed.), *Welfare States in Transition.* London: Sage.

Castles, F.G. (2010) 'The English-speaking countries'. In: F.G. Castles, S. Leibfried, J. Lewis and H. Obinger. Oxford: Oxford University Press.

Castles, F.G. and Mitchell, D. (1991) *Three Worlds of Welfare Capitalism or Four?* Discussion Paper No. 21, Public Policy Program. Canberra: Australian National University.

Catling-Paull, C., Dahlen, H. and Homer, C.C.S.E. (2011) 'Multiparous women's confidence to have a publicly-funded homebirth: a qualitative study', *Women and Birth,* 24 (3): 122–128.

Catling-Paull, C., Foureur, M.J. and Homer, C.S.E. (2012) 'Publicly-funded home-birth models in Australia', *Women & Birth,* 25 (4): 152–158.

Commonwealth of Australia (2009) *Improving Maternity Services in Australia; the Report of the Maternity Services Review (1–74186–833–5)* [online]. Available from: www.ag.gov.au/cca. Accessed 2 September 2014.

Department of Foreign Affairs and Trade (DEFAT) (2013) *Australia in Brief.* Canberra: DEFAT.

Dahlen, H.G., Barclay, L.M. and Homer, C.S. (2010) 'The novice birthing: theoris-ing first-time mothers' experiences of birth at home and in hospital in Australia', *Midwifery,* 26 (1): 53–63.

Department of Health (2012) *Postnatal Care Program Guidelines for Victorian Health Services.* Melbourne: Victorian State Government.

Department of Human Services (2014) *Social and Health Related Payments and Services.* Canberra: Australian Government.

Esping-Andersen, G. (1990) *Three Worlds of Welfare Capitalism.* Cambridge: Polity Press.

Fisher, C., Hauck, Y. and Fenwick, J. (2006) 'How social context impacts on women's fears of childbirth: a Western Australian example', *Social Science and Medicine,* 63 (1): 64–75.

Geohive (2014) *Urban/Rural Division of Countries for the Year 2010* [online]. Available from: www.geohive.com/earth/pop_urban2.aspx. Accessed 20 May 2014.

Greenville, J., Pobke, C. and Rogers, N. (2013) *Trends in the Distribution of Income in Australia.* Canberra: Australian Government.

Hastie, C. (2006) 'Midwifery: women, history and politics', *Birth Issues,* 15 (1): 11–17.

Hastie, C. (2008) *Submission to National Maternity Services Review* [online]. Available from: www.healthh.gov.au/internet/main/publishing.nsf/Content/maternityservicesreview-180. Accessed 2 September 2014.

Health Workforce Australia (2013) *Australia's Health Workforce Series – Health Workforce by Numbers.* Adaelaide: Health Workforce Australia.

International Monetary Fund (2014) *IMF Reports and Publications by Country* [online]. Available from: www.imf.org/external/country/AUS/index.htm. Accessed 20 May 2014.

Janssens, S., Wallace, K.L. and Chang, A.M.Z. (2008) 'Prepartum and intrapartum caesarean section rates at Mater Mothers' Hospital Brisbane 1997–2005', *Australian and New Zealand Journal of Obstetrics and Gynaecology,* 48 (6): 564–569.

Jordan, R.G. and Murphy, P.A. (2009) 'Risk assessment and risk distortion: finding the balance', *Journal of Midwifery & Women's Health,* 54 (3): 191–200.

Kitzinger, S., Green, J.M., Chalmers, B., Keirse, M.J.N., Lindstrom, K. and Hemminki, E. (2006) 'Why do women go along with this stuff?', *Birth: Issues in Perinatal Care,* 33 (2): 154–158.

Klein, M.C., Sakala, C., Simkin, P., Davis-Floyd, R., Rooks, J.P. and Pincus, J. (2006) 'Roundtable discussion: part 2. Why do women go along with this stuff?', *Birth: Issues in Perinatal Care,* 33 (3): 245–250.

Laws, P.J., Tracy, S.K. and Sullivan, E.A. (2010) 'Perinatal outcomes of women intending to give birth in birth centers in Australia', *Birth: Issues in Perinatal Care,* 37 (1): 28–36.

Li, Z., Zeki, R., Hilder, L. and Sullivan, E. (2013) *Australia's Mothers and Babies 2011.* Perinatal Statistics Series No. 28. Catalogue No. PER 59. Canberra: Australian Insitute of Health and Welfare .

MacColl, M. (ed.) (2009) *The Birth Wars – the Conflict Putting Australian Women and Babies at Risk.* St Lucia: University of Queensland Press.

McIntyre, M., Chapman, Y. and Francis, K. (2011a) Hidden costs associated with the universal application of risk management in maternity care. *Australian Health Review,* 35 (2): 211–215.

McIntyre, M., Francis, K. and Chapman, Y. (2011b) 'Shaping public opinion on the issue of childbirth: a critical analysis of articles published in an Australian newspaper', *BMC Pregnancy and Childbirth,* 11: 47. doi:10.1186/1471-2393-11-47.

McIntyre, M., Francis, K. and Chapman, Y. (2011c) National Review of Maternity Services 2008; women influencing change. *BMC Pregnancy and Childbirth,* 11: 53. doi:10.1186/1471-2393-11-53.

McIntyre, M., Francis, K. and Chapman, Y. (2012a) 'The struggle for contested boundaries in the move to collaborative care teams in Australian maternity care', *Midwifery,* 28 (3): 298–305.

McIntyre, M., Francis, K. and Chapman, Y. (2012b) 'Primary maternity care reform: whose influence is driving chamge?' *Midwifery*, 28 (5): e705–e711.

Muir, S. (2007) *Rural/Urban Divide Information and Statistics Project* [online]. Available from: www.dpi.nsw.gov.au/__data/assets/pdf_file/0003/206580/urban-rural-divide.pdf. Accessed 20 June 2014.

Munro, S., Kornelsen, J. and Hutton, E. (2009) 'Decision making in patient-initiated elective cesarean delivery: the influence of birth stories'. *Journal of Midwifery & Women's Health*, 54 (5): 373–379.

National Consensus Framework for Rural Maternity Services (2008) *National Consensus Framework for Rural Maternity Services* [online]. Brisbane: Australian College of Rural and Remote Medicine. Available from: www.acrrm.org.au/files/uploads/pdf/advocacy/Rural-Maternity-Services_National-Consensus-Framework.pdf. Accessed 20 June 2014.

National Health and Medical Research Council (2012) *Clinical Practice Guidelines: Antenatal Care – Module I* [online]. Canberra: Commonwealth of Australia. Available from: www.health.gov.au/internet/main/publishing.nsf/content/015FBFD D266795DBCA257BF0001A0547/$File/ANC_Guidelines_Mod1_v32.pdf. Accessed 20 May 2014.

National Rural Health Alliance (2008) *The Importance of Birthing in the Bush. Submission to National Maternity Services Review* [online]. Available from: http://ruralhealth. org.au/sites/default/files/submissions/sub-08-10-30.pdf. Accessed 2 September 2014.

Newman, L. (2009) 'The health care system as a social determinant of health: qualitative insights from South Australian maternity consumers', *Australian Health Review*, 33 (1): 62–71.

Office of the Fair Work Ombudsman (2012) *Fair Work*. Canberra: Australian Government.

OECD (2013) *Country Statistical Profile: Australia 2013* [online]. Paris: OECD. Available from: www.oecd-ilibrary.org/docserver/download/191100011e1t005.pdf?e xpires=1398430564&id=id&accname=freeContent&checksum=C17AF99E29B45 932FE419689D9A2F5CC. Accessed 20 May 2014.

Purcal, N. (2008) 'The politics of midwifery education and training in New South Wales during the last decades of the 19th century', *Women and Birth*, 21 : 21–25.

Reiger, K. (2006) 'A neoliberal quickstep: contradictions in Australian maternity policy', *Health Sociology Review*, 15 (4): 330–340.

Roberts, C.L., Ford, J.B., Algert, C.S., Bell, J.C., Simpson, J.M. and Morris, J.M. (2009) 'Trends in adverse maternal outcomes during childbirth: a population-based study of severe maternal morbidity', *BMC Pregnancy and Childbirth*, 9: 7–17.

Schwartz, H. (1998) 'Social democracy going down or under: institutions, internationalized capital, and indebted states', *Comparative Politics*, 30 (3): 253–272.

Titmuss, R.M. (1987) 'Developing social policy in conditions of rapid change: the role of social welfare'. In: B. Abel-Smith and K. Titmuss (eds), *The Philosophy of Welfare: Selected Writings of Richard M. Titmuss*. London: Allen & Unwin.

6 Scotland

Helen Cheyne

Background

Scotland is one of the four countries that make up the UK. Scotland is a relatively small country, both geographically (with a land mass of only 78,770 km^2) and in terms of population. The UK population is approximately 63.7 million (UK National Statistics 2014), with only 5,313,600 people living in Scotland (General Register Office for Scotland 2013). The majority of the population lives in the historically industrialised areas of the central belt, which includes Scotland's largest cities of Glasgow and Edinburgh. There is a distinct urban/rural divide, with 82 per cent of the population living in only 6 per cent of the land area (Scottish Government 2012). However, Scotland also has significant rural and remote rural communities, including the northern and western islands, where populations have been growing over the last fifteen years (Scottish Government 2012). In 2014 Scotland faced a period of unprecedented political and social uncertainty as the people decided in a referendum whether they wished to remain as part of the UK or to become an independent country.

The UK was formed through the unions of the four countries of England, Scotland, Wales and Northern Ireland; the political union of Scotland and England took place in 1707. Historically, the four countries of the UK have maintained many distinct social, political and cultural characteristics. For example, each retained responsibility for issues such as health, education and justice, allowing these to develop distinct national characteristics. There was movement towards greater political autonomy for Scotland, Wales and Northern Ireland throughout the final decades of the twentieth century. Following a referendum in 1997, the then Labour government pledged to devolve political powers to each of the three 'Celtic' countries of the UK and, in 1999, the act of devolution established the National Welsh Assembly Government, the Scottish Executive and Parliament and the Northern Ireland Executive. Devolution is a process of the decentralisation of government and, through this process, a range of powers, previously held by the UK Parliament, were transferred to the elected administrations in each of the devolved countries (GOV.UK 2013).

The scope of devolved powers varies between the countries, but each includes responsibility for health, social work, education and justice, while the UK Parliament retains UK-wide responsibility for policy in areas such as defence, foreign affairs and trade. England does not have a devolved administration and therefore the UK Parliament retains responsibility for all legislation relating to England. Devolution in the UK has been described as a natural experiment (Bevan 2010), the longer term implications and outcomes of which are now unfolding.

Scotland as a welfare regime

The provision of welfare varies extensively between different countries, but typologies have been put forward to categorise countries into distinctive welfare state regimes or family types. Esping-Andersen (1990) categorised the UK as belonging to a liberal regime, characterised by residual welfare provision. In the liberal regime (the UK, the USA, Ireland, Canada and Australia), state provision of welfare is minimal; social transfers are modest with strict entitlement criteria and a tendency to stigmatise recipients. In this model, the dominance of the market is encouraged. The typical liberal welfare regime minimises the decommodification effects of the welfare state and a division exists between those who rely on state aid and those who are able to afford private provision.

Sullivan (2002) and Tannahill (2005) argued that Scotland's National Health Service (NHS) post-devolution reflects Scotland's 'communitarian' values and demonstrates the continuation of an existing characteristic of Scottish welfare. Mooney and Poole (2004), on the other hand, argued that in key areas of policy, such as welfare-to-work, New Labour policies in Scotland were identical to those of the UK Parliament. Mooney and Scott (2012) identified four factors that they conclude are attributes of post-devolution Scotland: the maturation of the institutions of a devolved government; changes in the UK Government; the economic crisis that has developed since 2008; and the victory of the Scottish National Party in the 2011 elections.

Some commentators have explored whether devolution has provided for significant social policy innovation in Scotland, Wales and Northern Ireland since 1999 (Stewart 2004; Mooney and Scott 2005; Birrell 2009; Greer 2009; Mooney and Wright 2009; Keating 2010). Scott and Wright (2012) argue that devolution has been viewed as an avenue to enhance and innovate social policy differentiation; for some it offers the opportunity to enhance social democracy and expand welfare, while for others it represents a race to the bottom.

Health care system

The NHS was formed in 1948 with the aim of providing health care for all and is funded through general taxation. The founding principal of the

NHS was that health care would be provided free at the point of delivery, based on clinical need rather than on the ability of individuals to pay (Rivett 1998). Although this principle still underpins the NHS UK-wide, health care is currently provided against a political and social background that is increasingly diverse as the effects of devolution become increasingly apparent, having an impact much more profound than was anticipated at its introduction (Greer 2004; Brimelow 2011; Royal College of Midwives Communities 2011).

Pre-devolution, UK health policy was determined centrally, with relatively minor differences between the four countries (Connolly *et al.* 2011). It was initially assumed that health policy across the four countries would remain broadly similar following devolution (Greer 2004). However, this has not proved to be the case, as each country has developed unique features with increasing divergence in policies. Although the overall aspirations of the NHS to provide universal, safe and effective health care remain, the means of achieving these aims are increasingly different. In particular, the philosophy underpinning health policy within Scotland has been described as directly opposite to that adopted in England (Winchester and Storey 2008). For example, in England the principle of competition within an internal market underpins the structure of the NHS. There is a strong emphasis on consumer choice, explicit competition between service providers, target setting and payment-by-results. In contrast, within Scotland the NHS is managed centrally by the Scottish Government. The system is explicitly designed to prevent inter-organisation competition and has eschewed the market-driven approach, aspiring to ideals of collaboration and co-operation between health care providers.

This thread of collaboration rather than competition, and a sustained focus on the reduction of health inequalities, has characterised Scottish health policy since devolution. In 1997 the Scottish Government White Paper Designed to Care; Renewing the National Health Service in Scotland (Scottish Executive 1997) outlined the planned post-devolution changes in the NHS in Scotland, launching the objective of reducing health inequalities and improving the poor health record of the Scottish people, who are typically at the bottom of international league tables for conditions such as coronary heart disease and cancer. The Designed to Care report established the principles of nationwide NHS policy and planning, the reduction of the internal market, the introduction of health improvement programmes and greater emphasis on primary care. Following devolution, the newly established Scottish Executive (later to be renamed the Scottish Government) produced Our National Health: a Plan for Action, a Plan for Change (Scottish Executive 2000). This set out a plan for the reformation of the NHS in Scotland, abolishing the internal market and establishing the principle of collaboration rather than competition within the NHS (a key difference from policy in England). The focus was on public health initiatives with the aim of reducing health inequalities and improving the health of the population. With the publication of Better Health, Better Care: Action Plan (Scottish Government 2007), the balance of care moved further towards outpatient, community-based care, adopting the principle of 'mutuality' where patients and the public are seen as 'co-owners' of the Scottish NHS.

The Scottish Government is currently funded by an annual block grant from the UK Government of approximately £26 billion (Deener and Philips 2013). The Scottish Government has the autonomy to decide how to allocate funds from this grant, including what proportion to allocate to health. In 2011–2012, health spending accounted for 34 per cent of the overall Scottish Government budget (Steel and Cylus 2012), estimated to be 10 per cent of the GDP (the GDP specifically for Scotland is considered by some researchers to be uncertain because of disagreement about the apportioning of North Sea oil revenues; Deener and Philip 2013). Health spending across the UK accounts for 9.4 per cent of GDP, which is slightly above the OECD average of 9.3 per cent (OECD 2013); spending increased by an average of 5.7 per cent per year from 2000 to 2009 before decreasing by 2.5 per cent in 2010 and 1.1 per cent in 2011. In Scotland, the per capita public spending on health was £2,072 per year in 2012 (Steel and Cylus 2012) and was 8.9 per cent above the UK national average in 2011 (Deener and Philip 2013), although this gap has narrowed significantly from 18.9 per cent in 2002–2003.

The private sector accounts for less than 1 per cent of health care in Scotland (Timmins 2013) and is mainly focused on areas such as care of the elderly and hospice care, as well as some small private hospitals providing medical and surgical facilities (Steel and Cylus 2012). The people of Scotland are entitled to health care that is, for the most part, free at the point of delivery, with the exception of dental and ophthalmic care, some aspects of which must be paid for directly. Prescription charges were abolished in 2011. Payment for care for the elderly and for those with long-term conditions is more complex; personal care (e.g. personal hygiene) is free, whereas other aspects of care require payment (Timmins 2013).

Health care is delivered through a partnership between the Scottish Government and NHS Scotland. The Scottish Government currently comprises six directorates, each with a remit to work towards achieving strategic objectives that reflect the overarching ambitions to address the causes of Scotland's long-standing health and social problems and to make Scotland 'wealthier and fairer, healthier, safer and stronger, smarter, greener' (Scottish Government 2014a). Progress towards the achievement of these objectives is monitored through the National Performance Framework, Scotland Performs (Scottish Government 2014a), which comprises targets, outcomes and indicators of progress towards achieving the strategic objectives. Through the Health and Social Care Directorate, the Scottish Government has responsibility for the provision of the overall strategic direction, policy and monitoring of health care across Scotland (Scottish Government 2014a).

Although the overall direction is provided by government, health care is delivered through NHS Scotland, an organisation consisting of fourteen regional NHS Boards that provide health care services within distinct geographical areas (Scottish Government 2014b). In addition, there are seven special NHS Boards, including all-Scotland service providers such as the Scottish Ambulance Service, which provides pre-hospital emergency care, and NHS 24, which provides telephone-based advice and information. The special NHS Boards also include NHS Education for Scotland, which provides ongoing education and training of NHS staff, and NHS Health Scotland, which provides health education and health promotion. Also under the umbrella of NHS Scotland is Health Care Improvement Scotland (described as a public health body), which is responsible for the development and implementation of consistent, evidence-based care guidance across all NHS Boards, as well as having a governance function through the regular inspection of services.

The NHS Boards have responsibility for planning, commissioning and providing local health care. They are directly accountable to Scottish Government ministers and are supported by the Health and Social Care Directorate, with monitoring through the Scotland Performs reporting framework (Scottish Government 2014a). The NHS Boards are required to report on progress towards achieving a set of performance targets known as the HEAT targets (Health Improvement, Efficiency, Access and Treatment), which address the National Performance Framework outcomes and indicators. This structure forms a 'warp and weft' within which the overarching strategic direction, policy and monitoring is provided by the national government, with devolved planning, organisation and delivery of local services through NHS Boards. This is supported by the cross-cutting provision of national care guidance and governance, education and health promotion. The structure aims to ensure the national implementation of health policy, a shared overall direction of travel in achieving national objectives, a reduction in variations in health care provision and standards across the NHS Boards, as well as uniformity of the pay, conditions and education of NHS staff.

Within the NHS Boards, Community Health Partnerships (CHPs) provide the link between health and social care (Community Health Partnerships 2014). The CHPs develop local community health services and aim to ensure the integration of health and social care services. Single outcome agreements between the Scottish Government and the CHPs outline how both will work towards improving outcomes for people within local contexts in line with the Scottish Government National Outcomes. Scotland is currently undergoing a significant reform of public services, moving towards the full integration of health and social care services. The Adult Health and Social Care Bill will see CHPs replaced by Health and Social Care Partnerships.

These will produce joint outcome agreements between the Health Boards (traditionally responsible for health care) and local authorities (responsible for social care), aiming to facilitate a further shift in the balance of care from hospital to community-based settings (Scottish Government 2014c). Several NHS Boards and local authorities are in the process of integration; however, it is not yet clear how these new configurations will operate in practice. Full integration will involve a wide spectrum of disciplines and agencies, each with their own theoretical approaches and distinct terminology. There are currently competing understandings of some of the core concepts of care between the medical and social models and these are likely to pose significant challenges to the successful integration of health and social care services. Maternity care may provide an exemplar. Midwives have traditionally had a public health role and so the principals of the integration of the health and social models of care are consistent with their core values and practice. However, midwives are now required to undertake a wide range of assessments and interventions during routine antenatal care. These include clinical assessments, the assessment of well-being using a strengths- or assets-based approach, screening and sensitive questions about health behaviours and mental health, and motivational interviewing to support changes in health behaviour. Concepts such as strengths-based approaches and ecological thinking (consistent with social care models) contrast with deficit-based approaches. Terms such as resilience, wellness and self-efficacy have been introduced, along with the more traditional concerns about the medical versus normality focused models of care. Although some midwives report better joined-up working across agency boundaries and increased problem-solving resources for working with families, they have also encountered challenges in integrating the range of clinical and social assessments required at antenatal booking and subsequent antenatal contacts (Cross *et al.* 2012).

Table 6.1 Human and physical resources in Scotland

	2011
Physicians per 100,000*	309
Nurses and midwives per 100,000*	947
Total available staffed hospital beds (total)**	16,230
Obstetric beds (total)**	822
Consultant obstetricians***	185 (2013)
	*March 2014***
Total number of nurses and midwifes**	67,074
Total number of midwives	3,686
Total number of medical staff	11,489

Notes
* Steel and Cylus (2012).
** ISD Scotland (2014).
*** Royal College of Obstetricians and Gynaecologists (2013).

Seventy per cent of the overall NHS expenditure is accounted for by staff costs and NHS Scotland directly employs the majority of health care workers (Steel and Cylus 2012) (Table 6.1). Nurses, midwives and doctors are employed directly by the NHS Boards; the exception is medical and dental practitioners providing primary care, who are directly reimbursed for contracted services provided to the NHS.

All nurses and midwives in the UK are required to be registered with the Nursing and Midwifery Council (NMC). This UK-wide body provides guidance and regulation for professional issues relating to nursing and midwifery, in particular the standards of conduct, performance and ethics for nurses and midwives, and the midwives rules and standards. All midwives are required to notify their intention to practice annually to the NMC and to have a named Supervisor of Midwives with additional NMC accredited training. The role of the Supervisor of Midwives is to provide professional support and guidance to midwives. Although this role is statutory and includes aspects of public protection through insuring compliance with NMC guidance and standards, the Supervisor of Midwives role is distinctly professional rather than managerial.

Pre-registration nursing and midwifery courses are commissioned by the Scottish Government and quality assured by the NMC (NHS Scotland 2014a), with all courses at degree level. Nursing students may undertake a three- or four-year degree programme. The majority of midwives entering the profession in Scotland do so as 'direct-entry', i.e. they are not registered nurses. Direct-entry pre-registration midwives undertake a three- or four-year degree programme, while those who are already registered nurses may undertake a shortened 18-month programme.

Medical students are required to undertake five years of study in a medical school accredited by the General Medical Council. In order to practice medicine in the UK, doctors must be registered with the General Medical Council and undergo a process of revalidation every five years. Revalidation was introduced by the General Medical Council in 2012 and aims to ensure that all doctors are up-to-date and fit to practice (General Medical Council 2014).

Demographic profile

The number of births in Scotland has risen slightly over the last ten years after a period of consistent decline through the previous decade. There are currently around 58,000 births annually (General Register Office for Scotland 2012). A history of industrialisation with crowded inner cities and poverty, compounded by a long process of industrial decline, has resulted in a legacy of health inequalities. As a result, Scotland has traditionally been regarded as one of the 'sick men' of Europe, with higher rates of cancer and cardiovascular disease and a lower life expectancy within distinct geographical areas and socio-economic groups than other parts of the UK and Western Europe. For example, Audit Scotland (2012) reported that the life expectancy for a woman living in one of the most deprived areas of Scotland was 76.8 years compared with 84.2 years in the most affluent areas (Table 6.2). These health inequalities have also impacted on maternal and child health. In 2011 the percentage of low birthweight babies was over twice as high in the most deprived areas of Scotland than in the areas of least deprivation. Only 15 per cent of women in the most deprived areas were exclusively breastfeeding their babies at six to eight weeks of age compared with 40 per cent in the most affluent areas (Audit Scotland 2012).

A reduction in health inequalities, an improvement in public health and, in particular, an improvement in infant and child health and well-being has consistently been the key driver of post-devolution health policy in Scotland. Multiple factors (including physical, social, contextual, behavioural and psychological factors) have an impact on health and well-being. The greatest potential for impact occurs pre-birth and in the early years of a child's life; impacts during this time have the greatest potential to promote lifelong well-being. At the same time, negative impacts at this stage may have long-term consequences for the health and well-being of individuals and society. Recognising this, the Scottish Government introduced Getting it Right for Every Child (GIRFEC), a

Table 6.2 Demographic profile (mid-year 2011–2012) of Scotland

Population*	5,313.600
Number of women*	2,736.460
Population aged 0–14 years*	854,752
Women of childbearing age (15–44 years)*	1,051.7
Population aged 65 years and above*	896,364
Population annual growth (%)*	0.3
Population density per square kilometre*	68 (range 9–3,407)
Urban population (%)***	82
Total fertility rate (births per woman)**	1.75 (2010)
Crude birth rate per 1,000 people**	10.9
Crude death rate for men per 100,000 people (2010)	785
Crude death rate for women per 100,000 people (2010)	552
Ethnic groups (breakdown) (% of population 2011)****	
African	0.6
Asian/Asian Scottish/Asian British	2.7
Caribbean or Black	0.1
Mixed/Multiple ethnic groups	0.4
Other ethnic groups	0.3
White	96

Notes
*　　General Register Office for Scotland (2013).
**　　UK National Statistics (2014).
***　　Scottish Government (2012).
****　　Scottish Government (2014e).

multi-agency integrated approach or framework for working with children and young people (Scottish Government 2014d). The GIRFEC approach aims to provide an integrated framework and common language for assessment and intervention for all health and social care agencies that interact with families, children and young people, including maternity services, social work, education, criminal justice and housing services. GIRFEC introduced a national practice model that focuses on well-being and a strengths- or assets-based approach aiming for early assessment, intervention and prevention. The Children and Young People (Scotland) Act (Scottish Parliament 2014) was passed by the Scottish Government in March 2014. This places many of the principles of GIRFEC in statute, including a definition of well-being, and makes explicit the responsibility of the government and all agencies within Scotland to protect the rights and well-being of children and young people. Some specific aspects of the Act include an increase in free childcare for all three- and four-year-old children and some vulnerable two-year-olds to around sixteen hours per week, free school meals for the first three years of primary school education and, more controversially, the appointment of a 'named person' for every child from birth to eighteen years old. The named person is likely to be a health visitor or teacher and they will have the responsibility to use the GIRFEC national practice model (Scottish Government 2014d) approach to identify, record and raise concerns about a child's well-being.

Maternity provision

The Winterton and Cumberledge reports (House of Commons Health Committee 1992; Department of Health 1993) advocated the principles of choice, continuity and control for women throughout pregnancy and childbirth. These seminal reports, although specifically applying to England, have provided a long-lasting, overarching philosophy for maternity provision across the UK. Within Scotland, maternity provision, over more than twenty years, has been underpinned by a series of government reports and policies that have recognised pregnancy and childbirth as a normal physiological event and endorsed midwifery care for all women through pregnancy, birth and the postnatal period (Scottish Office Home and Health Department 1993; Scottish Executive 2001; Scottish Executive Health Department 2002; Scottish Government 2011).

Midwife-led care was supported by the findings of two randomised controlled trials conducted in Scotland (Hundley *et al.* 1994; Turnbull *et al.* 1996) and is now expected to be the norm for women assessed as low risk within an integrated multidisciplinary/multi-agency maternity care service. Health policy has consistently supported the principle that women should be provided with informed choice for the place of birth, with the option of a home birth and for maternity care to be provided as close to the woman's home as possible (Scottish Office Home and Health Department 1993; Scottish Executive 2001; Scottish Executive Health Department 2002; Scottish Government 2011).

However, despite consistent policy endorsement for the principle of normal birth and midwife-led care, implementation in practice has been slow and inconsistent across the NHS Boards. Rising rates of routine medical intervention in pregnancy and birth, in particular caesarean sections, have been a cause for concern. In response, the Scottish Government developed and led a national maternity care programme that aimed to maximise the opportunities for women to have as natural a birth experience as possible, reduce routine interventions and provide woman-centred care. This programme, entitled Keeping Childbirth Natural and Dynamic (KCND) introduced national pathways for maternity care (Healthcare Improvement Scotland 2009). The pathways comprise risk assessment tools and care pathways for antenatal, intrapartum and postnatal care. Using a traffic light approach, healthy women identified as being at low risk of experiencing medical or obstetric complications based on a set of screening criteria receive midwife-led care (green pathway), while those identified as being at higher risk (red pathway) receive maternity team care led by an obstetrician. An 'amber' category triggers referral for medical assessment, but not necessarily a transfer to obstetric-led care. The KCND programme aimed to progress the implementation of specific practices considered to support normal birth – for example, the discontinuation of routine electronic foetal heart monitoring on admission in labour and the establishment of the midwife as the first point of professional contact for pregnant women.

Maternity care is currently provided through an integrated network of seventeen consultant-led maternity units (some with integral midwife-led birth units) and twenty-one community midwife-led units and birth centres. Although the nomenclature has varied over time, the distinction essentially relates to the levels of care provided and the profession providing the lead care role. Consultant-led units provide multi-professional team care to women considered to be either high or low medical, social or obstetric risk. Obstetricians provide the clinical lead role. Midwife-led units are generally smaller maternity units in which midwives provide the lead professional role. Midwife-led units many be geographically distinct or co-located with consultant-led maternity units and, in general, aim to provide care to healthy women assessed as being at low risk of developing obstetric or medical complications.

Maternity services have evolved from the traditional UK model of shared maternity care in which women's care was divided between the general practitioner (GP or family doctor) and hospital-based obstetric consultant, with midwives providing in-hospital care, care during labour and birth, and community-based postnatal care. Current maternity policy recommends community-focused, midwife-led antenatal care for healthy women experiencing uncomplicated pregnancies, whereas a multidisciplinary maternity team care (i.e. obstetrician, midwife, anaesthetist and others) is recommended for those with more complex needs (Scottish Government 2011). The particular role of the GP is in providing continuing general medical care to the mother, as required, throughout pregnancy and for the family following the birth.

Maternity entitlements

Almost all working women in Scotland are entitled to twelve months of maternity leave irrespective of their length of employment. There are some exceptions – for example, policewomen. Women may decide when to start their period of leave at any time after 29 weeks of pregnancy and how long their leave will last, although a compulsory period of two weeks of leave after childbirth is statutory. The first twenty-six weeks of leave is Ordinary Maternity Leave, after which time women are entitled to return to their original job. An additional period of twenty-six weeks leave, known as Additional Maternity Leave, may follow immediately, after which women are entitled to return to their original or similar job. Women's terms and conditions of employment are not affected by maternity leave. Fathers may be entitled to a period of one or two weeks of paternity leave depending on their length of service with their employer (Citizens Advice Bureau 2014).

Childbirth in Scotland

Antenatal care

Early and direct access to maternity care is a key priority for maternity care in Scotland and is the focus of the only national HEAT target relating to maternity care (Scottish Government 2014a). The target states that an initial assessment of health, obstetric and social needs (known as the booking assessment) will be undertaken by twelve weeks of pregnancy for 80 per cent of women in each socio-economic group by March 2015. This target has already been surpassed in almost all NHS Boards (Cheyne *et al.* 2014). However, despite government policy supporting the midwife as the appropriate first point of professional contact, the majority of women still directly contact their GP, who then makes a referral to maternity services. Once a woman is 'in' the maternity care system, the majority of her care will be provided by midwives. A recent national survey of women's experiences of maternity care (Cheyne *et al.* 2014) found that almost all women (98 per cent) reported that they saw a midwife for their antenatal check-ups, while 12 per cent also saw a GP and 37 per cent saw a hospital doctor.

In most cases a midwife undertakes the initial antenatal booking assessment and streams the woman to the appropriate care pathway according to the KCND guidance (Healthcare Improvement Scotland 2009). Women are offered an ultrasound scan for pregnancy dating and nuchal fold screening for Down's syndrome between eleven and fourteen weeks of pregnancy and another scan between eighteen and twenty-one weeks of pregnancy with the aim of detecting structural anomalies in the foetus (NHS Scotland 2014b).

A woman who is identified as at low risk at the first assessment, and who remains so throughout pregnancy, would be expected to receive between seven and ten antenatal visits (depending on her parity), with her care provided by a midwife, according to the 'green pathway' schedule of care. Women who are allocated to the 'red pathway' will also receive the majority of their care from a midwife, but the lead professional will be an obstetrician. A national audit of maternity care conducted in 2010 found that 60 per cent of women were identified as low risk at booking and just over half remained so, or had been reassessed as low risk, by the end of their antenatal care (Cheyne *et al.* 2013a).

A national core syllabus for parent education was implemented across the NHS Boards in 2011. The syllabus was developed by Healthcare Improvement Scotland, NHS Education for Scotland and NHS Health Scotland with the aim of providing consistent parent education that is 'universally applicable but targets the needs of vulnerable and socially excluded parents' across all NHS Boards (NHS Health Scotland 2011).

Intrapartum care

Although maternity policy explicitly endorses a woman's choice of a home birth, in practice only around 1.5 per cent of women give birth at home. The large majority (96 per cent) give birth in a consultant-led maternity unit, with the remainder giving birth in a community midwife-led unit or birth unit (Cheyne *et al.* 2014). In practice, women's options are limited by the maternity facilities within their local area. Not all NHS Boards have the full range of maternity units and, although cross-Board travel is possible, in most cases this would involve considerable travel for pregnant women and their families. Their choice of place of birth is also influenced by women's own perceptions of safety. A study conducted in Scotland found that some women will opt to travel from their local area to give birth in a consultant-led unit that they perceive as safer, even where a local community midwife-led maternity unit is available (Pitchforth *et al.* 2009).

Current care guidance indicates that women should be advised to remain at home until labour has become established (Healthcare Improvement Scotland 2009). Women are usually advised to contact the unit by telephone when they think that labour has started. Based on this telephone consultation, women will either be advised to attend the hospital for a full assessment or to remain at home. This gate-keeping approach to hospital admission is not universally popular with women. Several studies have found that women are uncertain whether and when to contact the maternity unit when they think that they are in labour, and that they may feel that their experiences and concerns are not always taken seriously by staff when they seek admission (Green *et al.* 2012).

Once labour is established (currently considered to be when cervical dilatation has reached four centimetres), one-to-one care with a midwife throughout labour and birth is the standard for care across Scotland (Healthcare Improvement Scotland 2009). Considerable effort at government policy level has been exerted to reduce routine medical intervention in labour (Healthcare Improvement Scotland 2009). However, intervention rates have not noticeably reduced and the rate of caesarean section has continued to rise. A number of factors may be involved; almost 50 per cent of women are likely to be considered as higher risk by the time labour starts and these women are likely to receive interventions such as augmentation of labour, continuous electronic foetal monitoring and epidural anaesthesia. Around 24 per cent of women currently have their labour induced. This rate has remained relatively stable over the last twenty years after falling from its highest level of 47.5 per cent in 1976. Women who receive labour induction will also require continuous electronic foetal heart rate monitoring and are more likely to require epidural anaesthesia. The rate of planned caesarean section is now rising faster than that of unplanned/emergency caesarean section (Information Services Division Scotland 2013a). This may be accounted for by factors such as the virtual elimination of vaginal breech birth in favour of caesarean section for breech-presenting babies and by the low rate of vaginal birth following a primary caesarean section (Table 6.3).

Postnatal care

The majority of women leave hospital within two days of giving birth. A recent survey found that 63 per cent of women reported that they left the hospital within two days and 11 per cent of women reported going home within twelve hours of giving birth (Cheyne *et al.* 2014). Midwives are responsible for providing care for mothers following birth and for at least ten postnatal days. However, midwifery care can be extended as necessary until the end of the postnatal period (six weeks). Almost all women receive home visits from a community midwife, with the majority (76 per cent) reporting that they receive between three and six home visits, with transfer to the care of a health visitor at or soon after the tenth postnatal day. Midwifery care at this time is focused on monitoring the health and well-being of mother and baby, establishing infant feeding and providing parenting support and advice.

The breastfeeding rate in Scotland has remained relatively static over the last decade, despite considerable effort through the UNICEF Baby Friendly

Table 6.3 Birth interventions and outcomes for selected years in Scotland*

Years			2000–2002	2003–2005	2006–2008
Maternal mortality***			10.08	13.07	11.39

Years	1971	1980	1990	2000+	2010#	2012#
Total live births#	87,335	68,892	65,973	53,076	58,791	58,027
Perinatal deaths per 1,000 live and stillbirths	24.5	13.1	8.7	8.4	6.9	6.5
Neonatal deaths per 1,000 live births	13.5	7.8	4.4	4.0	2.6	2.6
Infant mortality per 1,000 live births	19.9	12.1	7.7	5.7	3.7	3.7

Years	1976	1980	1990	2000	2010	2012
Induction (%)*	47.5	34.2	21.2	27.4	22.5	23.8
Forceps (%)*	13.4	13.7	11.2	7.1	9.7	9.7
Vacuum (%)*	0.6	0.4	1.2	5.3	2.9	3.1
Caesarean (%)*	8.7	11.5	14.6	20.7	26.6	29
Episiotomy (%)	–	–	–	–	23.6**	–

Notes

*** UK data for triennium, direct and indirect deaths per 100,000 maternities.

* ISD Scotland (2013a).

\# General Register Office for Scotland (2013).

** EURO-PERISTAT (2013).

+ The Still-Birth (Definition) Act 1992 re-defined stillbirths, from 1 October 1992, to include losses between 24 and 27 weeks gestation.

Initiative and other programmes to increase the numbers of women who initiate and continue to breastfeed. The European Perinatal Health Report (EURO-PERISTAT 2013) indicates that Scotland has lower rates of breastfeeding at forty-eight hours following birth than any of the other UK countries and has one of the lowest reported rates in Europe. In 2012–2013, only 47.1 per cent of babies were breastfed at around ten days of age; this figure includes the 35.2 per cent of babies who were exclusively breastfed and 11.9 per cent who were receiving mixed breast and formula feeding. By around six to eight weeks of age, 36.5 per cent of babies were breastfed (26.2 per cent exclusively with 10.3 per cent mixed) (Information Services Division Scotland 2013b). There is considerable variation in breastfeeding rates between different socio-economic groups – for example, only 15 per cent of women from the most deprived areas breastfed at six to eight weeks compared with 40 per cent in the most affluent areas (Audit Scotland 2012). Despite policy and even legislative support of breastfeeding (Scottish Parliament 2005), the rate of exclusive breastfeeding appears to be resistant to change. Almost all women report being given the opportunity to have a period of direct skin-to-skin contact with their baby immediately following the birth, a practice recommended by the UNICEF Baby Friendly Initiative; however, a significant proportion of women report receiving inconsistent feeding advice and that they do not always receive the support and encouragement they require from midwives and other health professionals (Cheyne *et al.* 2014).

The number of maternal deaths in Scotland and across the UK is low and the maternal death rate is not reported specifically for Scotland. Scottish data on maternal mortality contributes to a UK-wide audit and enquiry into all maternal deaths during pregnancy and up to one year after childbirth; this has been reported on a triennial basis since 1985 (Weindling 2003). In the most recently reported triennium (2006–2008) there were 261 maternal deaths reported as directly or indirectly related to pregnancy and childbirth in the UK, with 107 direct deaths. The overall maternal mortality rate was 11.39 per 100,000 maternities and the direct death rate was 4.67 per 100,000 maternities, a decrease in direct deaths from the rate in the previous triennium of 6.24 per 100,000 maternities in 2003–2005 (Centre for Maternal and Child Enquiries 2011). The most recent enquiry reported that sepsis was the leading cause of direct maternal death (1.13 per 100,000 maternities), with cardiac disease the leading cause of indirect death (2.31 per 100,000 maternities) (Centre for Maternal and Child Enquiries 2011). There was an ongoing audit of severe maternal morbidity reported by all of the seventeen consultant-led maternity units in Scotland between 2003 and 2014, undertaken by Healthcare Improvement Scotland. The rate of severe morbidity in 2011 was 7.3 women per 1,000 births, with major obstetric haemorrhage the most frequently recorded event (5.93 per 1,000 births) (Healthcare Improvement Scotland 2013).

A current major focus of NHS Scotland activity is the Scottish Patient Safety Programme (Healthcare Improvement Scotland 2014). The Patient Safety Programme was launched in 2008 as a major government-led, Scotland-wide, initiative with the aim of improving the safety and reliability of health care and the reduction of avoidable harm. The programme is co-ordinated by Healthcare Improvement Scotland supported by NHS Education for Scotland and the NHS Scotland Quality Improvement Hub among others (Healthcare Improvement Scotland 2014). It has adopted a Quality Improvement approach to service change and is partnered with the US-based Institute of Healthcare Improvement. The Institute of Healthcare Improvement approach involves national 'learning events', local quality champions, 'action periods' of data collection and change activities focused on key topics within all NHS Boards (Healthcare Improvement Scotland 2014). The programme involves every NHS Board. Initially focused on acute care, the programme has subsequently been extended to include mental health, primary care and maternity and child care. The Maternity and Children Quality Improvement Collaborative was launched in 2013 with strands of quality improvement work in maternity, neonatal and paediatric care (Healthcare Improvement Scotland 2014). Within the maternity strand targets have been set to increase the percentage of women who are satisfied with their maternity care to 95 per cent by 2015 and to reduce avoidable harm in women and babies by 30 per cent within the same timescale. In this context, avoidable harm is defined specifically as related to stillbirth and neonatal death, postpartum haemorrhage, non-medically indicated elective deliveries (induction of labour and caesarean section) and reduction of harm associated with smoking during pregnancy.

Consumer involvement

A central aspect of Scottish Government policy is a commitment to mutuality and this encompasses involvement, responsiveness and access (Scottish Health Council 2010). Public Partnership Forums operate within each CHP and have a role in providing a link between local communities and the CHPs, influencing the provision of local health services. NHS Boards have a responsibility to ensure the involvement of maternity service users through the Maternity Service Liaison Committees (MSLCs). The MSLCs were first established in 1984 and have traditionally been the forum through which maternity service users and other stakeholder representatives are enabled to work with maternity service providers to influence the development of services at a local level (Scottish Health Council 2010). Although MSLCs are the mainstay of formal service user involvement in NHS Boards, concerns have been raised about their representativeness and whether involvement is meaningful or tokenistic.

The Scottish Government established a programme of service user surveys in 2009 through the Better Together Patient Experience Programme (Scottish Government 2008). National surveys of patients' experiences of hospital inpatient and GP care have been undertaken through this programme. In 2013 a national survey of women's experience of maternity care was carried out as part of this programme (Cheyne *et al.* 2014). The questionnaire asked about women's experience of antenatal care, care during labour and postnatal care in hospital and at home in the six weeks following birth. It included questions about specific aspects of the experience and process of care, as well as the overall rating of care quality at each stage. The survey found that the majority of women rated the care they received very highly and, in particular, the policy targets. However, some significant concerns were raised in relation to antenatal access to services and the provision of skin-to-skin contact after birth – for example, only just over half of the women reported that they were given a choice of place of birth and 20 per cent of women reported that they were left alone during labour when this concerned them. Postnatal care was most poorly rated, with deficits reported in continuity of care, provision of support, and information and advice.

A number of service user organisations provide advice and support to women and families and operate as advocacy or lobbying groups for maternity care. Some, such as the SANDS, the Stillbirth and Neonatal Death charity, represent specific service user needs. Others, such as the National Childbirth Trust (NCT), operate as more general information and support organisations for parents. The NCT operates UK-wide, providing a range of services, including antenatal, postnatal and parenting courses, and local support groups for mothers and families. In recent years online support organisations such as Netmums have been established. Dr Foster – Birth Guide is an independent online information resource that provides detailed information on individual hospital services and outcomes, including caesarean section rates.

Risk and rights

Childbirth is typically considered to be the time of highest risk for mother and baby and, at the same time, a normal life event considered as an expression of wellness rather than ill health. This paradox is reflected in maternity care that endorses pregnancy and childbirth as normal, reduces routine interventions and offers a choice of place of birth for women, but only within a tight system of risk screening and gate-keeping for low-tech models of care, midwife-led maternity units and home birth. The assumption underpinning risk screening in pregnancy is that some women are more likely than others to experience pregnancy complications and that these women may be prospectively identified during the antenatal period on the basis of specific factors or criteria. Risk is the probability or likelihood that an event will occur given a particular situation or condition; a risk factor is a characteristic that is associated with a particular health condition on the basis of epidemiological evidence. The risk factor may not be causal of the condition; its association may be weak or strong or it may merely be a marker of some other causative factor (Walker *et al.* 1998; Petts *et al.* 2001; Burt no date). Although antenatal risk screening is now mandatory, the predictive value of antenatal risk assessment tools has consistently been found to be poor (Enkin *et al.* 2000). Risk assessment tools form part of the Scotland-wide maternity pathways in which a list of around fifty risk criteria are used to stream women to green (midwife-led) or red (consultant-led) care pathways. These criteria comprise a variety of factors and characteristics, clinical and psychosocial, drawn from clinical opinion, craft knowledge and epidemiology; many are socially constructed. The use of these criteria typically result in women being labelled as high or low risk and this often appears to be considered a diagnosis in itself, as health professionals may refer to a woman as having been 'diagnosed' as high-risk. There are negative consequences associated with their use. For example, identifying that a woman has risk factors is likely to trigger additional tests and interventions. Risk assessment is used to gate-keep access to midwife-led care and home birth and so is likely to constrain women's choice of place of birth. There is evidence that women are concerned about the effects of risk screening and about the way health professionals communicate with them about risk. A consultation project with twelve diverse groups of mothers living in Scotland, which aimed to identify women's priorities for maternity care research, found that questions about the proliferation of risk screening, the impact of risk screening on women and risk communication were among the top ten priority issues for research (Cheyne *et al.* 2013b).

Within the Scottish Government and NHS Scotland, maternity and early years care is seen as one of the vehicles through which ambitions to improve the long-term health, well-being and prosperity of the population may be achieved. This is evidenced by the sustained focus on the implementation of maternity care policies and government-led strategies for maternity care, most recently through legislation in relation to the early years through the Children and Young People (Scotland) Act (Scottish Parliament 2014). By proxy, it would seem that maternity care is also seen as a key priority area and this appears to be the case as demonstrated by policy drivers for early and universal access to maternity care. However, there are some potential risks. The Children and Young People (Scotland) Act legislation is very new (April 2014) and it is not as yet clear how its influence will unfold in practice. For example, there may ultimately be conflicts between the prioritisation of the rights and welfare of the child and those of the mother. Examples of such conflict have been reported elsewhere, e.g. court-enforced caesarean section (*Telegraph* 2013). Vigilance will be required in case similar unintended consequences arise as a result of early years legislation.

Within Scotland, maternity policy appears to pursue parallel and, on the surface, mutually exclusive views of pregnancy and childbirth. This is the childbirth paradox: on one hand, pregnancy and childbirth are endorsed as normal physiological life events and, at the same time, they are viewed as a time of increased risk and danger. This manifests as the promotion of women's choice of home birth and support of community midwife-led maternity units, while simultaneously ensuring that all consultant-led maternity units are co-located with hospitals where full adult intensive care facilities are available and by mandating extensive lists of risk criteria that gate-keep women's access to more normal birth options. Midwives work within the area of tension created by this paradox and are required to hold both perspectives as true, bridging the social and medical models of childbirth. This creates tensions as, for example, midwives may feel both protected and proscribed by risk assessment criteria and care pathways (Cheyne et al. 2013a). A key driver for the NHS across Scotland is the recently initiated Patient Safety Programme. The maternity care strand of this programme (Maternity and Children's Quality Improvement Collaborative) was launched in March 2013. It remains to be seen what the impact of this strong focus on safety will be on the perceptions of care providers of childbirth as a normal or risky event.

The traditional shared care roles, where antenatal care was divided between the GP and hospital-based obstetrician with midwives providing a subsidiary role, no longer predominate. Midwives now provide the majority of antenatal care for all women and take the lead professional role for women deemed to be at low risk of medical or obstetric complications, although the criteria by which the level of risk is determined is largely outside the control of midwives. In general, obstetricians have been supportive of midwives assuming increased responsibility for the care of healthy pregnant women. In some areas GPs have largely withdrawn from maternity care. This has sometimes caused strains in the relationships between primary care and maternity services, and some GPs have expressed concerns about the loss of skills.

Conclusion

Maternity care is a universal service that all women resident in Scotland are entitled to receive. Since devolution, the direction of the NHS in Scotland has consistently been towards mutuality, collaboration and co-operation. The Scottish Government provides a strong policy direction for maternity services, largely directed at the key aspirations of reducing the effects of social inequalities on health, reducing the occurrence of adverse events and improving safety. There is a unified, pan-Scotland approach to health service delivery, with all NHS Boards working towards the achievement of outcomes in line with the *Scotland Performs* framework; collaboration rather than competition characterises the relationship between service providers. Maternity services have been the focus of much Scottish Government policy since devolution in 1999. The balance of policy direction has generally been towards supporting the principles of childbirth as normal, with midwifery care for every woman within a multi-professional framework. Although some tensions have arisen between professional groups, there has been general support for the concepts of normality and midwifery care. Despite this, intervention in labour is common and the caesarean section rate continues to rise.

Useful web sites

General Medical Council	www.gmc-uk.org/
National Childbirth Trust	www.nct.org.uk/
Netmums	www.netmums.com/
Stillbirth and Neonatal Deat	www.uk-sands.org/

References

Audit Scotland (2012) *Health Inequalities in Scotland.* Edinburgh: Audit Scotland. Available from: www.audit-scotland.gov.uk/docs/health/2012/nr_121213_health_inequalities.pdf. Accessed 19 June 2014.

Bevan, G. (2010) Impact of devolution of health care in the UK: provider challenge in England and provider capture in Wales, Scotland and Northern Ireland? *Journal of Health Services Research and Policy,* 15 (2): 67–68.

Birrell, D. (2009) *The Impact of Devolution on Social Policy.* Bristol: Policy Press.

Brimelow, A. (2011) *Devolution Points Way to Different Types of NHS* [online]. Available from: www.bbc.co.uk/news/health-13122448S. Accessed 19 June 2014.

Burt, B.A. (no date) *Definitions of Risk* [online]. Available from: www.nidcr.nih.gov/NR/rdonlyres/59E8463F-469F-4D06-95C3-CB877673DC98/0/Brian_Burt_Risk.pdf. Accessed 19 June 2014.

Centre for Maternal and Child Enquiries (2011) 'Saving mothers' lives: reviewing maternal deaths to make motherhood safer: 2006–2008. The Eighth Report on Confidential Enquiries into Maternal Deaths in the United Kingdom', *British Journal of Obstetrics and Gynaecology,* 118 (Suppl 1): 1–203.

Cheyne, H., Abhyankar, P. and McCourt, C. (2013a) 'Empowering change: realist evaluation of a Scottish Government programme to support normal birth', *Midwifery,* 29 (10): 1110–1121.

Cheyne, H., McCourt, C. and Semple, K. (2013b) 'Mother knows best: developing a consumer led, evidence informed, research agenda for maternity care', *Midwifery,* 29 (6), 705–712.

Cheyne, H., Skar, S., Paterson, A., David, S. and Hodgkiss, F. (2014) *Having a Baby in Scotland 2013: Women's Experiences of Maternity Care, Volume 1: National Results.* Edinburgh: Scottish Government/NHS Scotland. Available from: www.scotland.gov.uk/Publications/2014/01/8489. Accessed 19 June 2014.

Citizens Advice Bureau (2014) *Advice Guide: Self Help from Citizens Advice. Maternity Leave* [online]. Available from: www.adviceguide.org.uk/scotland/work_s/work_time_off_work_s/maternity_leave.htm. Accessed 15 June 2014.

Community Health Partnerships (2014) [online]. Available from: www.chp.scot.
nhs.uk/.

Connolly, S., Bevan, G. and Mays, N. (2011) *Funding and Performance of Healthcare Systems in the Four Countries of the UK Before and After Devolution. A Longitudinal Analysis of the Four Countries, 1996/97 2002/03 and 2006/07 Supplemented by Cross-sectional Regional Analysis of England 2006/07.* London: The Nuffield Trust.

Cross, B., Cheyne, H. and The Scottish Midwifery Research Collaboration (2012) *Right From the Start. A Scoping Study of the Implementation of the GIRFEC Practice Model Within Maternity Care in Three Contrasting Sites Across Scotland.* Available from: www.nmahp-ru.ac.uk/files/2012/08/GIRFEC-Scoping-Study-Right-from-the-StartAUG2012final.pdf. Accessed 19 June 2014.

Deener, B. and Philips, D. (2013) *Government Spending on Public Services in Scotland: Current Patterns and Future Issues.* Institute of Fiscal Studies Briefing Note BN140 [online]. Available from: www.ifs.org.uk/publications/6858.

Department of Health (1993) *Changing Childbirth: Report of the Expert Maternity Group (Cumberlege Report).* London: HMSO.

Enkin, M., Keirse, M., Neilson, J., Crowther, C., Duley, D., Hodnett, E. *et al.* (2000) *Guide to Effective Care in Pregnancy and Childbirth.* Oxford: Oxford University Press.

Esping-Andersen, G. (1990) *The Three Worlds of Welfare Capitalism.* Cambridge: Polity Press.

EURO-PERISTAT (2013) *The European Perinatal Health Report 2010* [online]. Available from: www.europeristat.com/reports/european-perinatal-health-report-2010.html. Accessed 19 June 2014.

General Medical Council (2014) *Revalidation* [online]. Available from: www.gmc-uk.org/doctors/revalidation.asp. Accessed 19 June 2014.

General Register Office for Scotland (2012) *Vital Events Reference Tables 2012. Section 4 Stillbirths and Infant Deaths* [online]. Available from: www.gro-scotland.gov.uk/statistics/theme/vital-events/general/ref-tables/2012/section-4-stillbirths-and-infant-deaths.html. Accessed 19 June 2014.

General Register Office for Scotland (2013) *Mid-2011 and Mid-2012 Population Estimates Scotland. Population Estimates by Sex, Age and Administrative Area* [online]. Available from: www.gro-scotland.gov.uk/statistics/theme/population/estimates/mid-year/2012/index.html. Accessed 19 June 2014.

GOV.UK (2013) *Devolution of Powers to Scotland, Wales and Northern Ireland* [online]. Available from: www.gov.uk/devolution-of-powers-to-scotland-wales-and-northern-ireland. Accessed 19 June 2014.

Green, J.M., Spiby, H., Hucknall, C. and Foster, H.R. (2012) 'Converting policy into care: women's satisfaction with the early labour telephone component of the All Wales Clinical Pathway for Normal Labour', *Journal of Advanced Nursing,* 68 (10): 2218–2228.

Greer, S.L. (2004) *Four Way Bet: How Devolution Has Led to Four Different Models for the NHS* [online]. Available from: www.ucl.ac.uk/constitution-unit/S. Accessed 19 June 2014.

Greer, S.L. (ed.) (2009) *Devolution and Social Citizenship in the UK.* Bristol: Policy Press.

Healthcare Improvement Scotland (2009) *Keeping Childbirth Natural & Dynamic (KCND)* [online]. Available from: www.healthcareimprovementscotland.org/default.aspx?page=12536. Accessed 19 June 2014.

Healthcare Improvement Scotland (2013) *Scottish Confidential Audit of Severe*

Maternal Morbidity: Reducing Avoidable Harm. 9th Annual Report [online]. Available from: http://file:///C:/Users/hlc1/Downloads/2013–08–09%20Final%20 9th%20annual%20SCASMM%20report%20(2).pdf. Accessed 19 June 2014.

Healthcare Improvement Scotland (2014) *Scottish Patient Safety Programme* [online]. Available from: www.healthcareimprovementscotland.org/our_work/patient_ safety/spsp.aspx. Accessed 19 June 2014.

House of Commons Health Committee (1992) *Second Report on Maternity Services (Winterton Report).* London: Department of Health.

Hundley, V.A., Cruickshank, F.M., Lang, G.D., Glazener, C.M.A., Milne, J. M., Turner, M. *et al.* (1994) 'Midwife managed delivery unit: a randomised controlled comparison with consultant led care', *BMJ*, 309 (6966): 1400–1404.

Information Services Division Scotland (2013a) *Births in Scottish Hospitals* [online]. Available from: www.isdscotland.org/Health-Topics/Maternity-and-Births/Births/. Accessed 19 June 2014.

Information Services Division Scotland (2013b) *ISD Breastfeeding Statistics Financial Year 2012/13* [online]. Available from: http://isdscotland.scot.nhs.uk/Health-Topics/Child-Health/Publications/2013–10–29/2013–10–29-Breastfeeding-Summary.pdf?38851565123. Accessed 19 June 2014.

Information Services Division Scotland (2014) *Workforce* [online]. Available from: www.isdscotland.org/Health-Topics/workforce/. Accessed 19 June 2014.

Keating, M. (2010) *The Government of Scotland after Devolution*, 2nd edn. Edinburgh. Edinburgh University Press.

Mooney, G. and Poole, L. (2004) 'A land of milk and honey?', Social policy in Scotland after devolution', *Critical Social Policy*, 24 (4): 458–483.

Mooney, G. and Scott, G. (eds) (2005) *Exploring Social Policy in the 'New' Scotland.* Bristol: Policy Press.

Mooney, G. and Scott, G. (2012) *Social Policy and Social Justice in Scotland.* Bristol: Policy Press.

Mooney, G. and Wright, S. (2009) 'Introduction: social policy in the devolved Scotland: towards a Scottish welfare state?', *Social Policy and Society*, 8 (3): 361–365.

NHS Health Scotland (2011) *Scottish Antenatal Parent Education. Core Syllabus for Professional Practice to Support Education for Pregnancy, Birth and Early Parenthood Pack* [online]. Available from: www.healthcareimprovementscotland.org/pro-grammes/reproductive,_maternal__child/parent_education/parent_education_ syllabus.aspx. Accessed 19 June 2014.

NHS Scotland (2014a) *Setting the Direction for Nursing and Midwifery Education in Scotland* [online]. Available from: www.scotland.gov.uk/settingthedirectionsum-mary. Accessed 19 June 2014.

NHS Scotland (2014b) *Your Guide to Screening Tests During Pregnancy* [online]. Available from: www.healthscotland.com/documents/3985.aspx. Accessed 19 June 2014.

OECD (2013) *Health at a Glance. OECD Indicators* [online]. Available from: http:// dx.doi.org/10.1787/health_glance-2013-en. Accessed 19 June 2014.

Petts, J., Horlick-Jones, T. and Murdock, G. (2001) *Social Amplification of Risk: the Media and the Public Contract.* Research Report 329/2001. Sudbury: HSE Books.

Pitchforth, E., Teijlingen, E. van, Watson, V., Tucker, J., Kiger, A., Ireland, J. *et al.* (2009) '"Choice" and place of delivery: a qualitative study of women in remote and rural Scotland', *Quality & Safety in Health Care*, 18 (1): 42–48.

128   H. Cheyne

Rivett, G. (1998) *From Cradle to Grave: Fifty Years of the NHS.* London: King's Fund.

Royal College of Midwives Communities (2011) *One NHS, or Four? RCM Communities* [online]. Available from: http://community.rcm.org.uk/blogs/one-nhs-or-four. Accessed 20 June 2014.

Royal College of Obstetricians and Gynaecologists (2013) *RCOG Census Report 2012* [online]. Available from: www.rcog.org.uk/our-profession/good-practice/medical-workforce-census. Accessed 20 June 2014.

Scottish Executive (1997) *Designed to Care – Renewing the National Health Service in Scotland.* Edinburgh: Scottish Executive.

Scottish Executive (2000) *Our National Health: a Plan for Action, a Plan for Change.* Edinburgh: Scottish Executive.

Scottish Executive (2001) *A Framework for Maternity Services in Scotland.* Edinburgh: Scottish Executive.

Scottish Executive Health Department (2002) *Report of the Expert Group on Acute Maternity Services (EGAMS). Implementing a Framework for Maternity Services in Scotland* [online]. Available from: www.scotland.gov.uk/library5/health/egas.pdf. Accessed 19 June 2014.

Scottish Government (2007) *Better Health, Better Care: Action Plan* [online]. Available from: www.scotland.gov.uk/Publications/2007/12/11103453/0. Accessed 19 June 2014.

Scottish Government (2008) *Better Together: Scotland's Patient Experience Programme: Building on the Experiences of NHS Patients and Users.* Available from: www.scotland.gov.uk/Publications/2008/11/20095545/0.

Scottish Government (2011) *A Refreshed Framework for Maternity Services in Scotland.* Edinburgh: Scottish Government. Available from: www.scotland.gov.uk/Publications/2011/02/11122123/2. Accessed 19 June 2014.

Scottish Government (2012) *Rural Scotland Key Facts. People and Communities, Services and Lifestyle, Economy and Enterprise* [online]. Available from: www.scotland.gov.uk/Publications/2012/09/7993. Accessed 19 June 2014.

Scottish Government (2014a) *Scotland Performs* [online]. Available from: www.scotland.gov.uk/About/Performance/scotPerforms. Accessed 19 June 2014.

Scottish Government (2014b) *Directorates* [online]. Available from: www.scotland.gov.uk/About/People/Directorates. Accessed 19 June 2014.

Scottish Government (2014c) *Integration of Adult Health & Social Care Integration Bill – Programme for Government 2012–13* [online]. Available from: www.scotland.gov.uk/About/Performance/programme-for-government/2012–13/Adult-Health-Bill. Accessed 19 June 2014.

Scottish Government (2014d) *Wellbeing* [online]. Available from: www.scotland.gov.uk/Topics/People/Young-People/gettingitright. Accessed 19 June 2014.

Scottish Government (2014e) *Summary: Ethnic Group Demographics* [online]. Available from: www.scotland.gov.uk/Topics/People/Equality/Equalities/DataGrid/Ethnicity/EthPopMig. Accessed 19 June 2014.

Scottish Health Council (2010) *Good Practice in Service User Involvement in Maternity Services: Involving Women to Improve Their Care* [online]. Available from: www.maternityservices.scot.nhs.uk/wp-content/uploads/MaternityServicesAction.pdf. Accessed 20 June 2014.

Scottish Office, Home and Health Department (SOHHD) (1993) *Provision of Maternity Care in Scotland: a Policy Review.* Edinburgh: SOHHD.

Scottish Office, Department of Health (1997) *Designed to Care; Renewing the National Health Service in Scotland.* London: The Stationery Office.

Scottish Parliament (2005) Breastfeeding etc. (Scotland) Act 2005 [online]. Available www.legislation.gov.uk/asp/2005/1/contents. Accessed 19 June 2014.

Scottish Parliament (2014) *Children and Young People (Scotland) Bill* [online]. Available from: www.scottish.parliament.uk/parliamentarybusiness/Bills/62233.aspx. Accessed 19 June 2014.

Scott, G. and Wright, S. (2012) 'Devolution, social democratic visions and policy reality in Scotland', *Critical Social Policy*, 32 (3): 440–453.

Steel, D. and Cylus, J. (2012) 'United Kingdom (Scotland): health system review', *Health Systems in Transition*, 14 (9): 1–150.

Stewart, J. (2004) *Taking Stock*. Bristol: Policy Press.

Sullivan, M. (2002), 'Health policy: differentiation and devolution.' In: J. Adams and K. Schmuecker (eds), *Devolution in Practice*. London: Institute for Public Policy Research, pp. 60–68.

Tannahill, C. (2005), 'Health and health policy'. In: G. Mooney and G. Scott (eds), *Exploring Social Policy in the 'New' Scotland*. Bristol: Policy Press, pp. 99–219.

Telegraph (2013) [online]. Available from: www.telegraph.co.uk/news/uknews/law-and-order/10503079/Alessandra-Pacchieri-Pitiful-tale-of-a-mother-and-her-lost-child.html. Accessed 19 June 2014.

Timmins, N. (2013) *The Four UK Health Systems. Learning From Each Other*. London: The Kings Fund. Available from: www.kingsfund.org.uk/publications/four-uk-health-systems-june-2013. Accessed 19 June 2014.

Turnbull, D., Holmes, A., Shields, N., Cheyne, H., Twaddle, S., Gilmour, W.H. *et al.* (1996) 'Randomised, controlled trial of efficacy of midwife-managed care', *The Lancet*, 348 (9022), 213–218.

UK National Statistics (2014) *Gateway to UK National Statistics. Population*. London: Office for National Statistics. Available from: www.statistics.gov.uk/hub/population/. Accessed 15 May 2014.

Walker, G., Simmons, P., Irwin, A. and Wynne, B. (1998) *Public Perceptions of Risks Associated with Major Accident Hazards*. Sudbury: HSE Books.

Weindling, A.M. (2003) 'The confidential enquiry into maternal and child health (CEMACH)', *Archives of Disease in Childhood*, 88: 1034–1037.

Winchester, N. and Storey, J. (2008) *Devolved Governance Systems*. NHS/SDO Project Working Paper, No. 2/2008. Milton Keynes: Open University. Available from: www7.open.ac.uk/oubs/research/pdf/SDO_Project_07_2.pdf. Accessed 19 June 2014.

www.parliament.uk (2014) *Living Heritage. Act of Union 1707* [online]. Available www.parliament.uk/about/living-heritage/evolutionofparliament/legislative-scrutiny/act-of-union-1707/. Accessed 19 June 2014.

7   Canada

Louise Marie Roth and Amanda M. Lubold

Background

Canada is a high-income country with an advanced industrial economy and the ninth highest per capita income in the world (Marchildon 2013). Canada was founded on its rich natural resources and developed into an advanced economy through global trade networks (Easterbrook 1959). Canada has maintained a strong economic performance throughout the global recession that began in 2008, largely because its banking sector is highly regulated (Henderson 2010). Canada also has relatively low income inequality and ranks highly on international measurements of education, government transparency, civil liberties, quality of life and economic freedom (Heritage Foundation 2014; International Monetary Fund 2013; OECD 2009).

Originally composed of French and English colonies, Canada became a self-governing confederation in 1867 when the British North America Act joined English-speaking Upper Canada (Ontario), French-speaking Lower Canada (Québec) and other British territories in Eastern Canada (the Maritime Provinces) (Bothwell 1996). Canada gained independent nation status in 1931, but remains a member of the British Commonwealth (Hail and Lange 2010). Consequently, Canada's governmental structure and model of citizenship resemble other English-speaking Commonwealth countries, such as the UK, Australia and New Zealand. Canada is a constitutional monarchy with a parliamentary system and also a federation with two constitutionally recognised orders of government: a central federal government and ten provincial governments (Marchildon 2013). The three sparsely populated northern Canadian territories are separate from the provincial government system.

Canada as a welfare regime

In his classic work, Esping-Andersen (1990) identified three welfare state regimes based on the national arrangements of markets, the state and families: social democratic, conservative and liberal regimes. He classified

Canada with the USA and the UK in the liberal regime, which provides limited social welfare programmes to citizens. Other scholars have grouped countries into four welfare families, including an English-speaking family that includes Canada, Australia, New Zealand, Ireland, the UK and the USA (Castles and Mitchell 1993). In both classifications, Canada falls among the English-speaking countries that provide relatively few social supports and financial benefits to citizens, preferring instead for the markets to provide these supports and benefits (Castles and Mitchell 1993; Esping-Andersen 1990). Accordingly, Canada's social spending, welfare programmes and labour market are primarily market-based, with relatively few regulations affecting wages and earnings. Market-based welfare states are characterised by inequality in training and educational resources, which traditionally target the top third of wage-earners in Canada (Myles 1998). Low income workers in Canada earn about 40 per cent of the median wage, compared with an average of 63 per cent in other high-income OECD countries (Myles 1998). This difference between Canada and other developed nations relates directly to the differences in welfare regimes and the strategies for providing basic social services.

Canada's welfare state also developed within a strong history of federalism, in which the Constitution Act of 1982 allotted specific powers of legislation to the central federal government and the provincial governments (Banting 2004). Canada's welfare state programmes are a combination of shared-cost programmes, in which the federal government gives financial assistance to the provinces with specific terms attached, and joint-decision programmes that require agreement between both levels of government before any action is taken (Banting 2004).

Canada also differs notably from the other English-speaking, market-based welfare states in its development of a few robust, universal welfare programmes. The Great Depression in the 1930s created tremendous hardship for many working families, leading Saskatchewan's Co-operative Commonwealth Federation to introduce elements of a welfare state at the provincial level in the 1940s and 1950s (Mulvale 2008). This offered a prototype for future social programmes, such as the universal health insurance programme. In the 1960s and 1970s, the Canadian federal government introduced universal welfare programmes, including Medicare (single-payer, taxpayer-funded universal health care), the Canada Pension Plan and student loan programmes (Sarrouh 2002). Canada's pension system was initially a means-tested programme, but became increasingly universal over time (Myles 1998).

Health care system

Canada has a single-payer, publicly funded health care system that provides all Canadians with health care services, irrespective of their ability to pay (Myles 1998). Based on earlier initiatives in the provinces, in 1966

Lester B. Pearson's federal government introduced the Medical Care Act, which established a universal health care plan that combined federal funding with provincial administration of the Medicare system (Naylor 1986). The federal government passed the Canada Health Act in 1984, which prohibited user fees and extra billing by physicians (Naylor 1999; Stevenson *et al.* 1988). As a result, most health care services are free at the point of use, with no deductions or co-payments. The federal government maintains standards for the quality of care, but does not participate directly in providing care or collecting health information (Naylor 1986, 1999). Provincial Health Ministries issue health cards to all legal residents and everyone is entitled to the same level of care. The system emphasises preventive care and encourages individuals to have yearly check-ups. The federal government also negotiates drug prices with pharmaceutical suppliers, which controls the costs of drugs (Menon 2001; Wiktorowicz 2003).

Unlike the UK's National Health Service, which owns facilities and employs physicians directly, physicians in Canada are typically private, self-employed, fee-for-service practitioners (Hutchison *et al.* 2001; Naylor 1999). Canada's provincial health care plans pay health care providers according to a fee schedule that the provincial government negotiates with the medical association (Naylor 1999; Stevenson *et al.* 1988). As a result, physicians receive standard fee rates for services and cannot charge whatever they choose. Health care providers gain familiarity with the rules and claim procedures of the provincial insurer and individual patients are not involved in billing or in the filing of insurance claims. The Canadian health care system is cost-effective because it simplifies administration (Woolhandler and Himmelstein 1989). Canadians strongly support Canada's public health care system, with 91 per cent of Canadians indicating that they prefer it over the system in the USA (Abelson *et al.* 2004; Soroka 2011).

Health spending in Canada represents 11.2 per cent of the GDP, which is higher than the OECD average of 9.3 per cent, but slightly lower than some European countries, such as France, Germany and the Netherlands (OECD 2013). However, Canadian health care costs have risen faster than economic growth in recent years, primarily because of increases in the fees for services and the rising costs of hospital care (Canadian Institute for Health Information 2011a). Payments to physicians for clinical services increased by 6 per cent in 2010–2011, representing a slower growth than the previous two years (Canadian Institute for Health Information 2012).

The number of physicians in Canada has been rising, although the ratio of practising physicians to the population in Canada is below the OECD average of 3.1 (Canadian Institute for Health Information 2011b). The Canadian Medical Association estimates that there were 38,286 family physicians, 27,030 medical specialists and 9,455 surgical specialists in 2014 (Canadian Medical Association 2014). In 2012, family physicians (GPs) in Canada earned an average of US$255,881 and specialists' compensation averaged US$356,263 (Canadian Institute for Health Information 2012). GPs are the front line of the Canadian health care system, but there is a critical national shortage of GPs, with particularly high demand in rural areas (Canadian Medical Association 2014; Esmail 2011).

Other types of care providers, such as nursing professionals, offer alternatives to GPs for primary care, although their numbers are inadequate to fully meet the health care needs of all Canadians and the needs of the maternity care system in particular. The number of practising nurses in Canada is above the OECD average of 8.4 per 1,000 population, but the ratio of registered midwives is far below the OECD average of 69.8 per 100,000 women (Canadian Institute for Health Information 2011b). Hospital bed ratios are also lower than the OECD average (Canadian Institute for Health Information 2011b). Table 7.1 gives the ratios of health care practitioners and hospital beds to the population in Canada.

Canada's universities maintain seventeen accredited medical schools and Canada maintains its own professional associations and accreditation bodies for health care workers (American Board of Medical Specialties 2012). In Canada, private organisations provide accreditation to the professional schools, review standards of training and certification for foreign-trained physicians, and develop standards for licensure. The College of Family Physicians of Canada sets standards for the training, certification and continuing education of family physicians. The Royal College of Physicians and Surgeons of Canada sets the credentialing requirements for a variety of specialties, including obstetrics and gynaecology. The Royal College of Physicians and Surgeons of Canada is also the main body that accredits the physician residency programmes. Canadian medical and nursing schools also receive accreditation from American professional associations such as the American Board of Medical Specialties.

For nursing education, the Canadian Association of Schools of Nursing accredits Bachelor of Nursing Degree Programs and Bachelor of Science in Nursing Programs at over forty-six universities and community colleges across Canada (Canadian Association of Schools of Nursing 2014). Most

Table 7.1 Human and physical resources in Canada

Physicians per 1,000 population[a]	2.4
Nurses per 1,000 population[a]	9.4
Medical graduates per 100,000 population[b]	7.4
Nursing graduates per 100,000 population[b]	44.99
Total hospital beds per 1,000 population[b]	2.8
Curative (acute) care beds, per 1,000 population[b]	1.7
Gynaecologists and obstetricians per 100,000 women[a]	14.3
Registered midwives per 100,000 women [a]	4.5

Sources: a Canadian Institute for Health Information (2011b); b OECD (2011).

registered nurses hold a four-year baccalaureate degree and can pursue further education at masters or doctoral level. Some colleges in Canada also offer diploma programmes for Registered Practical Nurses or Licensed Practical Nurses after two years of study.

Midwifery in Canada is regulated at the provincial level and most provinces require midwives to be registered with the provincial College of Midwives, with exceptions for aboriginal midwives and healers in Ontario and British Columbia (Canadian Midwifery Regulators Consortium 2014). Most midwives graduate from one of seven four-year baccalaureate midwifery education programmes, so that most registered midwives in Canada have at least a baccalaureate degree (Canadian Association of Midwives 2014). These midwifery education programmes administer the provincial regulatory bodies' licensing exams (Canadian Association of Midwives 2014).

Demographic profile

Canada is the thirty-seventh most populous country in the world, with a population of approximately thirty-five million people (Statistics Canada 2013a). With 0.49 per cent of the world's population living in the second largest country by area, Canada's population density is among the lowest in the world. Canada's population is growing, largely fuelled by immigration, but its growth is slower than the average for the world population (OECD 2011). In 2011, approximately 81 per cent of Canada's population lived in urban areas (Statistics Canada 2012). Most of the population also lives within 150 km of Canada's southern border with the USA (Custred 2008). Table 7.2 gives the demographic profile of contemporary Canada.

Canada recognises English and French with equal status as its two official languages in all federal institutions and is one of the most multicultural and ethnically diverse nations in the world. Although aboriginal populations have inhabited Canada for thousands of years, today only 4.3 per cent of Canada's citizens identify themselves as aboriginal, falling in three broad groups: First Nations, Métis and Inuit (Hayes 2008; Marchildon 2013). Canada emphasises multicultural diversity (a cultural 'mosaic') rather than assimilation (a 'melting pot') (Esses and Gardner 1996; Gibbon 1938; Kelley and Trebilcock 2010). Large-scale immigration from many countries has generated a contemporary population that is racially diverse.

The health profile of Canadians with respect to life expectancy is similar to other English-speaking countries, except the USA (which fares worse). In 2012, Canada's life expectancy at birth was 80.4 years, with a life expectancy for men of 78.8 years and a life expectancy for women of 84.1 years (Bohnert 2013). Canada's fertility rate of 1.59 is considerably lower than the world average of 2.47 and falls below those of the USA (2.06) and the UK (1.90).

Table 7.2 Demographic profile of Canada

Population	35,158,300
Women	17,726,100
Population aged 0–14 years	5,674,100
Women of childbearing age (15–44 years)	7,030,600
Population aged 65 years or older	5,379,500
Population annual growth (%)	1.14
Population density per square kilometre	3.8
Total fertility rate (births per woman)	1.6
Crude birth rate per 1,000 people	11.0
Crude death rate per 1,000 people	7.4
Urban population (%)	80.8
Ethnic groups (%)	
White	86.0
Black	2.9
East Asian	4.8
Latin America	1.2
South Asian	4.8
South-east Asian	2.8
West Asian and Arab	1.8
Multiracial	0.5
Other	0.3
Aboriginal	4.3

Source: Statistics Canada (2013b).

Even though the overall health status of Canadians has improved over time, there are patterns of health disparities in Canada by income, rural location and aboriginal status (Frohlich *et al.* 2006; Wilkins *et al.* 2002). An urban/rural divide characterises health care access in Canada. The approximately 20 per cent of the Canadian population that lives in very rural areas experiences limited access to medical care because of the distance to the available facilities (PHAC 2009). Income disparities are related to the urban/rural divide because rural areas tend to be poorer; income inequality in health has grown since 2009 (Kondro 2012). However, the worst disparities exist between the aboriginal populations and the rest of the Canadian population (Frohlich *et al.* 2006; Tjepkema 2002). Aboriginal populations in Canada have considerably higher rates of type 2 diabetes, cardiovascular disease, hypertension, substance abuse, interpersonal and family violence, and HIV/AIDS (Gracey and King 2009). Aboriginal populations also have higher infant and maternal mortality rates, lower birthweights, and lower average life expectancy (Gracey and King 2009; King *et al.* 2009). A range of cultural factors, such as racism, loss of language and environmental dispossession, have contributed to health disparities by aboriginal status (King and Gracey 2009; Reading and Wien 2009; Richmond and Ross 2009).

Maternity provision

Maternity care is an essential, basic form of care that the Canadian health care system covers for all residents (Wrede *et al.* 2001). However, Canada has a relative shortage of obstetricians, gynaecologists and midwives compared with other OECD countries, especially in rural areas. In 2009, Canada had only 14.3 gynaecologists and obstetricians per 100,000 women (Table 7.1), which is well below the OECD average of 26.8 and ranks third from the bottom among OECD countries (OECD 2011). In December 2008, the Society of Obstetricians and Gynaecologists of Canada reported a critical shortage of obstetricians and gynaecologists, predicting a one-third reduction in practitioners within five years (Society of Obstetricians and Gynaecologists of Canada 2008b).

These reductions have coincided with fewer family physicians providing maternity care. All the major accreditation bodies require family physicians to have training and experience in low-risk obstetrics. Family physicians who provide intrapartum care have lower intervention rates and equal or better outcomes than obstetricians for low-risk patients (Iglesias *et al.* 1998). Among family physicians, 64 per cent reported involvement in some aspect of maternity care and family physicians are particularly important providers of maternity care in small towns and rural areas, where 27 per cent of family doctors provide intrapartum care, compared with only 12 per cent in urban areas (Canadian Institute for Health Information 2007). However, many family physicians do not attend births because of the associated higher insurance premiums and liability risks (Woodward and Rosser 1989). The growing shortage of providers in rural areas increases the risk of adverse events because of the distance providers and clients have to travel to receive care and obtain access to specialised equipment (PHAC 2009).

To meet the maternity care needs of the Canadian population, Canada's supply of registered midwives has increased, with an annual growth rate of 8.7 per cent per year between 2000 and 2009 (OECD 2011). Although this is the second highest growth rate in this period, Canada has the fewest midwives per 100,000 women of all the OECD countries, with only 4.5 midwives per 100,000 women in 2009 (OECD 2011). Among women who want midwifery care in Ontario, almost 40 per cent cannot find a midwife (Benoit *et al.* 2010). Universities with midwifery programmes also admit very few students for training because of the intensive faculty-to-student ratio required to train quality midwives, so the capacity of programmes for training registered midwives is too small to meet even the existing demand (Hawkins and Knox 2003). Legal and health insurance restrictions are partly responsible for the dearth of registered midwives in Canada, where the Medical Practitioners Act restricted maternity services to licensed members of the College of Physicians and Surgeons until the early 1990s (Benoit *et al.* 2005). Provincial health care plans did not reimburse 'alternative' health services such as midwifery before 1992, which effectively restricted maternity care to hospitals and licensed physicians (Benoit *et al.* 2005). Even today, only five provinces and one territory regulate and reimburse midwives (Hawkins and Knox 2003). In those jurisdictions, midwives receive payments from the provincial health plan for out-of-hospital births as well as hospital births and the health care system institutionalises obstetric back-up for midwifery care, thus reducing obstetric risk. In fact, efforts to improve the quality of maternity care in Canada explicitly include integrating different models of birth into the system and encouraging collaboration among nurses, midwives, family physicians and obstetricians (Peterson *et al.* 2007; Society of Obstetricians and Gynaecologists of Canada 2008b).

In its statement, A National Birthing Initiative for Canada, the Society of Obstetricians and Gynaecologists of Canada noted that societal and demographic shifts in Canada over the past twenty years (including a higher average age of women giving birth, a drop in the overall fertility rate, an increase in multiple births and an increase in the number of infants needing treatment in intensive care units) have increased risks for pregnant women and babies (Society of Obstetricians and Gynaecologists of Canada 2008b). In addition, the report noted a need to improve accountability for maternity services, as local changes in maternity care can occur without input or oversight from the regional or provincial governments. Thus the Society of Obstetricians and Gynaecologists of Canada aims to increase maternity care oversight at the national level.

Maternity entitlements

Maternity care has been universal in Canada since the adoption of a single-payer universal health care system, so all pregnant women are entitled to care that is free at the point of service in the antenatal, intrapartum and postpartum periods. In terms of other entitlements, Canada's parental leave policies underwent a major change at the beginning of 2001, when the employment compensation system extended the national paid parental leave policy from fifteen weeks to fifty weeks (Calder 2003). The parental leave provision is theoretically divided between both legal parents, although in practice mothers typically take all of the leave. This significant extension of Canada's maternity entitlement is funded through the employment insurance system that covers all wage-earners through payroll deductions. Funding through employment insurance limits eligibility to employees who have logged at least 700 hours of employment in a fifty-two week period, so that those who are self-employed, seasonal workers and many part-time employees are ineligible (Calder 2003). In addition, the parental leave entitlement is not fully paid. Workers who use the benefit only receive 55 per cent of their average insured earnings through the employment insurance system, although some employers top up their workers' compensation to 100 per cent with a Supplemental Unemployment Benefit (Calder 2003; Marshall 2010). The Supplemental Unemployment Benefit is a government initiative that allows employers to reduce the net earnings loss of their employees on leave (Marshall 2010).

Childbirth in Canada

Antenatal care

In Canada, 97 per cent of new mothers receive antenatal care (Canadian Institute for Health Information 2007). In the 2006–2007 Maternal Experiences Survey, a nationally representative survey of pregnant women, 94.9 per cent of Canadian pregnant women were found to have initiated prenatal care in the first trimester (PHAC 2009). The Society for Obstetricians and Gynaecologists of Canada recommends the following standards for prenatal care:

- visits with a health care provider every four to six weeks early in pregnancy
- visits every two to three weeks after thirty weeks of gestation
- visits every one to two weeks after thirty-six weeks of gestation.

This standard is supposed to apply to all mothers, regardless of whether their pregnancies are high risk or uncomplicated (PHAC 2009).

Nationally in 2006–2007, 58.1 per cent of women received prenatal care from an obstetrician/gynaecologist, 34.2 per cent from a family physician, 6.1 per cent from a midwife and 0.6 per cent from a nurse or nurse practitioner (PHAC 2009). Women with a university degree are more likely to seek care from a midwife than those with less education (8.9 per cent versus 3.9 per cent) (PHAC 2009). Many mothers in Canada start prenatal care with their family doctor or GP and then switch to an obstetrician/gynaecologist or other professional in the second or third trimester. In fact, only 19 per cent of family physicians who gave some aspect of maternity care actually attended births in 2001 (Canadian Institute for Health Information 2007). As with most health care in Canada, family physicians are the first line of defence for assessing and addressing risk and make referrals to specialists as needed (Canadian Institute for Health Information 2007).

Antenatal care providers address and discuss the risk associated with childbirth during the prenatal care period. Routine prenatal care includes an ultrasound scan during the second trimester, unless there are complications. In 2003, the Canadian Task Force on Preventative Health Care determined that there was sufficient evidence to support ultrasound screening in normal pregnancies.

Intrapartum care

Canada has historically had low infant and maternal mortality rates, but has lost ground in recent years compared with other developed nations. In 1990, Canada ranked fifth among peer countries, but most recently it has had the second highest infant mortality rate, only performing better than the USA (OECD 2013). In 2009, Canada's infant mortality rate was 5.1 deaths per 1,000 live births, above the OECD average of 4.4 deaths per 1,000 live births. Both infant and maternal mortality have been increasing in Canada since the mid-1990s and low income infants are particularly vulnerable (Lisonkova *et al.* 2011; Society of Obstetricians and Gynaecologists of Canada 2008b; Wilkins *et al.* 2000; WHO 2010). In 2009, 6.0 per cent of babies in Canada had a low birthweight (<2,500g), which is better than the OECD average of 6.7 per cent in 2009 and ranks twelfth among thirty-nine OECD countries (OECD 2011). However, the percentage of babies with low birthweight in Canada increased from 1980 to 2009 as a result of several common changes in Western nations: women giving birth at older ages, more multiple births and increases in the induction of labour and caesarean deliveries of premature or late preterm infants (OECD 2011).

For maternal mortality, Canada currently ranks thirty-fifth in the world, with twelve deaths for every 100,000 live births – a considerably lower rate than in the USA (WHO 2010). However, Canada has slipped from second to eleventh place in the world ranking among the OECD countries since 1990. Maternal morbidity, which refers to illness or injury arising from complications of pregnancy or delivery, has also been increasing in Canada over the last two decades (Wen *et al.* 2004). Examples of maternal morbidity include gestational diabetes, pre-eclampsia and haemorrhage; examples of severe morbidity include peripartum hysterectomy, renal failure, heart failure, stroke, pulmonary embolism and septic shock. Some maternal complications are a leading cause of neonatal mortality and morbidity. Table 7.3 gives Canada's maternal and neonatal mortality statistics from 1970 to 2010.

Canada's Western medical tradition includes a culture of birth that normalises medical interventions. Almost half of all vaginal births (47.9 per cent) occurred from a supine position (with the mother lying on her back), while 45.8 per cent of women were propped up, even though Health Canada recommends that women receive information about various birth positions so that they can make an informed choice about their preferred position (PHAC 2009). The supine position, although common in Western medical practice, is among the least desirable physiologically.

Epidural analgesia, induction and stimulation with Pitocin, and continuous electronic foetal monitoring are extremely common. Table 7.3 gives Canada's rates for some of these procedures over time, showing that the rates of induction and caesarean delivery have risen, while

Table 7.3 Birth interventions and outcomes in Canada for selected years

	1970	1980	1990	2000	2010*
Maternal mortality, per 100,000	20[a]	4.5[a]	6[b]	7[b]	12[b]
Perinatal deaths per 1,000 live and stillbirths[a]	21.8	10.9	6.8	6.2	6.1
Neonatal deaths per 1,000 live births[a]	13.5	6.7	4.6	3.6	3.7
Infant mortality per 1,000 live births[a]	18.8	10.4	6.8	5.3	4.9
Induction (% of deliveries)[c]		12	20.7	22.5	21.8[1]
Forceps (% of vaginal deliveries)		21.2[d]	11.2[d]	6.2[d]	3.7[e]
Vacuum (% of vaginal deliveries)		0.6[d]	6.8[d]	10.6[d]	9.8[e]
Caesarean[d]	6	16	19	25.6	26.6
Episiotomy (% of vaginal deliveries)[d]		66.8	51.5	24.1	21.8[2]

Sources: a Statistics Canada; b World Bank; c Public Health Agency of Canada; d Health Canada (2003); e Canadian Institute for Health Information (2007) (data for 2005–2006).

Notes
* Or the most recent available year.
1 2009.
2 2004.

episiotomy rates have declined. Induction is 'the artificial initiation of labour before its spontaneous onset' and Health Canada recommends induction only 'when the risk of continuing pregnancy is greater than the risk of induction' (Health Canada 2000). However, in 2004–2005, 28.1 per cent of deliveries in Canada were artificially induced (PHAC 2009). In the Canadian Maternity Experiences study, 44.8 per cent of women who gave birth vaginally or attempted to give birth vaginally reported that their maternity care professional tried to induce labour (Chalmers *et al.* 2012).

Electronic foetal monitoring during labour is also common, with 90.8 per cent of women in the Canadian Maternity Experiences study reporting that they had some form of electronic foetal monitoring (Chalmers *et al.* 2012; PHAC 2009). Evidence-based medicine recommends against the use of electronic foetal monitoring because it increases the odds of other interventions, such as anaesthesia, vacuum or forceps delivery and caesarean section (PHAC 2009). Finally, although Canadian guidelines recommend that epidural analgesia is not used as a first approach to pain management, 57.3 per cent of women had an epidural (Chalmers *et al.* 2012). As with most interventions, however, there is a large urban/rural divide, so that only 24.2 per cent of women in Yukon and 13.0 per cent in Nunavut reported receiving an epidural, compared with 66.7 per cent in Québec and 60.7 per cent in Ontario (PHAC 2009).

Episiotomies, a once-routine practice, have declined in Canada over time. An episiotomy is an incision made to increase the vaginal opening, but there is no evidence that the routine use of episiotomies is beneficial and there is substantial evidence that it causes lasting harm to the perineum (Klein *et al.* 1992). The pioneer of research rejecting routine episiotomy as an unnecessary intervention was the Canadian obstetrician Michael C. Klein. The rate of episiotomies in Canada has declined from 68.8 per cent of vaginal births in 1980 to 21.8 per cent in 2004 (PHAC 2008).

Although Canada has advanced medical technology and surgical techniques, some maternal outcomes are worsening and advanced technology and surgery may be a significant part of the problem (Davis-Floyd 2004; Morris 2013). Caesarean delivery can be life-saving, but is over-used in most Western medical contexts and is associated with substantial increases in maternal mortality and morbidity (PHAC 2008). Caesarean rates have risen dramatically in Canada, where 26.6 per cent of live births in 2009 involved a caesarean delivery, slightly above the OECD average of 25.8 per cent and considerably higher than the WHO's recommended upper limit of 15 per cent (Canadian Institute for Health Information 2012; OECD 2011; WHO 2009). After dropping slightly during the 1990s, caesarean rates in Canada increased by 3.1 per cent between 2000 and 2009 (OECD 2011). In efforts to reduce Canada's high rates of caesarean section, the Society of Obstetricians and Gynaecologists of Canada released a 2008 policy statement in support of normal childbirth (Society of Obstetricians and Gynaecologists of Canada 2008a).

In terms of the location of birth, the vast majority of women in Canada give birth in hospitals (98.6 per cent) with an obstetrician/ gynaecologist (69.9 per cent) or a family physician (14.6 per cent) (PHAC 2009; Statistics Canada 2013c). The Maternal Experiences Survey surveyed women who gave birth in 2006 about their births and found that 69.9 per cent had an obstetrician/gynaecologist as their primary birth attendant, while 14.6 per cent had a family physician (PHAC 2009). Women in rural areas were much less likely to have an obstetrician/gynaecologist and much more likely to have a family physician attend their births (PHAC 2009).

Once again, there are significant urban/rural disparities in intrapartum care. While only 2.5 per cent of women nationally had to travel more than 100 km to give birth, that rate was 40.3 per cent in the Northwest Territories, 37.9 per cent in Nunavut, and 23.0 per cent in the Yukon (PHAC 2009). Women in remote rural areas have been routinely airlifted to facilities since the 1970s. However, research has found that removing these women from their communities to give birth causes financial, psychological and other stress for the women and for their families (Canadian Institute for Health Information 2004). Consequently, public health efforts have focused on increasing access to registered midwifery services, especially in remote rural areas (PHAC 2009). The Society of Obstetricians and Gynaecologists of Canada supports the integration of regulated, publicly funded midwifery care in all provinces and territories, with special efforts to increase access in the three sparsely populated Canadian territories (PHAC 2009).

Postnatal care

Canadian hospitals, health centres, public health nurses and family physicians provide postnatal care to all pregnant women and new mothers, and the public health system pays for this care (PHAC 2009). In an effort to reduce costs, the length of postpartum stays for mothers in Canada has decreased over time. After a vaginal birth, 25.5 per cent of mothers in 2004–2005 stayed in the hospital for less than two days compared with only 3.7 per cent in 1991–1992. After a caesarean delivery, 52.5 per cent of mothers had hospital stays of less than four days in 2004–2005 compared with 2.7 per cent in 1991–1992 (PHAC 2009). At the same time, in an effort to improve maternal–child health, Provincial Ministries of Health have promoted the Baby-Friendly Hospital Initiative (BFHI), a WHO programme that aims to improve the care of pregnant women, mothers and infants and to encourage breastfeeding (Labbok 2012). The provinces of Québec and New Brunswick have mandated implementation of the BFHI and other provinces and territories are implementing strategies at local and regional levels (Breastfeeding Committee of Canada 2012). Ontario required all public health units to begin implementation of the BFHI in 2012 (Ministry of Health and Long Term Care 2012). By 2012, there were thirty-five Baby-Friendly Hospitals, birthing centres and community health services in four Canadian provinces (Breastfeeding Committee of Canada 2012). In addition, many Canadian hospitals have implemented some 'baby-friendly' practices, such as early skin-to-skin contact. Among Maternal Experiences Survey respondents, 71.9 per cent had skin-to-skin contact with their babies within five minutes of birth in 2006–2007 (PHAC 2009). A majority of women in Canada receive postnatal care after hospital discharge from health care providers and have contact with those providers through phone calls, home visits and clinic visits (PHAC 2009). In 2006–2007, 93.3 per cent of women who responded to the Maternal Experiences Survey reported that a health care provider contacted them at home after they gave birth.

In the immediate postnatal period, 87.3 per cent of mothers initiated breastfeeding in 2010 compared with 69.3 per cent in 1995. This rate is above the OECD average, but behind the Nordic countries (with initiation rates above 97 per cent) (OECD 2012). In terms of meeting the guidelines for duration of breastfeeding, 38.7 per cent of mothers were breastfeeding at 6 months in 2003, increasing to 54 per cent in 2009 (Statistics Canada 2014). Canada's breastfeeding rates have markedly increased over the past few decades, perhaps partly due to public health policy initiatives and the extension of paid parental leave (Breastfeeding Committee of Canada 2012; Ministry of Health and Long Term Care 2012).

Consumer involvement

The 2006–2007 Maternity Experiences Survey asked women where they obtained their most useful sources of pregnancy-related information and

32.2 per cent of women reported that the most useful sources were their health care providers (PHAC 2009). The second most useful source of information was books (22.3 per cent), followed by information from a previous pregnancy (17.1 per cent). Most mothers were satisfied with the information that they received about physical changes during pregnancy (92.8 per cent), emotional changes (89.4 per cent), the warning signs of pregnancy complications (83.7 per cent), the effects of medication on the foetus (93.9 per cent) and prenatal tests and procedures (91.8 per cent) (PHAC 2009). However, it may be misleading to view women's satisfaction with their birthing process as a measure of quality of care, as many women tend to rate their experience as positive no matter what type of birth experience they have, especially if they are first-time mothers (Davis-Floyd 2004; PHAC 2009).

Consumer involvement with maternity care delivery in Canada has focused largely around access to midwifery services. The push to include midwives in the maternity care system began in Ontario in the 1970s (Bourgeault 2000). Small grassroots feminist groups began to organise to support midwives and alternative birthing options. At that time, Canada had no officially recognised practice of midwifery and these groups consolidated to form the Ontario Association of Midwives in 1982 (Bourgeault 2000). A separate consumer advocacy group, the Midwifery Task Force of Ontario, was also included in a coalition to push for the representation of midwives in the health professions. These midwifery groups petitioned the Ontario Health Professions Legislation Review and, by 1993, 'midwifery in the province of Ontario had become fully integrated into the government-funded health care system' (Bourgeault 2000: 172–173).

From the success of integration in Ontario, other consumer groups and feminist organisations began to petition provincial governments across Canada. As of 2005, midwives can legally practice in five provinces and, in four of these provinces, midwifery services are provided as part of the government-funded health care system (Benoit *et al.* 2005). In the Maternal Experiences Survey, mothers who had prenatal care from a midwife or a family physician, as opposed to an obstetrician, reported that they were slightly more satisfied with their birth experience (PHAC 2009).

Risk and rights

In Canada, all residents have the right to health care coverage, including immigrants and other non-citizens. Thus the social welfare net in Canada covers maternity care services for all women, regardless of their economic or citizenship status. There are no differences in entitlements, but there is variation in access to care across regions. The Provincial Ministries of Health have closed many small-volume centres in remote or rural areas with limited access to tertiary care facilities, so pregnant women in these areas have no local care options. Rural women often have to travel long distances or be airlifted to major health centres. As aboriginal populations are more likely to live in remote regions, these problems disproportionately affect aboriginal women and the lack of local maternity services can isolate them from sources of family and community support at a time when it is especially important. It also poses significant problems for women without the financial means to travel to other communities to seek routine prenatal, intrapartum and postpartum care, thus limiting their ability to access the full range of available maternity care services to which they are entitled (Iglesias *et al.* 1998). Overall shortages of maternity care providers in Canada also aggravate rural/urban and aboriginal/non-aboriginal disparities. Decreases in the number of family physicians providing maternity care, scarcities of registered midwives and shortages of obstetricians mean that the potential risks of childbearing have increased in the Canadian system (Society of Obstetricians and Gynaecologists of Canada 2008b). Thus, although recipients of maternity care have a right to care at a macro-level, the risks are higher in some areas of Canada as a result of lack of access to care providers and facilities, especially if emergencies arise.

At the micro-level, women have different views about what they want from maternity care: some prefer obstetric care and others prefer midwives. However, the shortages of providers influence women's ability to realise their preferences. Most specifically, while their numbers are growing, the number of midwives in Canada is extremely low compared with other OECD countries and there are too few to meet the demands of women who prefer midwifery care, even in urban areas (Malott *et al.* 2009; Peterson *et al.* 2007). Family physicians in Canada also provide much less intrapartum care than in the 1970s, when over two-thirds practised obstetrics (Kidd 2013). Family physicians are increasingly reluctant to attend births in Canada, leading many women with low-risk pregnancies to obtain maternity care from obstetricians, who specialise in higher risk pregnancies and use more interventionist approaches to care, even in uncomplicated pregnancies and births.

At the meso-level (service provider level), the notions of risk in obstetrics are organised around complicated and often rare occurrences, with a view of every birth as a potential emergency (Simonds *et al.* 2007). Risk is not completely avoidable and some adverse outcomes cannot be anticipated in advance (Iglesias *et al.* 1998). Consequently, the Society of Obstetricians and Gynaecologists of Canada has developed guidelines and policy statements for the management of common maternity care issues, including group B streptococcal infections, HIV testing in pregnancy, induction of labour, dystocia and maternal/foetal transport (Iglesias *et al.* 1998; Society of Obstetricians and Gynaecologists of Canada 2008a). These guidelines all operate within a medical model that focuses on solving problems and curing disease (Davis-Floyd 2004; Simonds *et al.* 2007).

Canadian maternity care is based on a Western medical tradition of physician-attended hospital birth, in which obstetricians maintain authoritative knowledge (Jordan 1992; Davis-Floyd 2004). The medical model of birth as a risky medical event defines all pregnancies as low risk or high risk (but none as no risk). The obstetrical society (the Society of Obstetricians and Gynaecologists of Canada) plays a dominant role in maternity care policy and provider supply within the Canadian health care system (Sandall *et al.* 2009). Obstetrical organisations can limit the availability of midwifery care to maintain a centralised power structure within the health care system; this has happened in other countries and historically in Canada (Sandall *et al.* 2009). Before the 1990s, midwives were virtually regulated out of existence in Canada through the Medical Practitioners Act, which restricted maternity care provision to licensed members of the College of Physicians and Surgeons (Benoit *et al.* 2005). Provincial health care plans also did not traditionally reimburse 'alternative' providers such as midwives and the integration of midwives into the Canadian maternity care system has been gradual and piecemeal across provinces (Benoit *et al.* 2005). Thus, until the 1990s, legal and reimbursement practices enshrined medical dominance over Canada's maternity care services (Benoit *et al.* 2005). This history helps to explain why Canada has such a small number of registered midwives (OECD 2011).

More recently, however, the Society of Obstetricians and Gynaecologists of Canada has recognised the need to include midwives in solutions to the shortage of maternity care providers. Family physicians in Canada often prefer not to practise obstetrics because of its around-the-clock time demands, concerns about malpractice suits and the cost of legal protection, and monetary reimbursements that are inadequate to offset these drawbacks, leading to a growing shortage of birth attendants (Kruse *et al.* 1990). The publication A National Birthing Initiative for Canada (Society of Obstetricians and Gynaecologists of Canada 2008) called for an increase in maternity care providers, including registered midwives. Although obstetricians still maintain power over midwives in health care settings where the two professions collaborate and the Society of Obstetricians and Gynaecologists of Canada establishes the standards for maternity care in Canada, there is a growing recognition of the need for collaboration among maternity care providers to meet Canada's maternity care needs.

Labour and delivery nurses are also important providers in Canada's maternity care system and are especially important in under-served rural areas (Davies and Medves 2004). As Table 7.1 shows, there is a substantially larger supply of nurses in Canada than of physicians, with nurses per 1,000 population exceeding the OECD average (OECD 2011). Although nurses have less power to establish guidelines for maternity care and typically serve below obstetricians in the maternity care hierarchy, nurses are more likely to be at the bedside of pregnant women during the intrapartum and postpartum periods. Nurses are particularly important members of collaborative teams that offer low-risk, minimally interventionist approaches to labour and birth in rural settings (Davies and Medves 2004). Rural care strategies are most effective when physicians and nurses mutually respect each other's contributions to a maternity support team (Davies and Medves 2004; Iglesias *et al.* 1998).

While maternity care in rural areas tends to be minimally interventionist, most urban maternity care settings involve the standard technologies of the Western obstetric model. In these settings, technology plays a large role in the delivery of maternity care and the definition and management of obstetric risk. With increased technology, there appears to be more interventions into pregnancy and birth. For example, Canadian antenatal care guidelines support one ultrasound scan at eighteen to nineteen weeks, but the average number of foetal ultrasound scans for women giving birth in Canada in 2006–2007 was 3.1 (PHAC 2009). There also remains no consensus and inadequate data to determine the effectiveness of prenatal ultrasound scans for foetal health (PHAC 2009). The use of ultrasound scans in early pregnancy to determine gestational age often influences later decisions about induction and intrapartum care. Thus the dates produced by ultrasound technology can override a woman's embodied understanding of when she conceived and lead to the use of additional technologies to induce labour at a date earlier than full term, then encouraging the use of further technologies to manage labour and delivery. Second trimester ultrasound scans can also set off false alarms that encourage prenatal chromosome testing in otherwise normal pregnancies. Chromosome testing, especially among mothers over the age of thirty-five years, is another important source of technological management of pregnancy. These interventions may occur because more women are 'high-risk', because medicalised birth gives rise to many opportunities to find pathology, or some combination of these reasons. Technological methods for gaining access to information about the foetus also aggravate a growing tendency to erase the pregnant woman from view and to view foetuses and pregnant women as separate, rather than connected, beings.

Technology is also a prominent feature of intrapartum care in Canada. Most urban hospitals adopted electronic foetal monitoring as a standard technological tool for labour management in the 1970s and 1980s, despite clinical trials that showed no benefit to foetal or maternal outcomes (Bassett *et al.* 2000). This affects the vast majority of women in Canada who give birth in hospitals with standardised protocols that include the management of labour with continuous electronic foetal monitoring. The prevailing view of birth in hospitals also focuses on managing all births as potential emergencies, which leads to high caesarean delivery rates – another form of technological intervention. While caesarean surgery has become safer over time, the current rate of over 26 per cent of births in Canada leads to increased risks to babies and mothers. Now that the risks of the over-use of caesarean delivery are better understood and documented, public health agencies and associations of care providers are increasingly recognising the rights of women to have a vaginal birth after caesarean section and not to be pressured into a caesarean delivery for their first birth.

Conclusion

Canada's maternity care system offers universal benefits and currently engages in efforts to improve maternity care access and public health, despite challenges with delivering care in remote areas. While Esping-Andersen (1990) classified Canada as a 'liberal' welfare regime with limited regulation of wages and earnings, Canada has some universal welfare programmes that resemble those of more generous welfare states. These include a universal, taxpayer-funded health insurance system and paid parental leave for all wage-earners. Health care, including maternity care, is free at the point of delivery and all Canadian residents are eligible for services, regardless of their ability to pay. Almost all pregnant women in Canada receive antenatal care and the vast majority initiate care in the first trimester. Public investment in postnatal care and paid parental leave encourage breastfeeding and promote the implementation of the Baby-Friendly Hospital Initiative.

Canadian maternity care follows a Western medical model. Most births take place in hospital and electronic foetal monitoring, induction and caesarean section are common. The majority of pregnant women receive care from an obstetrician/gynaecologist and a declining number of family practice doctors provide maternity care. Historically, the health care system did not recognise midwives and Canada's growing number of registered midwives is too small to meet the current demand. Contemporary public health initiatives aim to integrate various types of maternity care providers into the system, but long-term shortages and a lack of legal recognition for midwives in some provinces continue to present barriers.

Disparities between urban and rural areas represent Canadian maternity care's greatest challenge. As most practitioners and facilities are in urban areas, a lack of local providers and the need to travel long distances are barriers to care for women in rural areas. These disparities particularly affect aboriginal populations, who are more likely to live in remote areas. Consequently, recent public health efforts have aimed to improve access to care in sparsely populated areas.

References

Abelson, J., Mendelsohn, M., Lavis, J.N., Morgan, S.G., Forest, P. and Swinton, M. (2004) 'Canadians confront health care reform', *Health Affairs*, 23 (3): 186–193.
American Board of Medical Specialties (2012) *Accredited Medical Schools (U.S. and Canadian)* [online]. Available from: www.abmsdirectory.com/pdf/Resources_directory_MedSchools.pdf. Accessed 20 February 2014.

Banting, K.G. (2004) 'Canada: national-building in a federal welfare state'. In: H. Obinger, S. Leibfried and F.G. Castles (eds), *Federalism and the Welfare State: New World and European Experiences*. New York: Cambridge University Press, pp. 89–137

Bassett, K.L., Iyer, N. and Kazanjian, A. (2000) 'Defensive medicine during hospital obstetrical care: a byproduct of the technological age', *Social Science & Medicine*, 51 (4): 523–537.

Benoit, C., Wrede, S., Bourgealt, I., Sandall, J., De Vries, R. and Teijlingen, E.R. van (2005) 'Understanding the social organization of maternity care systems: midwifery as a touchstone', *Sociology of Health and Illness*, 27 (6): 722–737.

Benoit, C., Zadoroznyj, M., Hallgrimsdottir, H., Treloar, A. and Taylor, K. (2010) 'Medical dominance and neoliberalisation in maternal care provision: the evidence from Canada and Australia', *Social Science & Medicine*, 71 (3): 475–481.

Bohnert, N. (2013) *Mortality: Overview, 2008 and 2009*. Statistics Canada Catalogue No. 91–209-X. Ottawa: Statistics Canada.

Bothwell, R. (1996) *History of Canada Since 1867*. East Lansing, MI Michigan State University Press.

Bourgeault, I.L. (2000) 'Delivering the "new" Canadian midwifery: the impact on midwifery of integration into the Ontario health care system', *Sociology of Health and Illness*, 22 (2): 172–196.

Breastfeeding Committee of Canada (2012) *The Baby-Friendly Initiative (BFI) in Canada*. Status Report, February 19, 2012 [online]. Available from: www.breastfeedingcanada.ca/documents/BFI_Status_report_2012_FINAL.pdf. Accessed 24 February 2014.

Calder, G. (2003) 'Recent changes to the maternity and parental leave benefits regime as a case study: the impact of globalization on the delivery of social programs in Canada', *Canadian Journal of Women and the Law*, 15: 342–366.

Canadian Association of Midwives (2014) *Midwifery Practice – Midwifery Education* [online]. Available from: www.canadianmidwives.org/midwifery-education.html. Accessed 20 February 2014.

Canadian Association of Schools of Nursing (2014) *Accredited Canadian Nursing Education Programs* [online]. Available from: www.casn.ca/vm/newvisual/attachments/856/Media/AccreditedCanadianNursingEducationPrograms.pdf. Accessed 20 February 2014.

Canadian Institute for Health Information (2004) *Giving Birth in Canada: Providers of Maternity and Infant Care*. Ottawa, ON: Canadian Institute for Health Information.

Canadian Institute for Health Information (2007) *Giving Birth in Canada: Regional Trends from 2001–2002 to 2005–2006*. Ottawa, ON: Canadian Institute for Health Information.

Canadian Institute for Health Information (2011a) *Health Care Cost Drivers: the Facts*. Ottawa, ON: Canadian Institute for Health Information.

Canadian Institute for Health Information (2011b) *Learning from the Best: Benchmarking Canada's Health System*. Ottawa, ON: Canadian Institute for Health Information.

Canadian Institute for Health Information (2012) *National Physician Database, 2010–2011 – Data Release*. Ottawa, ON: Canadian Institute for Health Information.

Canadian Medical Association (2014) *Number of Physicians by Province/Territory and Specialty, Canada, 2014*. Canadian Medical Association Masterfile, January 2014 [online]. Available from: www.cma.ca/multimedia/CMA/Content_Images/ Inside_cma/Statistics/01Spec&Prov.pdf. Accessed 20 February 2014.

Castles, F.G. and Mitchell, D. (1993) 'Worlds of welfare and families of nations'. In: F. G. Castles (ed.), *Families of Nations: Patterns of Public Policy in Western Democracies*. Dartmouth: Aldershot, pp. 93–128.

Chalmers, B., Kaczorowski, J., O'Brien, B. and Royle, C. (2012) 'Rates of interventions in labour and birth across Canada: findings of the Canadian Maternity Experiences Survey', *Birth*, 39 (3): 203–210.

College of Family Physicians of Canada (2014) *Certification Examination in Family Medicine* [online]. Available from: www.cfpc.ca/Home/. Accessed 20 February 2014.

Custred, G. (2008) 'Security threats on America's borders'. In: A. Moens and M. Collacott (eds), *Immigration Policy and the Terrorist Threat in Canada and the United States*. Vancouver, BC: The Fraser Institute, pp. 95–112.

Davies, B.L. and Medves, J.M. (2004) 'Sustaining rural maternity care – don't forget the RNs', *Canadian Journal of Rural Medicine*, 10 (1): 29–35.

Davis-Floyd, R.E. (2004) *Birth as an American Rite of Passage: with a New Preface*. Oakland, CA: University of California Press.

Easterbrook, W.T. (1959) 'Recent contributions to economic history: Canada', *Journal of Economic History*, 19: 76–102.

Esmail, N. (2011) 'Canada's physician supply', *Fraser Forum*, March/April: 12–18.

Esping-Andersen, G. (1990) *The Three Worlds of Welfare Capitalism*. Cambridge: Polity Press and Princeton: Princeton University Press.

Esses, V.M. and Gardner, R.C. (1996) 'Multiculturalism in Canada: context and current status', *Canadian Journal of Behavioural Science*, 28 (3): 145–152.

Frohlich, K.L., Ross, N. and Richmond, C. (2006) 'Health disparities in Canada today: some evidence and a theoretical framework', *Health Policy*, 79 (2–3): 132–143.

Gibbon, J (1938) *The Canadian Mosaic*. Toronto: McClelland & Stewart.

Gracey, M. and King, M. (2009) 'Indigenous health part 1: determinants and disease patterns', *Lancet*, 374: 65–75.

Hail, M. and Lange, S. (2010) 'Federalism and representation in the theory of the founding fathers: a comparative study of US and Canadian constitutional thought', *Publius: the Journal of Federalism*, 40 (3): 366–388.

Hawkins, M. and Knox, S. (2003) 'Midwifery care continues to face challenges', *Canadian Women's Health Network*, 6: 2–3. Available from: www.cwhn.ca/en/ node/39533. Accessed 20 February 2014.

Hayes, D. (2008) *Canada: an Illustrated History*. Madiera Park, BC: Douglas & McIntyre.

Health Canada (2000) *Perinatal Health Indicators for Canada: a Resource Manual*. Ottawa, ON: Minster of Public Works and Government Services Canada.

Health Canada (2003) *Canadian Perinatal Health Report*. Ottawa, ON: Minster of Public Works and Government Services Canada.

Henderson, D.R. (2010) *Canada's Budget Triumph*. Working Paper No. 10–52, September 30, 2010. Fairfax, VA: Mercatus Center, George Mason University. Available from: http://mercatus.org/sites/default/files/publication/Canada's%20 Budget%20Triumph.WP__0.pdf. Accessed 18 February 2014.

Heritage Foundation (2014) *2014 Index of Economic Freedom* [online]. Available from: www.heritage.org/index/. Accessed 18 February 2014.

Hutchison, B., Abelson, J. and Lavis, J. (2001) 'Primary care in Canada: so much innovation, so little change', *Health Affairs*, 20 (3): 116–131.

Iglesias, S., Grzybowski, S., Klein, M.C., Gane, G.P. and Lalonde, A. (1998) 'Rural obstetrics: joint position paper on rural maternity care', *Canadian Family Physician*, 44 (Apr): 831–843.

International Monetary Fund (2013) *World Economic Outlook: Canada. October 2013 data* [online]. Available from: www.imf.org/external/pubs/ft/weo/2013/02/weodata/weorept.aspx. Accessed 18 February 2014.

Jordan, B. (1992). *Birth in Four Cultures: a Crosscultural Investigation of Childbirth in Yucatan, Holland, Sweden, and the United States*. Long Grove, IL: Waveland Press.

Kelley, N. and Trebilcock, M.J. (2010) *The Making of the Mosaic: a History of Canadian Immigration Policy*, 2nd edn. Toronto: University of Toronto Press.

Kidd, M. (2013) 'Family practice versus specialist care for low-risk obstetrics: examining patient satisfaction in Newfoundland and Labrador', *Canadian Family Physician*, 59 (10): e456–e461.

King, M., Smith, A. and Gracey, M. (2009) 'Indigenous health part 2: the underlying causes of the health gap', *Lancet*, 374: 76–85.

Klein, M.C., Gauthier, R.J., Jorgensen, S.H., Robbins, J.M., Kaczorowski, J., Johnson, B., Corriveau, M., Westrich, R., Waghorn, K. and Gelfand, M.M. (1992) 'Does episiotomy prevent perineal trauma and pelvic floor relaxation?', *The Online Journal of Current Clinical Trials*, 6,019 words.

Kondro, W. (2012) 'Health disparities among income groups becoming more pronounced', *Canadian Medical Association Journal*, 184 (13): e695–e696.

Kruse, J., Phillips, D. and Wesley, R.M. (1990) 'Withdrawal from maternity care: a comparison of family physicians in Ontario, Canada, and the United States', *Journal of Family Practice*, 20 (3): 336–341.

Labbok, M.H. (2012) 'Global baby-friendly hospital initiative monitoring data: update and discussion', *Breastfeeding Medicine*, 7 (4): 210–222.

Lisonkova, S., Rouleau, J., Liu, S., Liston, R.M., Joseph, K.S. and Maternal Health Study Group of the Canadian Perinatal Surveillance System (2011) 'Temporal trends in maternal mortality in Canada I: estimates based on vital statistics data', *Journal of Obstetrics and Gynaecology Canada*, 33 (10): 1011–1019.

Malott, A.M., Davis, B.M., McDonald, H. and Hutton, E. (2009) 'Midwifery care in eight industrialized countries: how does Canadian midwifery compare?', *Journal of Obstetrics and Gynaecology Canada*, 31 (10): 974–979.

Marchildon, G.P. (2013) 'Canada: health system review', *Health Systems in Transition*, 15 (1): 1–179.

Marshall, K. (2010) 'Employer top-ups,' *Perspectives*, Statistics Canada – Catalogue No. 75–001-X. Available from: www.statcan.gc.ca/pub/75–001-x/2010102/pdf/11120-eng.pdf. Accessed 20 February 2014.

Menon, D. (2001) 'Pharmaceutical cost control in Canada: does it work?' *Health Affairs*, 20 (3): 92–103.

Ministry of Health and Long Term Care (2012) *Technical Document: Public Health Accountability Agreement Indicators 2011–13*. Public Health Division/Health Promotion Division, December 14, 2012. Catalogue No. 017285. Toronto, ON: Queen's Printer for Ontario.

Morris, T. (2013) *Cut it Out: the C-Section Epidemic in America*. New York: NYU Press.

Mulvale, J.P. (2008) 'Basic income and the Canadian welfare state: exploring the realms of possibility', *Basic Income Studies*, 3 (1).

Myles, J. (1998) 'How to design a 'liberal' welfare state: a comparison of Canada and the United States', *Social Policy and Administration*, 32 (4): 341–364.

Naylor, C.D. (1986) *Private Practice, Public Payment: Canadian Medicine and the Politics of Health Insurance 1911–1966*. Montreal, QC: McGill-Queen's University Press.

Naylor, C.D. (1999) 'Health care in Canada: incrementalism under fiscal duress', *Health Affairs*, 18 (3): 9–26.

OECD (2009) *Comparing Countries' and Economies' Performances, PISA 2009 Results*. Paris: OECD Publishing.

OECD (2011) *Health at a Glance 2011: OECD Indicators*. Paris: OECD Publishing. Available from: http://dx.doi.org/10.1787/health_glance-2011-en. Accessed 20 February 2014.

OECD (2012) *OECD Family Database*. Paris: OECD Publishing. Available from: www.oecd.org/social/family/database. Accessed 21 February 2014.

OECD (2013) *OECD Factbook 2013: Economic, Environmental and Social Statistics*. Paris: OECD Publishing.

Peterson, W.E., Medves, J.M., Davies, B.L. and Graham, I.D. (2007) 'Multidisciplinary collaborative maternity care in Canada: easier said than done', *Journal of Obstetrics and Gynaecology Canada*, 29 (11): 880–886.

Public Health Agency of Canada (PHAC) (2008) *Canadian Perinatal Health Report, 2008*. Ottawa, ON: PHAC.

Public Health Agency of Canada (PHAC) (2009) *What Mothers Say: the Maternal Experiences Survey*. Ottawa, ON: PHAC.

Reading, C. and Wien, F. (2009) *Health Inequalities and Social Determinants of Aboriginal People's Health*. Prince George, BC: National Collaborating Centre for Aboriginal Health.

Richmond, C. and Ross, N.A. (2009). 'The determinants of First Nation and Inuit Health: a critical population health approach', *Health & Place*, 15 (2): 403–411.

Sandall, J., Benoit, C., Wrede, S., Murray, F.S., Teijlingen, E.R. van and Westfall, R. (2009) 'Social service professional or market expert? Maternity care relations under neoliberal healthcare reform', *Current Sociology*, 57: 529–553.

Sarrouh, E. (2002) Social Policies in Canada: a Model for Development. Social Policy Series, No. 1. New York: United Nations.

Simonds, W., Rothman, B.K. and Norman, B.M. (2007) *Laboring on: Birth in Transition in the United States*. New York: Taylor & Francis.

Society for Obstetricians and Gynaecologists of Canada (2008a) 'Joint Policy Statement on Normal Childbirth', *Journal of Obstetrics and Gynaecology Canada*, 30: 1163–1165.

Society of Obstetricians and Gynaecologists of Canada (2008b) *A National Birthing Initiative for Canada: an Inclusive, Integrated and Comprehensive Pan-Canadian Framework for Sustainable Family-centered Maternity and Newborn Care*. Ottawa, ON: Society of Obstetricians and Gynaecologists of Canada.

Soroka, S.N. (2011) *Public Perceptions and Media Coverage of the Canadian Healthcare System: a Synthesis*. Ottawa, ON: Canadian Health Services Research Foundation.

Statistics Canada (2012) *The Canadian Population in 2011: Population Counts and Growth*. Catalogue No. 98–310-X20111001.

Statistics Canada (2013a) *Population by Year, by Province and Territory*. CANSIM Table 051–0001.

Statistics Canada (2013b) *Births and Total Fertility Rate, by Province and Territory (Fertility Rate)*. CANSIM Table 102–4505.

Statistics Canada (2013c) *Live Births and Fetal Deaths (Stillbirths), by Place of Birth (Hospital and Non-hospital), Canada, Provinces and Territories, Annual.* CANSIM Table 102–4516.

Statistics Canada (2014) *Breastfeeding Practices by Age Group.* CANSIM Table 105–0501.

Stevenson, H.M., Williams, A.P. and Vayda, E. (1988) 'Medical politics and Canadian Medicare: professional response to the Canada Health Act,' *The Milbank Quarterly,* 66 (1): 65–104.

Tjepkema, N. (2002) 'The health of the off-reserve Aboriginal population', *Supplement to Health Reports,* 13: 73–88.

Wen, S.W., Rusen, I.D., Walker, M., Liston, R., Kramer, M.S., Baskett, T., Heaman, M., and Liu, S. (2004) 'Comparison of maternal mortality and morbidity between trial of labor and elective cesarean section among women with previous cesarean delivery', *American Journal of Obstetrics and Gynecology,* 191 (4): 1263–1269.

Wiktorowicz, M.E. (2003) 'Emergent patterns in the regulation of pharmaceuticals: institutions and interests in the United States, Canada, Britain, and France', *Journal of Health Politics, Policy and Law,* 28 (4): 615–658.

Wilkins, R., Berthelot, J. and Ng, E, (2002) 'Trends in mortality by neighbourhood income in urban Canada from 1971 to 1996', *Supplement to Health Reports,* 13: 1–12.

Wilkins, R., Houle, C., Berthelot, J.-M. and Ross, N. (2000) 'The changing health status of Canada's children', *Isuma,* 1: 57–63.

Woodward, C.A. and Rosser, W. (1989) 'Effect of medicolegal liability on patterns of general and family practice in Canada', *Canadian Medical Association Journal,* 141 (4): 291–299.

Woolhandler, S. and Himmelstein, D.U. (1989) 'A National Health Program: northern light at the end of the tunnel', *JAMA,* 262 (15): 2136–2137.

WHO (2009) *Monitoring Emergency Obstetric Care: a Handbook.* Geneva: WHO.

WHO (2010) *Trends in Maternal Mortality: 1990 to 2008 Estimates Developed by WHO, UNICEF, UNFPA and the World Bank.* New York: WHO.

Wrede, S., Benoit, C. and Sandall, J. (2001) 'The state and birth/the state of birth: maternal health policy in three countries' In: R. De Vries, S. Wrede, E. van Teijlingen and C. Benoit (eds), *Birth by Design: Pregnancy, Maternity Care and Midwifery in North America and Europe.* New York: Routledge.

8 Japan

Rieko Kishi Fukuzawa and Naonori Kodate

Background

Japan is an island nation in East Asia and consists of four main islands and forty-seven administrative divisions (prefectures). Although Japan's total land area is similar to that of Germany, the population of Japan is one and a half times larger. Until 2010, Japan's economy had been the second largest in the world for forty-two years and the nation once achieved the status of an 'all middle-class' society. Japanese women live the longest in the world, with a life expectancy at birth of 86.41 years in 2012 (Ministry of Health, Labour and Welfare 2014a).

The size of the Japanese population has been in decline since 2006 as a result of the ageing of the population combined with a diminishing birth rate as Japanese women have chosen, for various reasons, to have fewer pregnancies. The proportion of the population aged sixty-five years and older was 24.1 per cent in 2012. This increasingly older population has led to an increase in the cost of health care and welfare in Japan. The total fertility rate in Japan was 1.41 in 2012 (Ministry of Health, Labour and Welfare 2014a).

The distribution of Japan's population is increasingly skewed in terms of geography. Younger people tend to live in the urban areas, whereas older people tend to live in rural areas. The elderly dependency rate in rural regions in 2010 was 44.3, while that in urban regions was 32.7 (OECD 2014a).

Only 1.7 per cent of the total population is non-Japanese (OECD 2014a). However, these data are based on nationality rather than ethnic background. Of foreign nationals, 32 per cent are from China, followed by Korea (26.0 per cent), the Philippines (10.0 per cent) and Brazil (9.5 per cent). The total number of registered foreign nationals in 2013 was more than two million (Ministry of Justice 2013).

Japan is prone to natural disasters, most notably earthquakes. Recent examples include the Great Hanshin Earthquake in 1995 and the so-called Triple Disaster of 2011, during which both a tsunami and an earthquake threatened the safety of Japanese citizens, followed by dangerous conditions at the nuclear plant in Fukushima. All of these incidents seriously affected people's lives and the Japanese economy.

These changes in population and the concurrent economic stagnation have affected Japanese society significantly, particularly with regard to social policies. The ensuing effects have reshaped maternal and infant health care in Japan.

Japan as a welfare regime

Japan is an outlier in the classical welfare typology proposed by Esping-Andersen (1990), in which he classified Japan as employing a conservative welfare model with some characteristics of the liberal welfare state (Esping-Andersen 1997, 1999).

However, universal health care access has been provided in Japan since 1961. This universal health insurance coverage was introduced to ensure that all people living in Japan, regardless of citizenship or age, would receive at least partly subsidised health care. In the 1970s, the central government, led by the Liberal Democratic Party, took a step towards introducing free health care services for the elderly as a result of pressures from local government policy initiatives. Medical services for those older than seventy years of age became free of charge in 1973, but, as a result of soaring costs, the scheme was abolished in 1983.

The Japanese welfare state today is a hybrid of liberal and conservative regimes, with a strong flavour of familialism (male breadwinner model). Taxes have been kept low and, as a result, wages and employment levels have been maximised; there is universal health coverage based on the social insurance model. There has been a strong division of gender roles in the labour market and the labour force participation rate among women is one of the lowest in the advanced industrial economies (World Economic Forum 2013).

The Japanese welfare state was later classified as an East Asian or developmental regime (Holiday 2000; Aspalter 2006; Lee and Ku 2007). Social policy has long been regarded as secondary to the country's primary goal of economic growth. Social investment is seen as a key productive factor for economic growth and the enhancement of political stability and governmental legitimacy. However, economic disparities among the population have been widening in recent decades. The Gini coefficient, an indicator of economic disparity, was 0.33 for Japan in the late 2000s, above the average of other OECD countries (OECD 2011). The percentage of people living with less than 50 per cent of the median equivalised household income was 15.7 per cent compared with an average of 11.1 per cent for other OECD countries (OECD 2011). In the Japanese welfare state, employment status determines the compensation packages for employees. According to a survey by the National Tax Agency in 2012, regular (full-time) employees receive better compensation, whereas non-regular (part-time or temporary) employed people receive less (National Tax Agency 2014). In recent years the proportion of part-time and temporary workers has increased; this trend has mainly affected young people, most of whom are of reproductive and childrearing age.

The gender gap is another unresolved problem in Japan that affects young people's lives. The wide difference in income between men and women was highlighted by the National Tax Agency survey. When including those with only temporary or part-time employment, income among female workers was only 53.3 per cent of that of male workers (National Tax Agency 2014). This figure has remained constant at around 50 per cent since the 1980s. The majority of women leave work as a result of pregnancy and childbirth, but even for those who do return to work, their employment tends to be on a part-time or temporary basis.

Health care system

Western medicine and nursing are currently predominant in the Japanese health care system. The Ministry of Health, Labour and Welfare controls and regulates licences and practices for health care providers, including doctors, nurses and nurse-midwives, while controlling national health care policy in Japan.

The medical insurance system includes employer-provided health insurance for regular employees, national health insurance for non-regular/temporary employees and independent workers, and health insurance system coverage for those aged seventy-five years or older.

The source of finance for medical care in Japan takes three different forms: taxes (income, corporate and consumption taxes, general government revenues), health insurance premiums and co-payments. Despite this hybrid use of 'single-payer' and 'universal' elements, it is strongly geared towards the former, as the national government itself is by far the largest single insurer. The Government-Managed Health Insurance is designed for the small business sector, whereas the Society-Managed Health Insurance is for large firms and the Citizens' Health Insurance is aimed at those who are unemployed. On the payment side, outpatient care is covered by a fee-for-service system, whereas inpatient care is paid for by patients through a mixture of *per diem* and fee-for-service billing. As a result, 20–30 per cent of the total fee is paid by patients as a co-payment.

Individuals can freely choose their providers and institutions according to their preferences, such as geographical convenience or reputation, regardless of their type of insurance or other socio-economic status. An ambulance car service is free for life-threatening events, including childbirth in an emergency.

In Japan, the government uses financial incentives to support all types of providers through a centrally controlled fee schedule. This has been successful in achieving a universal health service across the country and in containing the overall spending levels (Campbell and Ikegami 1998).

However, Japan's total annual health care spending has been steadily increasing, both in actual amount and as a percentage of the GDP. According to the Ministry of Health, Labour and Welfare, the total national health expenditure in 1965 was 1.1 trillion yen (US$10,792 using June 2014 rates), but 37.4 trillion yen in 2010 (US$366,931) (Ministry of Health, Labour and Welfare 2011a). Based on the System of Health Accounts (health expenditure estimates) initially introduced in 2000, the total expenditure on health was 5.9 per cent of GDP in 2000, 6.5 per cent of GDP in 2005 and 7.8 per cent of GDP in 2010 (Ministry of Health, Labour and Welfare 2011a).

Japan had fewer physicians per capita (2.2) than most other OECD countries (OECD average 3.2) in 2011 (Table 8.1), despite having the highest number of hospital beds of all the OECD countries (OECD 2013a). In addition, the Japanese health care system is characterised by a tolerance for lengthy hospital stays as well as a high availability of diagnostic technologies such as computed tomography scanners and magnetic resonance imaging units (OECD 2013a).

Non-national public hospitals are under different jurisdictions. Hospitals at the prefectural and municipality levels fall under the governance of the Ministry of International Affairs and Communications and teaching hospitals fall under the Ministry of Education, Culture, Sports, Science and Technology. The Ministry of Education controls the professional education of all doctors, nurses and nurse-midwives in Japan. Professional organisations and their branches set standards for health care and take leadership in advanced practices.

Medical schools have adopted a six-year programme that includes a clinical practicum. At the end of the final year students take a National Medical Licensing Examination. After licensing, all clinical doctors undergo a two-year residency. To become specialised in a particular field,

Table 8.1 Human and physical resources in Japan

Physicians per 1,000 population[a]	2.21
Nurses per 1,000 population[a]	10
Medical graduates per 100 000 population[a]	5.88
Nursing graduates per 100 000 population[a]	39.33
Total hospital beds per 1,000 population[a]	13.4
Curative (acute) care beds per 1,000 population[a]	7.95
Obstetricians and gynaecologists per 1,000 population[a]	0.08
Nurse-midwives per 1,000 population[a]	0.21
Paediatricians per 1,000 population[a]	0.12
Public health nurses per 1,000 population[b]	0.35
Pharmacist, per 1,000 population[a]	1.54

Sources: a OECD 2014b; b MCHWA 2013.

such as obstetrics or neonatology, the corresponding academic societies certify and register doctors who meet the required criteria acquired during an additional three years, as well as the specialised knowledge and skills required for their selected area of specialisation.

Higher education in nursing has developed rapidly in the past few decades in Japan, in part to help meet the persistent need for health care providers due to the shortage of physicians. Nurse-midwives and public health nurses are required to obtain the same licence as all nationally registered nurses before pursuing specialisation.

When required, disciplinary measures are undertaken by the Medical Ethics Council (*Idō Shingikai*); this occurs when clinical errors are reported. The Medical Ethics Council has the power to revoke health practitioners' professional licences or to put restrictions in place if there are questions about a practitioner's fitness to practises.

Demographic profile

The Japanese population is currently shrinking. In 2010, there were 2.8 young working people for each elderly person. The figure is estimated to further decrease to 2 in 2022 and 1.3 in 2060 (National Institute of Population and Social Security Research 2012).

The total fertility rate in 2012 was 1.41, with 1,037,231 babies born during that year. These numbers have increased slightly since 2006 as the children of the baby boomers have reached reproductive age (Ministry of Health, Labour and Welfare 2014a) (Table 8.2).

Among those of childbearing age, the number of people who remain unmarried or who delay marriage is increasing. According to a survey by the Cabinet Office in 2013, 85 per cent of unmarried people between the

Table 8.2 Demographic profile of Japan

Population[a]	127,520,000
Females[a]	64,630,000
Population aged 0–14 years[a]	13.0%
Women of childbearing age (15–44 years)[a]	22,130,000}
Population aged 65 years and older[a]	24.1%
Life expectancy at birth[a]	Men: 79.94 years
	Women: 86.41years
Population annual growth (%)[b]	–0.2014728
Population density per square kilometre[b]	341.38
Fertility rate, total (births per woman)[a]	1.41
Birth rate, crude (per 1000 people)[a]	8.2
Death rate, crude (per 1000 people)[a]	10.0
% urban population[c]	91.3%
Non-Japanese ethnicity[b]	1.7% of total population

Sources: a MHLW (2014a); b OECD (2014a); c Index Mundi (2013).

ages of twenty and thirty-nine years of age stated that they wished to marry, but cited financial reasons for their single status (Cabinet Office 2014). In 1947 the average age at first marriage was 26.1 years for men and 22.9 years for women. These numbers have continuously increased since then and in 2012 were 30.6 years for men and 29.2 years for women (Ministry of Health, Labour and Welfare 2014a). The average age at which mothers gave birth to their first child was 25.7 years in 1975 and had increased to 30.3 years in 2012 (Ministry of Health, Labour and Welfare 2014a).

The proportion of households with two breadwinners has also increased from 61 per cent in 2005 to 68 per cent in 2010 (Ministry of Health, Labour and Welfare 2014a). However, this lifestyle is commonly regarded as too stressful. Unmarried people attribute the reasons for the decreased number of children and delayed childbearing to inadequate arrangements in the Japanese work environment for employees with children (56.4 per cent) and to the high expense of children's education (51.9 per cent) (Cabinet Office 2014). These reasons were cited more frequently than their own health concerns as parents-to-be (47.4 per cent).

The marriage rate among couples with children is very high in Japan. The percentage of children born outside marriage was only 2.2 per cent in 2012 (Ministry of Health, Labour and Welfare 2014a). The divorce rate peaked in 2002 and then gradually decreased to 235,000 cases in 2012, or 1.87 per 1,000 individuals. In 2010, 36 per cent of divorced women were without a job and 56 per cent had children less than twenty years old (Ministry of Health, Labour and Welfare 2014a). Poverty among single mothers has become a pressing social problem.

The proportion of international marriages is small in Japan, totaling only 3.5 per cent in 2012 (Ministry of Health, Labour and Welfare 2014a). About half of spouses who are not Japanese are from Korea or China.

Maternity provision

In Japan, pregnancies were historically regarded as good fortune and childbirth as risking mothers' lives to have babies. Health care services for normal pregnancy and childbirth are not covered by public health insurance, based on the view that pregnancy and childbirth are not diseases. Therefore women have to pay 100 per cent of their maternity health care costs, although some fees are covered by other systems, such as the lump sum birth allowance. When pregnancy, childbirth or the postpartum process are medically diagnosed as abnormal, however, such as when childbirth is complicated and results in a vacuum, forceps or caesarean delivery, they are covered by medical insurance and the clients pay only the 30 per cent co-payment.

Parents may freely choose where to deliver their babies. Thus pregnant women have the option of delivering either at their home, in a midwifery centre or in a clinical setting based on their own needs and preferences and those of their families, as well as factors of geographical convenience (Kobayashi and Watanabe 2008). In 2011, 98.8 per cent of women gave birth in medical institutions, 1 per cent in midwifery centres and only 0.2 per cent at home or other non-institutional settings (Mothers' & Children's Health & Welfare Association 2013). The number of obstetrical institutions providing intrapartum care in Japan in 2014 was 2,875 (Japan Council for Quality Health Care 2014a).

Women generally prefer larger hospitals for the sense of security offered and the availability of advanced medical services, including neonatal intensive care units, especially older mothers and those who conceived through fertility treatment. However, in local areas, obstetric wards in large hospitals are closing and becoming less available as the number of children decreases, leading to a shortage of obstetricians. In contrast, the midwifery centres providing intrapartum care are mostly in urban areas. Consequently, although in theory women in Japan have the freedom to choose their place of delivery, in reality they are faced with limited choices, especially in rural areas. A system of family practitioners has not yet developed in Japan, particularly in the area of obstetrics.

There were 15.6 obstetricians/gynaecologists and 40.1 nurse-midwives per 100,000 women in 2011, falling far below the OECD averages of 27.3 and 69.9, respectively (OECD 2013b) (Table 8.1). The shortage of maternity health care providers is currently a critical social concern in Japan. The average annual growth rate for obstetricians/gynaecologists during 2000–2011 has declined to minus 0.5 per cent (OECD 2013b). From 2006 to 2012, the number of licensed obstetricians/gynaecologists increased by about 800, the majority of whom were women. Female obstetricians are generally preferred by patients, but young female obstetricians may have difficulties with their own work/life balance as a result of the heavy load in intrapartum units (Ministry of Health, Labour and Welfare 2014d).

In addition, the majority (64 per cent) of the recent increase in obstetricians/gynaecologists occurred in urban areas, while they are decreasing in rural regions, especially in Fukushima prefecture (Japan Society of Obstetrics and Gynecology Medical Reform Committee 2014). Thus the geographically uneven distribution of maternity care resources continues. Doctors in Japan are assigned from their alumni medical departments to affiliated hospitals. As medical departments increasingly do not have enough obstetrician members to dispatch, significant numbers of obstetric wards are closing, in particular in rural areas in Japan.

Obstetrics is known to have a high risk of litigation with frequent after-hours and emergency services on weekends and at night. Some doctors avoid obstetrics as their specialisation and some obstetricians/gynaecologists avoid providing intrapartum care services and change their specialty to fertility treatment.

Of all births in Japan in 2011, 52 per cent took place in hospital (defined as facilities with >20 beds) and 47 per cent occurred in clinics (defined as <20 beds) (Mothers' & Children's Health & Welfare Association 2013). The number of deliveries in one month per institution in 2011 averaged 44.1 in hospitals and 30.4 in clinics – a relatively low number compared with other countries (Ministry of Health, Labour and Welfare 2014b). Some walk-in clinics also offer prenatal care. Most clinics have the capacity to provide high levels of perinatal care. For instance, both vaginal and abdominal ultrasonography are readily available, even in small clinics. These devices enable thorough ultrasound screening to detect abnormalities in unborn babies. Cardiotocography is also readily available and is usually used, at least intermittently, during labour and delivery.

Midwifery in Japan has several unique characteristics. First, midwives have the right to independently franchise and can thus work autonomously. In the 1960s, the traditional place of delivery shifted from the home to hospital. Before then, midwives provided services in their communities. Under the latest law in place since 2007, independent midwives must associate themselves specifically with a contract obstetrician and contract hospital, which must, in turn, have emergency neonatal services available. Before 2007, the specialty of the contract doctor was not designated. Against this backdrop, it is becoming increasingly difficult for midwives to run their business without having such contracts.

The second characteristic of midwifery in Japan is that midwives are not permitted to engage in any medical practice, such as prescribing medication, ordering tests or performing minor surgery (episiotomies or perineum suturing), except in emergency situations. Hence independent midwives can only feasibly care for low-risk women within the normal course of pregnancy and childbirth. However, this limitation has actually enabled true natural childbirth with no medical intervention and with professional midwives in attendance, in spite of the widespread availability of advanced medical technologies in Japan (Misago and Yoshimoto 2013).

Midwives' income is entirely from out-of-pocket payments. Natural childbirth usually takes place around midnight or in the early morning (Matsushima *et al.* 2003) and midwifery staff must therefore be available twenty-four hours a day, seven days a week. If a mother or baby is transferred to a hospital when the course of pregnancy or childbirth becomes abnormal, then the midwife's income decreases. Moreover, despite the fact that, in recent years, the total number of deliveries is decreasing, the number of so-called 'high-risk' pregnancies in Japan is increasing. Therefore the business of the midwifery centres is strained. The cost of prenatal check-ups is now covered by the government and information about prenatal issues is freely available via the internet. As a result, women increasingly take it for granted that prenatal services are free of charge and independent midwives providing consultation and educational support face difficulties in maintaining their businesses.

The risk of a pregnant woman is determined by risk screening based on the Midwifery Practice Guidelines (Japanese Midwives Association 2014). Once the pregnancy, childbirth, or postpartum course is determined to be abnormal, the midwife must transfer the mother and/or baby to the care of an obstetrician. These guidelines consist of two sections: (1) criteria for the receipt of midwifery care; and (2) a protocol for emergency situations (Japanese Midwives Association 2014). The earlier version allowed for midwives' independent, on-the-spot judgements about patients' eligibility for midwifery care, but the latest version requires collaborative decision-making with an obstetrician. In addition, as revised, the criteria for making these judgements have become more detailed and restrictive, and the collaboration increasingly regimented, with a resulting loss of autonomy on the part of midwives.

The total number of employed, practising nurse-midwives was 31,835 in 2012 and most were practising at medical institutions (Ministry of Health, Labour and Welfare 2013a). In medical institutions, nurse-midwives usually work as nursing staff, constantly collaborating with obstetricians/gynaecologists. The autonomy of midwives has been challenged, but, spurred on by the shortage of obstetricians, more autonomous/independent models of midwifery care, such as prenatal check-ups by nurse-midwives in hospitals and dedicated hospital midwifery centres, have been proposed and attempted in clinical settings.

Because Japan has maintained the world's best levels of perinatal outcomes over the past few decades (Table 8.3), safe childbirth has been taken for granted. However, 2006 was a critical juncture that revealed the deteriorating quality of the maternity health care system in Japan. Pregnant women who had difficulties in finding a place to give birth as a result of provider shortages became known as 'childbirth refugees' and the phenomenon drew social attention. Several shocking circumstances in different parts of the country were publicised by the media. For example,

Table 8.3 Birth interventions and outcomes for selected years in Japan

	1970	1980	1990	2000	2010*
Maternal mortality per 100,000 live births[a]	52.1	20.5	8.6	7.1	4.6
Perinatal mortality per 1,000 live and stillbirths[a]	21.3	11.6	5.7	3.8	2.9
Neonatal mortality per 1,000 live births[a]	8.7	4.9	2.6	1.8	1.1
Infant mortality per 1,000 live births[a]	13.1	7.5	4.6	3.2	2.3
Forceps[b]	–	–		–	0.5
Vacuum[b]	–	–	–	–	5.3
Caesarean[c]	–	7.3	10.0	15.2	19.2
		(1984)	(1990)	(2002)	(2011)

Sources: a OECD (2014c); b MHLW (2011b); c MCHWA (2013).

Note
* Or the most recent available year.

in large cities with limited obstetric hospitals, women had to make a reservation for childbirth services very early in their pregnancy, sometimes even before eight weeks. On small islands with no obstetric facilities, pregnant women had to move to the mainland in advance to wait for labour well before their due date, separating them from their families. In one city, a gynaecologist was arrested after the death of a woman from haemorrhage during a caesarean section, although a reconciliation process with the victim and her family was already underway. 'Unnatural deaths' became a focal point of the ensuing discussion and criticism and the public protested against the arrest. The gynaecologist was the only one working in the prefectural hospital (Shimuta 2011). The shortage of gynaecologists in Japan and the worsening working environment for doctors prompted public apprehension and led to an outcry (Leflar 2009; Kodate 2014). At a very large maternity hospital it was found that the shortage of nurse-midwives had led to illegal situations in which nurses regularly executed pelvic examinations of women in labour under the direction of obstetricians, in violation of regulations requiring doctors and nurse-midwives to perform all pelvic examinations.

Responding to the outburst of problems with the maternity care system, several measures were taken in the following few years. For example, to prevent possible medical disputes and improve the quality of obstetric care, in 2009 the Japan Obstetric Compensation System for Cerebral Palsy was introduced. The fund is managed by a third-party, non-profit organisation, the Japan Council for Quality Health Care. The programme's aim is to compensate families for any financial burden in cases of severe cerebral palsy related to childbirth, while assisting in the prevention of recurrences by analysing the causes of accidents (Japan Council for Quality Health Care 2014b). Most of the measures have taken place in the central, urban areas of the country, while the situation in rural areas remains unresolved or may still be deteriorating.

In summary, although public awareness has been raised due to the crises in 2006, and some measures have been adopted, conditions are not improving across the whole country.

Maternity entitlements

Guaranteed maternity leave in Japan covers a period of six weeks before the due date until eight weeks after the actual birth. The six-week prenatal leave is at the discretion of individual pregnant women, while the eight-week postnatal leave is mandated. During maternity leave, the employee salary is covered up to two-thirds (66 per cent) of the base salary by the social insurance programme. Child care leave starts when maternity leave ends and lasts until the day before the child's first birthday; it may be extended up to an additional six months. Until women return to the workplace, their employment insurance pays half of the base salary until the baby reaches 1 year old. Mothers are exempt from paying social premiums during maternity leave.

Overall, support for working parents has been enhanced in recent years. The levels and contents of maternity entitlements for employees, however, differ greatly from workplace to workplace, based on the employer, the size of company, the status of the employee and the overall macro-economic performance. In general, regular employees have better rights, whereas non-regular employees, such as part-time employees, have fewer rights. Mothers with small children tend to have limited opportunities to find jobs or become regular employees. Even when they have jobs, the number of daycare centres for babies is severely limited in some places, such as Tokyo. Therefore some mothers return to work before their babies reach one year of age so that they receive more access to daycare centres. Even though, theoretically, there is a parenting leave system of up to three years, mothers can only be paid during the first year, forcing many to return to work earlier than they might wish due to financial reasons.

By law, work arrangements for pregnant employees and working mothers are entrusted to the employees, such as decreasing their workloads by changing the work content or by shortening their working hours. Eighty-four per cent of working mothers took parental leave in 2012; in contrast, only 1.9 per cent of working fathers did so (Ministry of Health, Labour and Welfare 2012).

Childbirth in Japan

Antenatal care

Most Japanese women see an obstetrician/gynaecologist after confirming their pregnancy with a home pregnancy test kit. Obstetricians/gynaecologists provide a series of tests, such as urine human chorionic gonadotropin tests, Pap smears and obstetric risk screening, as well as infection screening. A vaginal ultrasound scan by an obstetrician/gynaecologist is usually used to find the foetal heart rate and confirm the pregnancy. Before receiving a positive confirmation of pregnancy, mothers must pay out-of-pocket for various blood tests, including tests for HIV and other infectious diseases.

Once pregnancy is diagnosed, women need to report their pregnancy to the local government and receive the Maternal and Child Health Handbook. Worldwide, it is rare that women are required to register their pregnancy with their government. Information about support services for mothers and their families is provided in the Handbook. In 2011, 87 per cent of pregnancies in Japan were registered before eleven weeks of gestation and the Handbook was provided accordingly. Very few women do not report their pregnancy or have prenatal check-ups before walking into a facility to give birth.

The Maternal and Child Health Handbook is designed to be a record of growth, development, health education and immunisation for the mother and baby from pregnancy through to the pre-school year. Pregnant women are required to bring the Handbook to all prenatal and infant check-ups. The records are regarded as a formal medical record. The Handbook was originally introduced in 1942 and became formalised in 1965 under the Maternal and Child Health Act. It has been translated into eight languages, including English, and is also distributed to foreign pregnant women living in Japan. The content is revised every ten years. As an important tool for pregnant women's self-care, the Handbook has also been adopted in other countries, particulary in developing countries in Asia, Africa, and Central and South America (Nakamura 2009). In 2014 a new taskforce was established to develop and disseminate a digital Handbook that computerises the information of each individual woman and her baby, while collecting data to be used in health education as a large national database.

The officially recommended frequency of prenatal check-ups is every four weeks until twenty-three weeks of pregnancy, biweekly from twenty-four to thirty-five weeks and every week from thirty-six weeks. More frequent visits are usually instructed by practitioners for women who are overdue to evaluate the well-being of the foetus. Support measures have recently increased as a result of the government's promotion of encouraging women to have more children. The financial cover for prenatal check-ups was only for a few visits before 2009, but prenatal check-ups are currently supported for a total of fourteen visits over the course of a woman's pregnancy, primarily through local government, but also with partial support from central government. Local governments also provide prenatal education for expectant parents. Women with high-risk pregnancies, such as pregnancy-induced hypertension, can have a thorough ultrasound examination for free and women older than thirty-five years at their due date can have one ultrasound examination for free.

Ninety-nine per cent of pregnant women visit obstetric institutions once they become pregnant, meaning that they choose obstetricians as their primary health provider. However, most obstetric institutions hire nurse-midwives as nursing staff and provide midwifery care for women in collaboration with obstetricians. Unlike in other nations, even when women are unfamiliar with the midwifery profession, they automatically meet midwives and receive midwifery care while receiving obstetric services. Nurse-midwives in Japan provide parenting education and consultation services and also assist in the provision of medical services by obstetricians/gynaecologists. Some hospitals/clinics provide more independent, midwifery-led prenatal check-ups. The level of autonomy and responsibility taken by nurse-midwives differs greatly depending on the style of collaborative relationship with their obstetrician colleagues as well as the needs of their clients.

Ultrasound examinations are routinely provided for low-risk pregnant women in Japan and women widely accept them. A recent issue of a health education manual targeting obstetricians instructed that five ultrasound scans during a pregnancy are sufficient; however, in reality, some obstetricians provide an ultrasound examination at every prenatal check-up. In recent years, three-dimensional (stereoscopic) or four-dimensional (video) ultrasound devices have become commonly available. Very few lay people or professionals question the safety of these uses of ultrasound for either the foetus or for pregnant women. Some experts believe that visualisation of the foetus can enhance maternal attachment to their unborn baby (Unno 2012).

The Japanese trend of longer hospitalisation, compared with other OECD countries, is also seen in prenatal care. Pregnant women judged as high-risk, including threatened miscarriage, threatened premature labour, or pregnancy-induced hypertension, tend to be hospitalised prenatally for weeks or months, during which time an intravenous drip of a tocolytic drug along with bed rest are often prescribed by obstetricians. Costs for abnormal (medically indicated) pregnancies are covered by medical insurance. The cost of expensive care, such as over 100,000 yen (US$979.5) per month, is reimbursed.

Intrapartum care

For those with health insurance, childbirth is paid in the form of a lump sum birth allowance of 420,000 yen (US$4,113) provided by the health insurance union, as stipulated by law. Out of this payment, 30,000 yen (US$294) is part of an insurance premium for the Japan Obstetric Compensation System for Cerebral Palsy. The cost of childbirth depends heavily on the place of delivery; in urban areas, for example, the lump sum birth allowance typically does not cover the total expense. Postpartum visits are also out-of-pocket. For poorer families, special support systems to cover delivery expenses are available.

In hospital births, the primary providers of intrapartum care with the most responsibility are obstetricians, while nurse-midwives and nursing staff often act as the main personnel in providing direct care for women and their families during labour and delivery. As with prenatal care, the level and content of autonomy and responsibility of nurse-midwives in providing midwifery care differs greatly by setting, depending on the style of their collaborative relationships with the obstetricians as well as the patients' preferences. In-hospital midwifery centres that provide nurse-midwife-led intrapartum care have recently been promoted as a way to resolve the shortage of obstetricians, advocate natural childbirth and to encourage nurse-midwives to practise autonomously (Japanese Nursing Association 2012).

Although this is not an all-encompassing sample, according to an official source, the caesarean section rate in Japan has been increasing steadily. Every three years the government statistical division collects one month of comparative data on the rate of caesarean sections. The rate was 7.3 per cent in 1984, 10.0 per cent in 1990, 15.2 per cent in 2002 and 19.2 per cent in 2011 (Mothers' & Children's Health & Welfare Association 2013). Of the caesarean rate of 19.2 per cent in 2011, 13.6 per cent occurred in clinics and 24.1 per cent in hospitals. In part, this correlates with the tendency for large hospitals with neonatal intensive care units to generally treat more high-risk women and their babies than clinics. In contrast, a national sample in 2010 revealed that the caesarean rate of the whole sample (of which 61 per cent were hospitals) was 26.7 per cent, while the forceps delivery rate was 0.5 per cent and the vacuum delivery rate was 5.3 per cent (Ministry of Health, Labour and Welfare 2011b). There is no official statistical data for the use of episiotomy or induction/augmentation of labour. The rate of post-date births (>42 weeks) was 0.3 per cent in 2012, having decreased from 4.4 per cent in 1980 (Ministry of Health, Labour and Welfare 2014a), implying that post-date births are likely to be managed and strictly prevented. The premature birth rate (<37 weeks) remains unchanged at around 5.7 per cent in 2012, having slightly increased from 4.1 per cent in 1980 (Ministry of Health, Labour and Welfare 2014a).

The management of multiple pregnancies and pregnancies with a breech presentation has become more defensive and these deliveries are currently often managed by caesarean section. Caesarean section, forceps and vacuum deliveries are regarded as abnormal (medically indicated) and the costs for these types of intrapartum care are covered by medical insurance with a concomitant lower co-payment for these women.

The use of pain medication for labour pain is very limited in Japan compared with other developed countries, in spite of the wide availability of medical technology and equipment and an overall increasing rate of medical intervention in childbirth. The rate of epidural use in Japan was only 2.6 per cent in 2008 (Terui *et al.* 2008). Most facilities provide no access to epidural pain relief for women in labour, even if requested, and epidural use at the woman's request is accessible in only 250 of a total of approximately 2,800 facilities in Japan (Terui *et al.* 2008). In normal labour and delivery, the cost of pain medication is entirely out-of-pocket.

The trends of medical intervention during labour and delivery tend to differ greatly by provider and institution, similar to those of other countries, and the public has little access to this fact-based information.

Many Japanese people prefer breastfeeding and almost all women initiate breastfeeding unless they have particular infectious conditions or are taking a contraindicated drug, such as for a psychiatric disease. In spite of this, according to government data from 2010, the rate of exclusive breastfeeding was only 54.3 per cent at discharge, while 39.0 per cent used mixed feeding (a combination of breastfeeding and formula) and 6.7 per cent used formula feeding only (Ministry of Health, Labour and Welfare

2011b). At one to two months postpartum, the rate of exclusive breastfeeding was 51.6 per cent, that of mixed feeding was 43.8 per cent and that of exclusive formula feeding was 4.6 per cent, revealing a slightly increased rate of exclusive breastfeeding compared with the 2000 data (Ministry of Health, Labour and Welfare 2011b). There are sixty-nine Baby-Friendly Hospitals where staff have been certified in the ten steps to successful breastfeeding supported by the WHO and UNICEF (Japan Breast Feeding Association 2014). In short, the environment in Japan allows for the coexistence of a preferred value of breastfeeding and the wide acceptance and practice of formula feeding. Many mothers add formula when health care providers point out insufficient weight gain in their babies. These judgements about the sufficiency or insufficiency of babies' weight gain are usually made based on the growth curve published by the government and included in the *Handbook*. The curve was developed based on a national sample of infants that included mixed-fed babies. A new growth curve based solely on exclusively breastfed infants was developed and published by Japanese researchers in an international journal in 2013 (Tanaka *et al.* 2013).

Postnatal care

In the second half of the twentieth century, maternal and neonatal mortality outcomes in Japan greatly improved to reach the highest levels in the world. During this period, tremendous changes took place in Japanese society. For example, the typical birth setting shifted from mothers' homes to medical institutions, perinatal health care services were medicalised, neonatal medicine greatly developed and became widely available, and the standard of life and literacy rates also significantly improved.

In Oriental medicine, postpartum care is regarded as critical for women's later health. At least one month of postpartum recovery is secured in neighbouring countries such as China and Korea, where special postpartum care facilities are widely developed. In Japan, although there are a few such specialised facilities that have developed in recent years, women stay in maternity hospitals/clinics for a longer period than in many other countries, typically four to six days after a vaginal delivery and one week to ten days after a caesarean section. This early postpartum period is very important as a recovery time for new mothers, as well as a time for newborn babies to adjust to their extra-uterine life and a time to learn to breastfeed. Recently, however, the length of postpartum hospitalisation has been gradually shortened.

Care-givers during the postpartum hospitalisation period include nurse-midwives, nurses, obstetricians and paediatricians when necessary. Above all, nurse-midwives autonomously provide care in breastfeeding support during hospitalisation. In Japan, nurse-midwives have developed unique breast massage techniques and instruct prenatal and postpartum women to regularly conduct breast massage (Kishi 2010). These practices have spread widely since the 1990s. In recent years, an increasing number of nurse-midwives as well as paediatricians have been trained and certified as International Board Certified Lactation Consultants. They bring Western knowledge to breastfeeding support and the traditional Japanese approach of breast massage appears to be becoming less mainstream.

Public health nurses and nurse-midwives working in local government agencies also lead initiatives in postpartum and infant health care services, such as home visits for all postpartum women within two months and infant check-ups. Infant check-ups are usually provided at 3–6 months and 9–11 months of age for free. A mass screening test for inborn errors of metabolism is free of charge. A thorough physical examination is provided at no charge for infants with a disease or developmental problems. Expenses for medical services for low birthweight infants are covered by the prefectural governments. Other health services can be provided at the discretion of each local government. Parents of children under the age of three years can receive a monthly stipend of 15,000 yen (US$147) to cover childcare costs, with decreasing monthly sums available through junior high school.

In Japanese culture, women usually return to their parents' homes for the months surrounding delivery so they can give birth at a clinic or hospital nearby and receive care from their own mothers. This is called *Satogaeri*. Combined with a shortage of maternity facilities in rural areas and the ageing of couples' parents, *Satogaeri* practices are now seen less frequently. Although more husbands can spend time with their new babies and help their wives directly than was historically customary, few husbands take paternity leave, resulting in new mothers spending the most time with their new babies with little support, in a nuclear family, especially in urban areas. This trend is referred to as the 'postpartum crisis' (Uchida and Tsuboi 2013). The need for postpartum care services by non-family members has been recognised and, in 2013, the central government announced a new policy strengthening postpartum care, including short-stay services in postpartum care centres in addition to previously existing promotions of marriage, pregnancy and childbirth (Prime Minister of Japan & His Cabinet 2013). Costs for those postpartum care centres are not covered by medical insurance and are therefore out-of-pocket. Women who are not affluent or experienced mothers or who also have to take care of older children have limited access to these facilities and services.

Consumer involvement

Influenced by traditional Shinto animism, Japanese people have a tendency to value, respect and defer to natural law, rather than to attempt to conquer it (Murakami 1994). In addition, reflecting the overall Japanese characteristics of thoroughness, seriousness and compliancy, most pregnant Japanese women attend all the recommended check-ups, attend parenting education classes and engage in healthy self-care behaviour, such as attending to their eating habits during pregnancy and breastfeeding (Kishi *et al.* 2010). Publications on health education are very effective in Japan as almost everyone is literate. However, most Japanese women only obtain maternity-related information in the Japanese language. Thus the language barrier is a challenge for Japanese pregnant women in making evidence-based and fully informed choices regarding their maternity health care as the most up-to-date evidence-based research is often available in English or is only available to those with access to specialised publications designed for health practitioners.

Japanese culture and society have been strongly influenced by Western countries, above all the USA after World War II. This influence can also be seen in maternity-related folk traditions, obstetrics, midwifery and nursing practices. As a result, current maternity care practices in Japan are a mixture of traditional Japanese and imported Western ideas. Moreover, these practices and care services differ by birth setting and by individual practitioner. However, this information is not widely available in the public domain and is therefore not shared by many users and/or practitioners. Therefore women tend to choose where to deliver their babies based on geographical proximity, size of hospital, word-of-mouth, reputation and other amenities such as the facilities, food provided during hospitalisation, aesthetic services and, in the case of experienced mothers, their past experiences with their providers or hospital (Tsukamoto and Sugiura 2006). Japanese women should be better informed, as conditions are sufficient for developing large perinatal databases similar to those many Western countries use to equip and assist women in making informed choices.

Voices from childbearing women have emerged from time to time. Most advocacy groups for pregnancy and childbirth were established in the 1990s. There was a subtle wave of feminism from the 1970s through to the 1990s that promoted respect for women's innate ability to give birth. Many independent nurse-midwives imported new knowledge from the West, such as the Lamaze method and the concept of active birth (Misago and Yoshimoto 2013). However, Japanese women hold traditional values of obedience and patience, passively leaving decisions about maternity care to others, including professionals and even public opinion. Some women have access to grassroots survey data published on women's experiences and the voices of other women regarding their childbirth and postpartum experiences (Group Kirin 1997; Kishi 2011).

REBORN is a group that champions, encourages and supports each woman in playing an active role in childbirth to maximise her potential for a satisfactory perinatal experience while also bridging the gap between lay women and professionals. The group was established on 3 November 1993 and is known as the good birth day (*ii-osan-no-hi*, a play on words in

Japanese). Every year, many childbirth-related events take place on this day nationwide. The Breastfeeding Support Network of Japan is an example of a group in Japan that promotes a society friendly towards breastfeeding.

An example of an advocacy group triggered by childbirth-related accidents or malpractice lawsuits is the Group to Investigate Harms of Oxytocic Drugs, which had 210 members in 2013. This group was established to promote safety in childbirth. They advocate the appropriate use of oxytocic drugs by means of informing society, working with policy-makers in government, holding events, providing consultations and regularly issuing newsletters.

In addition, the non-profit organisation Sudden Infant Death Syndrome Family Group is a volunteer support group run by surviving families and professionals for bereaved family members who have lost an infant to sudden death.

Risk and rights

Although Japan has a universal health insurance system and has fewer income disparities among its people than some other nations, the population structure is rapidly changing to one with fewer children and more elderly citizens. This has increased uncertainty around the country's future, including its economic and social stability. Other related social problems include poverty and work/life balance issues among people of childbearing age, as well as among women overall.

People in Japanese society take the safety of childbirth for granted because Japan has the world's best perinatal outcome statistics. They also trust medical technology, assuming that leaving their health to professionals is the safest route to take (Kanzaki and Kumabe 2005). As women become pregnant at an older age, any adverse outcome becomes unacceptable. People therefore tend to choose large hospitals where advanced medical technologies are more readily available. First-time mothers have limited information regarding choosing birth settings, whereas experienced mothers need to choose geographically closer institutions to arrive in time for delivery. Choices depend on individual women and families, as expenses for perinatal care are out-of-pocket. Therefore the high commodification of maternity services in Japan renders a pregnant woman a 'customer'. Each woman and her family members need access to high-quality and rich database systems to assist in informed choices for their best health and happiness.

Japanese women have a theoretical right to choose their birth place and their health care providers; however, they cannot make informed choices due to limited information on intervention rates and perinatal outcomes. Most publicly available information sources are provided by authoritative professionals and are more about the prevention and management of accidents or abnormalities than about well-being during pregnancy and delivery. It is possible that maternity health care providers are increasingly more risk-adverse and are changing their practices. For example, the caesarean section rate continues to rise. The recommendations by the recurrence prevention committee for the Japan Obstetric Compensation System for Cerebral Palsy under the Japan Council for Quality Health Care emphasised the possibility that vaginal birth after caesarean could be a cause of uterine rupture causing cerebral palsy to newborn babies (Japan Council for Quality Health Care 2014c). Many obstetric wards have an incident reporting system which is standardised across a hospital. Despite the popularity/initial promotion of early skin-to-skin contact (kangaroo care), it has been implicated in several medical malpractice suits as the cause of hypothermia or suffocation in newborn babies and therefore more providers have become conservative and cautious in promoting early skin-to-skin contact (Japan Society of Perinatal and Neonatal Medicine 2012).

The government has increased policies to promote a mother- and child-friendly society, but the situation has not yet improved. It seems that current social policies mainly focus on increasing the number of children and have not paid sufficient attention to meeting individual preferences or overall happiness from the perspective of childbearing women and their children. Suicide is the leading cause of death among women aged 15–34 years and the second highest cause of death among women aged 35–54 years (Ministry of Health, Labour and Welfare 2014a). Evidence-based care taking into account individuals' desires and intentions has not been granted as a human right, either at policy or consumer levels.

A variety of mechanisms for funding infertility treatment are available in Japan, such as subsidy systems at the national, prefectural and city level, with varying degrees of coverage depending on the financial situation of the governing body. These mechanisms primarily target more advanced types of treatment, including external or *in vitro* fertilisation, which might otherwise prove prohibitively expensive; simpler treatment options are generally left to out-of-pocket payments. Their access, however, is subject to certain restrictions, including income brackets and, potentially, the age of the mother-to-be.

For pregnant women, induced abortion is legal in Japan. This is currently supported under the Maternal Protection Act, adapted from the original Eugenic Protection Act, which stipulated that only healthy babies without disability or disease should be born. However, induced abortion is permitted only up until the twenty-second week of pregnancy and under two conditions. These are that the pregnant woman seeks to induce an abortion along with the consent of the husband: (1) having a physical or economic reason with potential implications for the mother's health; or (2) for pregnancies resulting from rape (Ministry of Health, Labour and

Welfare 2013b). The media has recently highlighted the increasing number of women electing to pursue induced abortion out of fear of foetal abnormalities, resulting in the ethical issues surrounding abortion gaining social attention. In Japan, ultrasound scans are a routine part of prenatal check-ups. Amniotic fluid tests are also available, but far more sensitive and less invasive blood tests for prenatal diagnosis have now been developed and are becoming widespread. Although these technologies are advanced, the 'soft' support services surrounding the tests, such as pre- and post-test counselling and education, still lag behind the technology and ethical issues have yet to be addressed. In particular, on receiving a tentatively positive result, there are no protocols in place to guide maternal decision-making regarding whether or not to terminate the pregnancy.

Power imbalances exist in both policy-making (government officials) and health care providers (clinicians). The government is male-dominated, although the current government is promoting an increase in female politicians, aiming at 'a proportion of women with administrative positions to 30 per cent by 2020' (Gender Equality Bureau Cabinet Office 2011); however, the proportion of female members in the Diet was only 8 per cent (39 of 480) in 2014, meaning that Japan ranks 127th out of 189 countries in female representation according to the Inter-Parliamentary Union (Asahi Shinbun 2014). The voters also must own up to this problem in Japan as young people, in general, are not interested in politics, with a concomitant low voting rate among the current childbearing generation (Ministry of Internal Affairs and Communications 2012). Therefore politicians prioritise their social policies and consequent budget allocations for the elderly population (Yoshida 2013).

Power imbalances are also reflected in the clinical settings of maternity health care services. The majority of direct care-givers in the field of maternal health care are female nursing staff: nurse-midwives and nurses in medical institutions, with public health nurses active in local government. However, actual decisions are made by senior male doctors. There is a system, in theory, supporting nurse-midwives' independent and autonomous practices for low-risk women, but, in reality, reflecting the traditional gender role of women in Japan, they are usually afforded limited autonomy and work under supervising obstetricians. When nurse-midwives run their own birth centres, they are required to collaborate closely with a contract obstetrician and a highly medically equipped hospital. Limited interdisciplinary collaborative relationships and limited income when running an independent birth centre outside the medical insurance system have been obstacles in the autonomous practice of nurse-midwives.

The disparity between urban and rural areas is a serious concern that may represent the overall problems gripping Japanese society. This problem has been overlooked due to the excessive concentration of the population and industry in the Tokyo Metropolitan area. Information publicised through the media is also skewed towards urban issues. The distribution of physicians is not based on each community area, but by university medical departments. The placement of physicians in scarcely populated areas tends to be insufficient, resulting in further deterioration in the maternity health care system in rural areas. Areas damaged by the tsunami in the Tohoku area in 2011 need assistance to recover their maternity health care systems.

In Japan, industry and government play important parts in the actual arrangements of the work environment of pregnant women and working mothers, including parental leave systems and decreased workload. In society, 'Maternity Mark' logos are distributed (Ministry of Health, Labour and Welfare 2014c) and courtesy seats are designed in buses and trains to encourage people to be compassionate and kind to pregnant women and mothers with small children. Clothes specially designed for breastfeeding women have been developed (Mo House 2014) and have become widely available. The placement of nursing rooms in shopping malls and dotted around cities is encouraged. In a highly commercialised society, many initiatives in Japan are taken by companies and networks of individuals rather than a raft of government policies. However, due to the prolonged economic depression, companies and individuals cannot be expected to succeed through their own efforts alone.

On the other hand, economic liberalisation has been promoted, such as that seen in the Trans-Pacific Partnership. Business firms entering the health care market affect ethical issues, especially when more aggressive styles of business, such as medical tourism seeking surrogate mothers and egg donors outside the country, are pursued.

Conclusion

The Japanese welfare state has always been centred on wage-earners and based on the traditional family structure with a single breadwinner, usually a father, in one household. Childcare was in the past supported within the family structure (e.g. grandparents) with clearly demarcated gender roles and has never been seen as a right. This is confirmed by the fact that maternity care has not been covered by the national health care insurance. In the clinical settings of maternity health care, the unique collaborative style between obstetricians and nurse-midwives also internalises the traditional gender role.

So far Japan has maintained one of the world's best perinatal outcomes with fewer disparities than other countries. However, as the current system causes more difficulties in meeting people's needs for health care within the country's changing population structures and dwindling economic conditions, already overstretched health care resources will be further challenged. When individual efforts by health care practitioners providing direct care for women and their families are not adequately supported, this could potentially pose great risks to maternity services at all (micro-, meso- and macro-) levels.

The involvement of the government in this policy area needs to increase. Sufficient attention should be paid to individual preferences or overall satisfaction from the perspective of childbearing women and their children, while being thoughtful about the best balance between the medicalisation of maternity health care and humanistic strategies for surrounding ethical issues. The development of quality databases is desirable, not only to provide rationales for policy-makers and professionals, but also to support individual women's informed decisions. Every effort should be made to stop and prevent economic disparities among people and the skewed distribution of resources between urban and rural areas from further deteriorating. Radical transitions need to take place to realise family-friendly working environments for all people to balance work and home life. The developmental welfare state in Japan is under strain and its ongoing transformations have many future implications for maternity services and policy.

Acknowledgements

The authors thank Ms Brett Iimura, Dr Tamami Satoh and Dr Kenji Takehara for their critical reviews of the manuscript.

Useful web sites

REBORN	www.web-reborn.com
Sudden Infant Death Syndrome Family Group	www.sids.gr.jp/sids.html

References

Asahi Shimbun (2014) *Nihon no josei kokkai giin hiritsu, senshinkoku de saitei: shuin 8%* (Japan's female representation the lowest among developed countries: 8% in the House of Representatives) [in Japanese] [online]. 5 March 2014. Available from: www.asahi.com/articles/ASG347QK1G34UHBI04H.html. Accessed 25 June 2014.

Aspalter, C. (2006) 'The East Asian welfare model', *International Journal of Social Welfare*, 15: 290–301.

Cabinet Office (2014) *Kazoku to chiiki ni okeru kosodate ni kansuru ishiki chousa. Policy on Cohesive Society* [in Japanese] [online]. Available from: www8.cao.go.jp/shoushi/shoushika/research/h25/ishiki/index_pdf.htm. Accessed 18 January 2014.

Campbell, J. and Ikegami, N. (1998) *The Art of Balance in Health Policy: Maintaining Japan's Low-cost Egalitarian System*. Cambridge: Cambridge University Press.

Esping-Andersen, G. (1990) *The Three Worlds of Welfare Capitalism*. Cambridge: Polity Press and Princeton: Princeton University Press.

Esping-Andersen, G. (1997) 'Hybrid or unique? The distinctiveness of the Japanese welfare state', *Journal of European Social Policy*, 7 (3): 179–189.

Esping-Andersen, G. (1999) *Social Foundations of Postindustrial Economies*. Oxford: Oxford University Press.

Gender Equality Bureau Cabinet Office (2011) *2020 nen 30% no mokuhyou no jitsugen ni mukete* (Towards the goal of 30% by 2020) [in Japanese] [online]. Available from: www.gender.go.jp/kaigi/renkei/2020_30/pdf/2020_30_all.pdf. Accessed 25 June 2014.

Group Kirin (ed.) (1997) *Watashi tachi no osan kara anata no osan he: anketo 493 nin no koe* yori (From our childbirth to your childbirths: survey of 493 women's voices) [in Japanese]. Tokyo: Medica Publication.

Holliday, I. (2000) 'Productivist welfare capitalism: social policy in East Asia', *Political Studies*, 48 (4): 706–723.

Index Mundi (2013) *Japan Demographics Profile 2013* [online]. Available from: www.indexmundi.com/japan/demographics_profile.html. Accessed 25 June 2014.

Japan Breast Feeding Association (2014) *Baby-Friendly Hospital ni tsuite* [in Japanese] [online]. Available from: www.bonyu.or.jp/index.asp. Accessed 25 June 2014.

Japan Council for Quality Health Care (2014a) *Kanyu jokyo* (Members) [in Japanese] [online]. Available from: www.sanka-hp.jcqhc.or.jp/search/kanyujokyo.php. Accessed 25 June 2014.

Japan Council for Quality Health Care (2014b) *Sanka iryou hoshou seido* (The Japan Obstetric Compensation System for Cerebral Palsy) [in Japanese] [online]. Available from: www.sanka-hp.jcqhc.or.jp/index.html. Accessed 25 June 2014.

Japan Council for Quality Health Care (2014c) *Dai 4-kai Sanka iryou hoshou seido Saihatsu boushi ni kansuru houkokusho: Sanka iryou no shitsu no koujou ni mukete* (The Fourth Japan Obstetric Compensation System for Cerebral Palsy Prevention of Recurrence Report: to improve the quality of obstetric care) [in Japanese] [online]. Available from: www.sanka-hp.jcqhc.or.jp/documents/prevention/pdf/Saihatsu_Report_04_All_1.pdf. Accessed 25 June 2014.

Japan Society of Obstetrics and Gynecology Medical Reform Committee (2014) *Wagakuni no sanfujinkai no doukou: Ishi, Shikaishi, Yakuzaishi chousa yori* (Trends in obstetricians and gynaecologists in Japan: survey of physicians, dentists and pharmacists) [in Japanese] [online]. Available from: http://shusanki.org/theme_page.html?id=250. Accessed 18 January 2014.

Japan Society of Perinatal and Neonatal Medicine (2012) *Souki boshi sesshoku jisshi no ryuiten* (Points of attention in early skin-to-skin contact) [in Japanese] [online]. Available from: www.jspnm.com/Teigen/docs/sbsv13_10.pdf#zoom=100. Accessed 25 June 2014.

Japanese Midwives Association (2014) *Josan gyomu gaidorain 2014* (Midwifery Practice Guidelines 2014) [in Japanese] [online]. Available from: www.midwife.or.jp/pdf/guideline/guideline.pdf. Accessed 25 June 2014.

Japanese Nursing Association (2012) *Josan jissen nouryoku kyouka to sono taisei seibi* (Enhancing nurse-midwives' clinical competencies and related systems development) [in Japanese] [online]. Available from: www.nurse.or.jp/home/innaijyosan/index.html. Accessed 25 June 2014.

Kanzaki, J. and Kumabe, M. (2005) *Omakase shinai iryou: Jiritsu shita kanja ni narutameni* (Don't leave your health to providers: towards becoming independent patients) [in Japanese] [online]. Tokyo: Keio University Press.

Kishi, R. (2010) *Integration of Breastfeeding Care by Nurse-Midwives in Japan* [online]. Available from: www.childresearch.net/papers/parenting/2010_01.html. Accessed 25 June 2014.

176   R.K. Fukuzawa and N. Kodate

Kishi, R. (2011) *Mothers' Voices* [online]. Available from: https://sites.google.com/ site/mothersvoicesjapan/. Accessed 25 June 2014.

Kishi, R., McElmurry, B.J., Vonderheid, S., Altfeld, S., McFarlin, B. and Tashiro, J. (2010) 'Japanese women's experiences from pregnancy through the early post-partum period', *Health Care Women International*, 32 (1): 57–71.

Kobayashi, M. and Watanabe, N. (2008) 'The sense, behaviors and standard of selection of women in childbed considering the difference of the place for child-birth and the existence of the experience of childbirth', *Niigata Seiryou Daigaku Kiyou*, 8, 9–20.

Kodate, N. (2014) 'Focusing events, priority problems and governance arrange-ments: regulatory reforms in health and eldercare sector in Sweden and Japan'. In: M. Hill (ed.), *Studying Public Policy: an International Approach*. Bristol: Policy Press.

Lee, Y.-J. and Ku, Y.-W. (2007) 'East Asian welfare regimes: testing the hypothesis of the developmental welfare state', *Social Policy & Administration*, 41 (2): 197–212.

Leflar, R.B. (2009) '"Unnatural death", criminal sanctions, and medical quality improvement in Japan', *Yale Journal of Health Policy Law and Ethics*, 1: 1–51.

Matsushima, N., Morita, N., Ogata, N., Saeki, K., Matsuda, R. and Kurumatani, N. (2003) 'Live birth distribution by time and place from 1981 to 1998 in Japan', *Japanese Journal of Hygiene*, 57: 674–681.

Ministry of Health, Labour and Welfare (2011a) *Kokumin iryouhi no gaikyou: Kekkano gaiyou* (Overview of national health expenditures: summary of results) [in Japanese] [online]. Available from: www.mhlw.go.jp/toukei/saikin/hw/k-iryohi/11/dl/kekka.pdf. Accessed 25 June 2014.

Ministry of Health, Labour and Welfare (2011b) *Heisei 22 nen nyuyouji shintai hatsuiku chousa houkokusho* (Infant Physical Growth Survey Report 2010) [in Japanese] [online]. Tokyo: Department of Equal Employment and Children and Home.

Ministry of Health, Labour and Welfare (2012) *Heisei 24 nendo koyou kintou kihon chousa* (Equal Employment Opportunity Survey 2012) [in Japanese] [online]. Tokyo: Department of Equal Employment and Children and Home.

Ministry of Health, Labour and Welfare (2013a) *Heisei 24 nen eisei gyousei houkokurei no gaikyou* (Overall Report on Public Health Administration 2012: employed health care providers) [in Japanese] [online]. Available from: www.mhlw.go.jp/ toukei/saikin/hw/eisei/12/dl/h24_gaikyo.pdf. Accessed 25 June 2014.

Ministry of Health, Labour and Welfare (2013b) *Botai hogo hou 14 jou* (Maternal Protection Act 14) [in Japanese] [online]. Available from: http://law.e-gov.go. jp/htmldata/S23/S23HO156.html. Accessed 25 June 2014.

Ministry of Health, Labour and Welfare (2014a) *Vital Statistics in Japan: Trends up to 2012*. Tokyo: Statistics and Information Department, Minister's Secretariat.

Ministry of Health, Labour and Welfare (2014b) *Heisei 25 nen wagakuni no hoken toukei* [in Japanese] [online]. Available from: www.mhlw.go.jp/toukei/list/130–25. html. Accessed 25 June 2014.

Ministry of Health, Labour and Welfare (2014c) *Maternity mark nit suite* (About the Maternity Mark) [in Japanese] [online]. Available from: www.mhlw.go.jp/stf/ seisakunitsuite/bunya/kodomo/kodomo_kosodate/boshi-hoken/maternity_ mark.html. Accessed 25 June 2014.

Ministry of Health, Labour and Welfare (2014d) *Josei ishi rishoku boushi fukushoku shien ni tsuite* (Turnover prevention and support for female physicians) [in

Japanese] [online]. Available from: www.mhlw.go.jp/seisakunitsuite/bunya/kenkou_iryou/iryou/kinkyu/rishoku_fukushoku/. Accessed 25 June 2014.

Ministry of Internal Affairs and Communications (2012) *Senkyo, seiji shikin* (Election and political funding) [in Japanese] [online]. Available from: www.soumu.go.jp/senkyo/senkyo_s/news/sonota/nendaibetu/. Accessed 25 June 2014.

Ministry of Justice (2013) *Zairyu gaikokujin toukei* (Statistics on foreign residents) [in Japanese] [online]. Available from: www.e-stat.go.jp/SG1/estat/List.do?lid=000001118467. Accessed 25 June 2014.

Misago, C. and Yoshimoto, B. (2013) *Joshi no idenshi* (The gene for girls) [in Japanese] [online]. Tokyo: Aki Shobo.

Mo House (2014) Available from: http://mo-house.net/. Accessed 25 June 2014.

Mothers' & Children's Health & Welfare Association (MCHWA) (2013) *Boshi hoken no omonaru toukei* (Maternal and child health statistics of Japan) [in Japanese]. Tokyo: MCHWA.

Murakami, Y. (1994) *Bunmei no nakano kagaku* (Science in civilisation) [in Japanese]. Tokyo: Seidosha.

Nakamura, Y. (2009) *Maternal and Child Health Handbook in Global Perspective.* WHO Association of Japan Library No. 39: 5–8. Available from: www.japan-who.or.jp/library/2009/book3901.pdf. Accessed 25 June 2014.

National Institute of Population and Social Security Research (2012) [online] Available from: www.ipss.go.jp/syoushika/tohkei/newest04/con2h.html. Accessed 25 June 2014.

National Tax Agency (2014) *Heisei 24 nenbun minkan kyuyo jittai toukei chousa* (Statistics on private salary 2012) [in Japanese] [online]. Available from: www.nta.go.jp/kohyo/tokei/kokuzeicho/minkan/top.htm. Accessed 25 June 2014.

OECD (2011) *Society at a Glance 2011: Equity Indicators* [online]. Available from: www.oecd.org/berlin/47570121.pdf. Accessed 25 June 2014.

OECD (2013a) *OECD Health Data 2013: How Does Japan Compare?* Paris: OECD Publishing.

OECD (2013b) *Health at a Glance 2013: OECD Indicators.* Paris: OECD Publishing.

OECD (2014a) *OECD Country Statistical Profiles: Japan.* Paris: OECD Publishing.

OECD (2014b) *OECD Health Data: Health Care Resources.* Paris: OECD Publishing.

OECD (2014c) *OECD Health Data: Health Status.* Paris: OECD Publishing.

Prime Minister of Japan & His Cabinet (2013) *Shoushika kiki toppa no tameno kinkyu taisaku* (Emergent strategies to resolve the crisis of declining numbers of children) [in Japanese] [online]. Available from: www.kantei.go.jp/jp/singi/koku-minkaigi/dai16/sankou1.pdf. Accessed 25 June 2014.

Shimuta, K. (2011) 'Wagakuni no shuusanki iryou taisei no arikata: Sanka iryou hoshou seido no gemjou to kadai (The obstetric care system in Japan: current situation and challenges of the Japan Obstetric Compensation System for Cerebral Palsy [in Japanese].' *Prefectural University of Kumamoto Administration Graduate Program Bulletin,* 8: 23–50.

Tanaka, H., Ishii, H., Yamada, T., Akazawa, K., Nagata, S. and Yamashiro, Y. (2013) 'Growth of Japanese breastfed infants compared to national references and World Health Organization growth standards', *Acta Pediatrica,* 102 (7): 739–743.

Terui, K., Ueyama, H., Oonishi, Y., Okutomi, T., Ono, K., Kawana, S. and Morisaki, H. (2008) *Zenkoku no bunben toriatsukai shisetu ni okeru masuika sinryou jittai chousa* (Survey on anaesthetic practices at facilities providing intrapartum care in Japan) [in Japanese]. Tokyo: Health Labour Sciences Research Grant Report Database, pp. 433–467.

Tsukamoto, E. and Sugiura, K. (2006) Shussan basho sentaku youin ni kansuru kenkyu (Study on factors influencing choice of birth place) [in Japanese]. *Mie Kangogaku shi*, 8, 43–53.

Uchida, S. and Tsuboi, K. (2013) *Sango kuraishisu* (Postpartum crisis) [in Japanese]. Tokyo: Popular Publishing.

Unno, N. (2012) *"Suitei taiji taiju to taiji hatsuiku kyokusen" hoken shidou manyuaru* (Health education manual on estimated fetus weight and fetus growth curve) [in Japanese]. Tokyo: Japan Association of Obstetrics and Gynecologists. Available from: www.jaog.or.jp/all/document/taiji_2012.pdf. Accessed 25 June 2014.

World Economic Forum (2013) *The Global Gender Gap Report 2013* [online]. Available from: www3.weforum.org/docs/WEF_GenderGap_Report_2013.pdf. Accessed 25 June 2014.

Yoshida, H. (2013) *A Study on the Effect of Low Voter Turnout of Younger Generation on the Generational Imbalance in the Fiscal Policy* [online]. Discussion Paper, Tohoku Economics Research Group. Available from: www.econ.tohoku.ac.jp/e-dbase/dp/terg/terg298.pdf. Accessed 25 June 2014.

9 Italy

Marina Scavini and Chiara Molinari

Background

The foundations of Italy as a nation were laid in 1861 when several independent states in the peninsula were united under the House of Savoy as a constitutional monarchy. After the end of World War II the monarchy transitioned into a parliamentary republic ratified by popular vote in 1946, when Italian women were entitled to vote for the first time. The Constitution, written in 1948, established a bicameral Parliament with a Chamber of Deputies and a Senate. The head of state is the President, who is elected for a seven-year mandate by a joint session of the Chamber and Senate, while the Prime Minister – usually the leader of the party with the largest representation in the Chamber of Deputies – heads the government. Italy is subdivided into twenty regions, five with an autonomous statute granting autonomy in legislation, administration and finance. The country is further divided into 110 provinces and 8,092 municipalities. In 1957, Italy was a founding member of the European Community, which became the European Union in 1993 (Mack Smith 1997). Italy is part of the Schengen Area and has been a member of the Eurozone since 1999.

According to the OECD, in 2011 Italy's economy was the sixth largest among the industrial economies. Its annual GDP accounts for 17.0 per cent of the European Union area total GDP; nevertheless, the per capita income is nearly 7 per cent lower than that in the European Union area (OECD 2013a). Italy has limited natural resources, with only small deposits of iron, coal and oil. Natural gas reserves are abundant in the Po Valley and offshore in the Adriatic Sea. Most commodities and over 75 per cent of the national energy needs have to be imported. The Italian economy today is based on small- and medium-sized enterprises, with a smaller number of large companies and international companies (OECD 2013b). Tourism is an important contributor to the Italian economy, with over forty-six million foreign visitors every year (World Travel and Tourism Council 2014). In 2013, agriculture employed 3.6 per cent of the country's workforce, industry 27.2 per cent and the service sector 69.1 per cent (ISTAT 2014a). Italy is still divided into an industrial north and a mainly agricultural south, creating a dual economy with 75 per cent of total GDP being produced in the centre and north and only 25 per cent in the south (ISTAT 2014b), with little change over the last two decades. Italy's economy has been profoundly affected by the global recession that began in 2008, with high unemployment, restrictions in the supply of credit and decreased expenditure, which have widened this north/south divide. Italy ranks around average in the international scoring of education, government transparency, civil liberties, quality of life and economic freedom (Heritage Foundation 2014; International Monetary Fund 2013; OECD 2009).

Italy as a welfare regime

Esping-Andersen (1990) classified Italy's welfare state in the conservative–corporatist model, characterised by the following features: an average strength of social entitlements (decommodification); the aim of rewarding work performance and status; the principle of subsidiarity (what individuals can accomplish by their own enterprise and industry should not be committed to the state); and married women ensuring the stability of the traditional family by renouncing work outside the home. Later, Italy's welfare state – together with those of Spain, Greece and Portugal – was classified as the Mediterranean model of welfare, which is a variant of the conservative–corporatist model characterised by lower social entitlements that are partly counterbalanced by a strong supportive role of family networks, fragmented welfare provision – with generous benefits to some and meagre benfits to others – and a health care system providing only partial coverage (Ferrera 1996). Accordingly, Italy's social spending and welfare programmes are primarily state-based, with a heavily regulated labour market.

The Italian welfare system is based on three main pillars.

1   Health care is provided through the National Healthcare System (Sistema Sanitario Nazionale, or SSN) to all Italian citizens and foreign legal residents, with co-payments for outpatient diagnostic procedures and laboratory tests, specialist care and drug prescriptions.
2   A variety of social services is provided to specific groups of individuals (e.g. public schools from elementary to university level, vouchers for textbooks and school meals, long-term care for elderly and disabled people, subsidised housing, maternity leave, and family benefits related to income and family size).
3   Retirement and unemployment benefits are provided through the Istituto Nazionale di Previdenza Sociale (Niero 1996).

The typology of such a welfare system tends to penalise individuals and families in unstable, non-traditional or part-time job situations. It provides little benefit for those outside the insurance model (the new poverty of immigrants, the self-employed and young people, who experience significant difficulties in entering the workforce) (Esping-Andersen 1990). This group has made up a significantly larger proportion of the population since the start of the global recession in 2008.

Health care system

Healthcare Reform (Law 833/78 1978) was introduced in 1978 and established in Italy a universal single-payer, publicly funded national health care system (SSN), the beneficiaries of which are all citizens and foreign legal residents of Italy (Lo Scalzo *et al.* 2009; Ministero della Salute 2014a). Since 1998 some basic services have also been extended to illegal immigrants. The Italian SSN provides full coverage for general practitioner care (adults), paediatric care (children up to fourteen years of age) and hospitalisations, and also coverage with a co-payment (Ticket Sanitario) for outpatient diagnostic procedures and laboratory tests, specialist care and drug prescriptions. Exemptions from co-payment are granted based on income or for selected diseases or conditions. It has been estimated that in 2012 the annual cumulative disbursement for co-payments of SSN beneficiaries amounts to €4 billion (that is, on average, about €65 per person) and this is expected to increase to €6.6 billion in 2014 (Dossier Ticket 2012, 2014). In a similar manner to the UK's National Health Service, the Italian SSN owns facilities and employs health care professionals – including physicians – directly. Furthermore, SSN beneficiaries may choose to receive their care through private hospitals and outpatient care facilities that have received accreditation from the SSN. In the early 1990s the central government transferred the responsibility of managing the provision of health care services for their residents to the nineteen Regions and two Autonomous Provinces (Trento and Bolzano) of Italy (Law 412/91 1991). Regions deliver health services (primary care, hospital care, public health, occupational health and health care related to social care) through their local health units, managed by a chief executive officer appointed by the governor of the Region. Furthermore, the Regions negotiate the purchase of health care services according to a standard fee-for-service from accredited private facilities, with direct billing to the Region. The Regions issue health cards (Carta Regionale dei Servizi) that entitle all residents to receive health services. SSN beneficiaries can also receive health services outside the region of residence without any additional charges. Italian citizens and foreign legal residents are also covered within the European Union for urgent medical care and for highly specialised care not available in Italy (Directive 2011/24/EU 2011). The system emphasises preventive care, with vaccinations and most screening tests (e.g. Pap smears, mammograms, colonoscopies and urological assessments) offered at no charge. In 2009 a survey documented that 88 per cent of the users of an

SSN hospital were either very satisfied or somewhat satisfied with the medical and nursing care received during hospitalisation, with higher percentages of satisfaction in northern Italy than in southern Italy (ISTAT 2009).

Each year the central government sets the amount of funding for health care. This funding comes from the income of SSN health care facilities (co-payments and payments of health care services by third parties), regional taxes and contributions from the special statute regions. Health care expenditure which exceeds that covered by these sources will come from national taxes. In Italy, health care expenditure as a percentage of GDP has increased from 7.3 per cent in 1988 to 9.2 per cent in 2012 (a per capita €2,171 purchasing power parity) (OECD 2013c), which is close to the OECD average of 9.3 per cent and similar to the spending of European countries such as the UK, Norway, Finland and Iceland (OECD 2013c).

The Ministry of Health maintains minimum standards of health care (Livelli Essenziali di Assistenza). However, individual regions may increase – but not lower – these minimum standards of care for their residents, provided that the required additional funding is allocated in the Region's health care budget. To contain pharmaceutical expenditure, the Ministry of Health negotiates drug prices with pharmaceutical suppliers and encourages the prescription of generic formulations when available. Despite several campaigns to inform the general public about the savings of using generic drugs, it is estimated that in 2013 Italians spent more than €850 million purchasing brand-name drugs (Assogenerici 2012).

Italian universities maintain forty medical schools with about 6,500–7,000 graduates every year, of which, in the last few years, about 60 per cent have been women (Ministero dell'Università e della Ricerca 2012). Since 1999, access to medical schools has been restricted by making it mandatory for each prospective medical student to pass an admission test. After obtaining their degree, medical graduates may apply to train in medical and surgical subspecialtes (four to six years with an entry salary of €18,600 per year) or to train as family practitioners (three years for a salary of €11,600 per year). The number of new positions for subspecialty training is set every year by central government (in 2012 the offer was for 5,000 positions) based on the available budget. In the last few years there has been a progressive decrease in opportunities for subspecialty training, resulting in more Italian medical graduates applying for training positions abroad, mainly in Europe, but also in North America. It has been estimated that the reduction in training opportunities will cause a significant shortage of subspecialty physicians in the near future, mainly in the areas of paediatrics, internal medicine, general surgery, psychiatry, public health, obstetrics and gynaecology, and radiology (Palermo *et al.* 2013). The number of positions for training family practitioners is set every year by the regions – which develop their own curricula – based on the available budget (in 2012 the offer was for 890 positions).

Italy maintains a professional association and accreditation body (Ordine dei Medici e degli Odontoiatri) for each province, which are federated into a national association and accreditation body of all physicians (Federazione Nazionale degli Ordini dei Medici Chirurghi e Odontoiatri). In Italy the Ministry of Education (Ministero dell'Istruzione, Università e Ricerca) provides accreditation to professional schools, including subspecialty training, reviews standards of training and certification for foreign-trained physicians, and develops standards for licensure. In 2010, according to the National Physicians' Pension Fund (Ente Nazionale Previdenza e Assistenza Medici 2012), there were 348,846 practicing physicians in Italy, of whom 37 per cent were women. The age distribution of physicians in Italy is skewed, with 42 per cent of practising physicians in the age group 50–60 years. In 2010, according to the Italian Ministry of Health, 107,448 physicians were employed by the SSN, of whom 37 per cent were women (Ministero della Salute 2013a). In 2011, there were 46,061 family practitioners and 7,716 family paediatricians (Ministero della Salute 2013b). In 2009 the physicians employed by the SSN earned an average of €63,000–93,000 depending on their experience and position (Ministero della Salute 2013c), while a family practitioner earned, on average, €85,000 (Ente Nazionale Previdenza e Assistenza Medici 2012). Despite the increasing number of women physicians practising within the SSN, it was recognised that they have fewer career opportunities than their male counterparts, with <15 per cent of the top medical positions being occupied by women (Ministero della Salute News 2011). Furthermore, average earnings are lower for Italian women physicians than for men in any age group (Ente Nazionale Previdenza e Assistenza Medici 2012).

In Italy, nursing education was traditionally provided through hospital-based programmes, but since 2004 nursing education has been moved to academic-based programmes (Ministero della Sanità 1994). Italian universities now maintain thirty-nine Schools of Nursing with three-year Bachelor of Science in Nursing Programmes and the possibility of then entering a two-year Degree of Science in Nursing Programme; graduates can then pursue further education at the master or doctoral level. Practising nurses are required to be registered with the provincial College of Nurses. In Italy, there are no nursing professionals, such as the nurse practitioners in the USA, offering an alternative to family practitioners for primary care in adults or to family paediatricians for the primary care of children and adolescents. The number of practising nurses in Italy is 6.3 per 1,000 population, well below the OECD average of 8.4 per 1,000 population (OECD 2013a). Foreign nurses represent over 10 per cent of the practising nurses in Italy (Fortunato 2012).

There are thirty-six Schools of Nursing providing a three-year Bachelor of Midwifery Programme in Italy. Midwives are required to be registered with the provincial College of Midwives. Midwifery graduates may pursue higher education through the master or doctoral programmes offered by

Table 9.1 Human and physical resources in Italy

Physicians per 1,000 population	4.1
Nurses per 1,000 population	6.3
Medical graduates per 100,000 population	11.0
Nursing graduates per 100,000 population	18.8
Total hospital beds per 1,000 population	3.4
Curative (acute) care beds per 1,000 population	2.8
Gynaecologists and obstetricians per 100,000 women	40.8
Registered midwives per 100,000 women	55.8

Source: OECD (2013c).

the Schools of Nursing. In Italy, the number of registered midwives is 55.8 per 100,000 women, lower than the OECD average of 69.8 per 100,000 women (Table 9.1). However, as midwives in Italy can also practise as nurses, this ratio is likely to be even lower.

Table 9.1 gives the ratios of health care practitioners and hospital beds to population in Italy.

Demographic profile

Italy is the fifth most populous country in Europe and the twenty-third most populous in the word, with a population of approximately sixty million inhabitants (United Nations Department of Economic and Social Affairs 2012; ISTAT 2014b). Italy's population is growing, largely fuelled by immigration and the high birth rate of immigrant women (ISTAT 2014b), but overall its growth is slower than the average for the world population (OECD 2013a). Italy's population density is one of the highest in Europe, with 35.4 per cent of the population living in predominantly urban areas. (ISTAT 2014b). Table 9.2 illustrates the demographic profile of contemporary Italy.

Italy recognises Italian as the official language, with 72.8 per cent of Italians exclusively or predominantly speaking Italian, 20 per cent alternating Italian with a local language, while only 5.4 per cent of Italians speak only a local language (ISTAT 2006). German and Ladin in the region of Trentino Alto Adige and French in Valle d'Aosta have equal status with the Italian language.

Immigration started in modern Italy in the 1970s. Since the early 1990s the number of immigrants entering the country has been increasing dramatically, with a peak in 2010 and a decrease thereafter, possibly because of the economic crisis (ISTAT 2014b). In 2012 there were 4.8 million foreign residents in Italy (7.4 per cent of the population), an increase of 8.3 per cent since the previous year (ISTAT 2014b). This increase is mainly due to immigration from foreign countries (321,000 individuals), but also to children born to foreign mothers (80,000 babies) (ISTAT 2014b). The most

Table 9.2 Demographic profile of Italy

Population	59,685,200
Women	30,795,600
Population aged 0–14 years	8,513,200
Women of childbearing age (15–44 years)	23,331,200
Population aged 65 years or older	12,301,500
Population annual growth (2002–2012) (%)	0.4
Population density per square kilometre	197.1
Total fertility rate (births per woman)	1.42
Crude birth rate per 1,000 people	9.0
Life expectancy at birth (years)	84.5 women; 79.4 men
Marriage rate per 1,000 people	3.5
Crude death rate (per 1,000 people)	10.3
Immigrant population (%)	7.4
Population living in predominantly urban areas (%)	35.4
Population living in intermediate areas (%)	43.7
Population living in predominantly rural areas (%)	20.9

Source: ISTAT (2014b).

represented countries of origin of the foreign residents of Italy are Romania (933,000), Albania (465,000), Morocco (427,000), China (223,000), Ukraine (192,000) and the Philippines (140,000). Naturalisation is increasing, although it remains a marginal phenomenon (65,400 foreign residents becoming Italian citizens in 2012) (ISTAT 2014c).

The health profile of Italy with respect to life expectancy is similar to other Western European countries. In 2012, Italy's life expectancy at birth was 79.4 years for men and 84.5 years for women, higher than the reported OECD average of 77.3 years and 82.8 years, respectively (OECD 2013a). Italy's fertility rate of 1.59 births per woman is considerably lower than the world average of 2.47 births per woman and falls below the USA (2.06 births per woman) and the UK (1.90 births per woman) (OECD 2013a).

Even though the overall health status of the country has improved significantly over the last century, there are persisting patterns of health disparities by income and by geographical area (the north/south divide) (Gonzales 2011). Unlike in countries such as Canada and the USA, an urban/rural divide does not affect health care access in Italy, as the distance to the next available medical facility is usually less than eighty kilometres. The greatest disparities in the quality of health care provided through the Italian SSN is by geographical area, with worsening in a variety of quality indicators moving from north to south in the peninsula. The 2014 report commissioned by the Ministry of Health to assess compliance with the essential levels of care and the quality of hospital services documented that southern regions – with the exception of Basilicata – were not fully compliant with the essential levels of care and that SSN hospitals in the south of Italy have the poorest performances (Ministero della

Salute 2014b), although positive changes were recorded compared with the previous report (Ministero della Salute 2012). The disparities in health care between southern and northern Italian regions reflect disparities in income, education and employment that the recent economic crisis has further exacerbated.

Maternity provision

In Italy, maternity care is included in the essential levels of care and is provided free of charge to all women, regardless of their nationality or immigration status. Foreign pregnant women who have entered the country without a visa may obtain a temporary visa (Permesso di Soggiorno) until six months after childbirth (Law 286/98 1998; DPR 394/99 1999).

The outpatient family services (Consultori Familiari) were instituted in 1975 (Law 405/75 1975) to provide a wide range of services to the family, including family planning, antenatal and postnatal maternity services, prevention of cervical and breast cancer, and assisted medical fertilisation (Law 40/04 2004). The outpatient family services are managed at the regional level. Health care professionals working at the outpatient family services are gynaecologists, paediatricians, midwives, nurses, nurse educators, psychologists and social workers. Women may also choose to receive private care during pregnancy, either by a hospital-based obstetrician or an obstetrician working in a private practice. The proportion of women selecting either form of care varies significantly among regions, probably depending on the level and quality of care provided by the local outpatient family services (Ministero della Salute 2010). The outpatient family services are the predominant source of antenatal maternity services to immigrant women and women of lower socio-economic status (Ministero della Salute 2010). Since 2000 the planning of the SSN has incorporated an ambitious project on maternal and child health (Progetto Obiettivo Materno-Infantile) (DM 24/04/2000 2000) that identifies the outpatient family services as the main provider of health care services to women and children. The Progetto Obiettivo Materno-Infantile promotes the integration of primary (health promotion, preventive services), secondary (specialist care, outpatient diagnostic procedures) and tertiary (complex care, diagnostics) health care services, the prioritisation of health care objectives, the empowerment of patients and families, an active offer of services tailored to the need of specific patient populations, planning and assessment of health care services and training of health care personnel. The Progetto Obiettivo Materno-Infantile details in the Pathway to Birth (Percorso Nascita) give the objectives, planning and assessment of the entire range of maternity services offered through the SSN.

In Italy in 2010 there were 531 hospitals with a birth centre (Punto Nascita) (Ministero della Salute 2013d). Of the 531 hospitals with a birth centre, 124 have a neonatel intensive care unit (103 of these are in hospitals with >1,000 deliveries/year) and 205 have neonatology divisions (136 of these are in centres with >1,000 deliveries/year). Women may choose to deliver their babies in a SSN hospital or a private hospital providing services to the SSN (88.2 per cent) or in a private clinic (in the latter case paying for their services out-of-pocket or through a private health insurance) (11.8 per cent) (Ministero della Salute 2013d). Of all the deliveries in 2010, 67.9 per cent occurred in hospitals with more than 1,000 deliveries/year (208 hospitals), 25 per cent in hospitals with 500–1,000 deliveries/year (188 hospitals) and 7.1 per cent in hospitals with less than 500 deliveries/year (135 hospitals). Smaller birth centres are not cost-efficient to manage and tend to have more caesarean deliveries than larger centres, probably because of staffing issues. Birth centres with more than 1,000 deliveries/year are predominantly in northern Italy, while medium and small birth centres are more common in central and southern Italy (Ministero della Salute 2013d). A 2010 agreement between the central government and the regions (Conferenza Stato Regioni 2010) proposed the progressive closure of smaller birth centres to improve cost-efficiency and safety and to decrease the number of caesarean sections, for which Italy rates first in Europe (37.5 per cent in 2012; OECD 2013c).

Since 1978, the voluntary interruption of pregnancy within ninety days of pregnancy has been legal in Italy (Law 194/78 1978), but can only be performed in an SSN facility. Abortion is included in the minimum standards of health care and is provided free of charge to all women, regardless of their nationality or immigration status (Law 286/98 1998; DPR 394/99 1999). In the case of severe foetal malformations or chromosomal/genetic diseases, voluntary interruption of pregnancy may also be performed at a later gestational age (until twenty weeks of gestation). Parental consent is required for minors to have an abortion, although minors denied parental consent may obtain authorisation for the procedure by a judge (Law 194/78 1978). Health care professionals have the choice to opt out and not provide professional services related to inducing an abortion, with the exception of providing care in the case of a medical emergency (Law 194/78 1978). Of the obstetric/gynaecology specialists working in SSN facilities, on average 69.3 per cent have opted out, making it difficult to guarantee access to the voluntary interruption of pregnancy in some regions (Ministero della Salute 2013e)

Every year in Italy, approximately 400 newborn babies are given up for adoption straight after birth. To prevent newborn babies from being abandoned in unsafe conditions, Italy has implemented the Secret Mother (Madre Segreta) programme, which guarantees anonymity to any woman who does not want to keep her newborn baby. The programme allows women not to be recorded with their names when entering a hospital for delivery (DPR 396/2000 2000) and takes care of the adoption of the newborn babies. Some hospitals and religious institutions provide monitored heated cribs, where an unwanted newborn baby can be safely abandoned and provided with care within minutes.

Maternity entitlements

Italy's maternity entitlements are funded through the Istituto Nazionale di Previdenza Sociale for all women who are employed and some of those who are self-employed. Part-time employees and seasonal workers may be eligible if they fulfil specific requirements (DLgs 151/2001 2001).

During pregnancy women cannot be employed in any activity that may endanger the pregnancy (e.g. exposure to radiation or toxic substances, physically demanding jobs or night shifts) and cannot be laid off work. Italy's maternity leave policies include five months of paid maternity leave (at 80 to 100 per cent of the current salary), two months before and three months after delivery. The maternity leave can be extended for an additional six months within the first three years of the baby's life, with a pay reduction of 70 per cent of the current salary. Maternity leave is granted to the father if the mother is deceased, or unable or unwilling to care for the newborn baby. Parental leave provisions entitle both legal parents to six months paid leave up to a combined ten months of paid leave between the two parents. Mothers typically take most of the leave so, to incentivise paternal leave, if a father takes all of his six months of leave, an additional month of leave will be granted. Single parents are entitled to ten months of paid parental leave. Similar entitlements are also granted in the case of adoption.

Childbirth in Italy

In Italy, information on pregnancy and delivery are collected for each birth through the Certificate of Delivery Assistance (CeDAP). The CeDAP is a nationwide mandatory questionnaire, completed by the midwife or physician attending the delivery, which collects information about the parents, the pregnancy, the delivery and the newborn baby (DM 349/2000). The CeDAP data are compiled at the regional level and then provided to the Ministry of Health, which, every two years, issues a report based on the analysis of CeDAP data to guide planning services to care for women at the time of delivery (Ministero della Salute 2013d). Data collected through the CeDAP is one of the most important sources of information about childbirth in Italy.

Antenatal care

The Istituto Superiore di Sanità has published updated guidelines for the prenatal care to be delivered through the SSN facilities (Ministero della Salute, Sistema Nazionale per le Linee Guida 2011), derived from those developed by the National Collaborating Centre for Women's and Children's Health (National Collaborating Centre for Women's and Children's Health 2008). According to these guidelines, during a normal pregnancy women should be offered no less than four visits with their health care provider and three ultrasound scans at ten to thirteen weeks of gestation (dating of pregnancy), twenty to twenty-two weeks (foetal morphology) and twenty-eight to thirty-two weeks (foetal growth).

The first visit is ideally planned before ten weeks of gestation to provide information on maternity services and entitlements, identify pregnancies at increased risk, offer screening for haemoglobinopathies, rhesus status, infectious diseases (e.g. HIV, rubella, syphilis and toxoplasmosis), provide information on screening and prenatal diagnosis of Down's syndrome and other chromosomal diseases, and offer a Pap smear if this has not been performed in the last three years. Furthermore, women are offered information on classes on pregnancy, types of delivery, breastfeeding, baby care and parenting (Corsi di Accompagnamento alla Nascita).

During the second trimester, pregnant women are checked for anaemia, hypertension, gestational diabetes (a 75 g oral glucose tolerance test is offered to women with risk factors), rubella and toxoplasmosis in serologically negative women. During the third trimester, pregnant women are checked for anaemia and are screened for vaginal beta-haemolytic streptococcus, toxoplasmosis, hepatitis B, hepatitis C and syphilis; rhesus-negative women receive anti-D prophylaxis. Preparation for labour and delivery is also discussed. Women with a breech presentation are offered external cephalic rotation to be performed after thirty-seven weeks of gestation. To limit the risks of an over-term pregnancy, induction of labour is offered to all women with an uncomplicated pregnancy from forty-one to forty-two weeks.

For pregnancies at increased risk (e.g. placenta previa, pre-gestational and gestational diabetes, hypertension, pre-eclampsia and other co-morbidities), the number and frequency of clinic visits and ultrasound scans are higher. According to the 2010 CeDAP Report, 98.1 per cent of women delivering a baby in Italy in 2010 received antenatal care (Ministero della Salute 2013d), with similar rates among Italian and immigrant women (98.3 and 97.4 per cent, respectively). Only 4.8 per cent of women initiated prenatal care after the first trimester – 2.9 per cent among Italian women and 13.8 per cent among immigrant women, possibly reflecting differences in both cultural practices and access to care (Ministero della Salute 2013d). Women younger than twenty years of age and women with a lower level of education were more likely to receive their first antenatal visit after the first trimester (Ministero della Salute 2013d). The majority of pregnant women attended more than the recommended four antenatal visits with their health care provider (84.8 per cent) and had more than the recommended three ultrasound scans during pregnancy (72.3 per cent), even when only women with a normal uncomplicated pregnancy were considered (Ministero della Salute 2013d). Significant regional differences were documented in the average number of visits and ultrasound scans during pregnancy (Ministero della Salute 2013d).

A 2010–2011 survey of 3,595 women in eleven regions of Italy documented that 61 per cent of immigrant women and 11 per cent of Italian women received antenatal care at an outpatient family services facility (Consultorio Familiare), while 23.1 per cent of immigrant women and 78.5 per cent of Italian women received antenatal care from private obstetricians/gynaecologists (either hospital-based or working in a private clinic), probably reflecting differences in socio-economic status (Istituto Superiore di Sanità 2012). The same survey reported that, among women experiencing their first pregnancy, 63.4 per cent of Italian women and 41 per cent of immigrant women attended educational classes on pregnancy, delivery and parenting. Attendance was considerably lower for subsequent pregnancies (Istituto Superiore di Sanità 2012).

In 2010, the overall proportion of pregnant women having an amniocentesis was 13.6 per cent, increasing to 38.7 per cent among those aged more than forty years (Ministero della Salute 2013d). The proportion of pregnant women having an amniocentesis shows significant geographical variations, being <12 per cent in southern regions (with the exception of Campania and Sardinia) and >25 per cent in Umbria and Valle d'Aosta.

Intrapartum care

The outcomes of pregnancies for selected years from 1970 to 2010 are shown in Table 9.3.

In Italy the maternal mortality ratio has decreased from ten deaths per 100,000 live births in 1990 to four deaths per 100,000 live births in 2010, a 65 per cent improvement over a twenty-year period. The maternal mortality ratio in Italy is lower than that of Canada (twelve deaths per 100,000 live births), the USA (twenty-one deaths per 100,000 live births) and is one of the lowest in Europe (WHO, UNICEF, UNFPA and the World Bank 2012). However, some evidence suggests that when the detection of maternal death relies only on the death certificate, the maternal mortality ratio is underestimated by 20 to >90 per cent. In fact, when a more accurate system of surveillance was set in place in five Italian regions (comprising 49 per cent of the women of childbearing age), a maternal mortality ratio of 11.8 deaths per 100,000 live births was estimated for the period 2000–2007 (Donati *et al.* 2011).

Infant mortality rates in Italy have been declining steadily over the last 40 years to 3.4 deaths per 1,000 live births in 2010, below the European Union and OECD averages of 4.2 and 4.1 deaths per 1,000 live births, respectively (OECD 2013c). Infant mortality rates in Italy are lower than in the USA (6.1 deaths per 1,000 live births), Canada (4.9 deaths per 1,000 live births) and the UK (4.3 deaths per 1,000 live births) (OECD 2013c).

Table 9.3 Birth interventions and outcomes for selected years in Italy

	1970*	1980*	1990*	2000*	2010*
Maternal mortality ratio, deaths per 100,000 live births	–	–	10.0[a]	4.0[a]	4.0[a]
					11.8[b]
Foetal deaths per 1,000 live births [c]	–	–	–	–	2.7
Neonatal deaths per 1,000 live births	–	–	6.3[c]	3.4[e]	2.4[e]
Infant mortality per 1,000 live births [f]	29.6	14.6	8.1	4.3	3.4
Induction of labor per 1,000 non-elective C-sections [c]	–	–	–	–	197
Caesarean per 100 deliveries	–	11.2[d]	22.4[d]	35.3[d]	37.5[c]

Sources: a WHO *et al.* (2012); b Donati *et al.* (2011); c Ministero della Salute (2013d); d XII Commissione Permanente, Igiene e Sanità (2012); e World Bank (2013); f OECD (2013c).

Note
* Or the most recent available year.

In 2011, 7.1 per cent of babies had a birthweight <2,500 g, slightly higher than the OECD average of 6.8 per cent and ranking twenty-fourth among thirty-nine OECD countries (OECD 2013c). The proportion of low birth-weight babies increased by 27 per cent from 1990 to 2011, probably due to changes common to Western nations, such as women giving birth at older ages, more multiple births as a result of assisted reproduction techniques and increased rates of induction of labour and caesarean deliveries of infants at premature or late preterm gestations (OECD 2013c).

Women deliver their babies in a SSN hospital (88.2 per cent), a private hospital providing services to the SSN (11.4 per cent) or in a private clinic (0.4 per cent) (Ministero della Salute 2013d). In the southern regions of Italy more women deliver in hospitals with <1,000 deliveries/year and in private hospitals providing services to the SSN than in the northern regions (Ministero della Salute 2013d). Hospitalisation for delivery in an SSN hospital or a private hospital providing services to the SSN is free of charge, whereas for delivery in a private clinic the services are paid out-of-pocket or through private health insurance. Only <0.1 per cent of deliveries occur outside hospital (Ministero della Salute 2013d) and these take place either at home or in one of the very few Case Maternità (the equivalent of Birth Centres in the UK and USA or the Maisons de Naissance in France). Only a few regions provide a partial reimbursement (about €800) of the expenses incurred by women who make the choice of delivering at home.

The rate of caesarean deliveries in Italy has risen dramatically, reaching 37.5 per cent in 2010, ranking first in Europe and well above the OECD average of 25.8 per cent (Ministero della Salute 2013d; OECD 2013c). The rate of caesarean delivery is higher among Italian (39.5 per cent) than immigrant (28.8 per cent) women (Ministero della Salute 2013d) and varies significantly among regions, with the southern regions having rates above 40 per cent (Ministero della Salute 2013d). Caesarean delivery rates are higher in private hospitals providing services to the SSN (58.3 per cent) and in private clinics (78.8 per cent) than in SSN hospitals (34.6 per cent). Although there is worldwide agreement that caesarean delivery can be life-saving, it is acknowledged that under non-emergency conditions caesarean sections are associated with a higher maternal mortality and morbidity than vaginal deliveries (Hall and Bewley 1999; Deneux-Tharaux *et al.* 2006). The WHO recommends that rates of delivery by caesarean section should not exceed 15 per cent of the total deliveries, although acknowledging that there is no evidence for an optimum percentage or range of percentages of caesarean deliveries (WHO, UNFPA, UNICEF and AMDD 2009). In efforts to reduce Italy's high rates of caesarean deliveries, the Istituto Superiore di Sanità released national guidelines for caesarean section delivery (Ministero della Salute, Sistema Nazionale per le Linee Guida 2012). Additional actions to reduce the high rates of caesarean deliveries include increasing the offer of educational classes and the presence of midwives in the care of pregnant women, making epidural analgesia more available in SSN hospitals, offering specific training to obstetricians/gynaecologists and specialists on the management of vaginal deliveries, and acting on the reimbursement policy (increasing the reimbursement for delivery without a differential between vaginal and caesarean delivery) (Conferenza Stato Regioni 2010). The progressive closure of smaller birth centres (< 1,000 deliveries/year) will also contribute to reducing the number of caesarean sections in line with the goal set by the Istituto Superiore di Sanità of less than 20 per cent, because in smaller centres elective caesarean delivery is often a consequence of staffing issues (Conferenza Stato Regioni 2010).

In 2010 the overall proportion of women who had a vaginal delivery after a caesarean section was 10.3 per cent, with higher proportions at SSN hospitals (11.2 per cent) than in private hospitals providing services to the SSN (6.6 per cent) or in private clinics (7.2 per cent).

A survey conducted across Italy in samples of 3,699 women in 2008–2009 and 3,594 women in 2010–2011 (response rate >95 per cent) interviewed after delivery provides data on the induction of labour, epidural analgesia and episiotomy among both Italian and immigrant women (Istituto Superiore di Sanità 2012). After excluding elective caesarean sections, the induction of labour increased from 18.3 per cent to 20.4 per cent among Italian women and decreased from 15.8 per cent to 9.5 per cent among immigrant women (Istituto Superiore di Sanità 2012). The overall increase in the induction of labour occurred despite WHO recommendations to limit the induction of labour to women with clear medical indications and when the expected benefits outweigh the potential harm (WHO, UNFPA, UNICEF and AMDD 2009). The use of epidural analgesia increased from 14.0 to 19.7 per cent among Italian women and from 3.3 to 6.6 per cent among immigrant women (Istituto Superiore di Sanità 2012). Although epidural analgesia has been included among the essential levels of care provided through the SSN since 2012, in 2014 only seventy-five hospitals in the country were offering epidural analgesia twenty-four hours a day, with the majority of facilities limiting the offer to week days and during the day. The use of episiotomy remains high, despite a decline from 45.5 to 41.7 per cent among Italian women and from 54.4 to 36.3 per cent among immigrant women (Istituto Superiore di Sanità 2012). Episiotomies, a once-routine practice, are now not recommended by the WHO because there is no evidence that their routine use is beneficial, while there is solid evidence that they cause lasting harm to the perineum (Klein *et al.* 1992; Woolley 1995).

Postnatal care

To reduce costs, the length of postpartum hospital stays for mothers in Italy has decreased over time. After a vaginal birth, the average hospital stay was 4.1 days in 1999 and 3.5 days in 2011, while after a caesarean delivery the average hospital stay was 6.4 days in 1999 and 4.7 days in 2011 (ISTAT 2000, 2013). After being discharged from hospital all new mothers receive postnatal care through the outpatient facilities of SSN hospitals or hospitals providing services to the SSN, through SSN outpatient family services or, if they chose, by private health care providers.

A survey conducted in 2004–2005 of 60,000 women who delivered in the previous five years showed that 81.1 per cent breastfed, with 65.4 per cent exclusively breastfeeding for some time (ISTAT 2006). The duration of breastfeeding was on average 7.3 months, a 1.2 month increase from the previous survey conducted in 1999–2000 (ISTAT 2006). In an effort to improve maternal–child health in the immediate postpartum period, in 2009 Italian regions started promoting the Baby-Friendly Hospital Initiative (Ospedale Amico dei Bambini programme), a WHO programme aiming to improve the care of pregnant women, mothers and babies and to encourage breastfeeding (Labbok 2012). By 2014, there were twenty Baby-Friendly Hospitals and local health communities in Italy (Bettinelli *et al.* 2012). A more recent survey conducted in the Lombardy region in 2012 of 1898 women who delivered at term after a normal pregnancy (Regione Lombardia Sanità 2012) showed that 95.6 per cent of mothers were breastfeeding at the time of hospital discharge (67.3 per cent exclusive breastfeeding), a rate above the OECD average, but behind the Nordic countries (with initiation rates above 97 per cent) (OECD 2014). As for the duration of breastfeeding, 67.8 per cent of mothers were breastfeeding at three months (47.3 per cent exclusive breastfeeding), 60.8 per cent at 5 months (27.0 per cent exclusive breastfeeding) and 32.2 per cent at 11 months (1.2 per cent exclusive breastfeeding). These proportions are higher than those recorded in 2006 when the Lombardy region started implementing programmes for health care providers and women to promote and sustain breastfeeding.

Consumer involvement

A survey conducted across Italy in a sample of 3,699 women in 2008–2009 and 3,594 women in 2010–2011 interviewed after delivery (response rate >95 per cent) provides data on women's satisfaction with maternal services (Istituto Superiore di Sanità 2012). The majority of women were satisfied with their delivery experience (82.4 per cent among Italian women and 83.9 per cent among immigrant women). However, satisfaction with their delivery experience was lower among women who had a caesarean delivery than among women who had a vaginal delivery. Epidural analgesia did not change the level of satisfaction among women who had a vaginal delivery. More than 90 per cent of women were satisfied with the care they received during labour and delivery. Both Italian and immigrant women rated the care by midwives as the best, compared with that by physicians and nurses

(Istituto Superiore di Sanità 2012). It is important to acknowledge that women's satisfaction with their delivery experience is not an adequate measure of the quality of care.

The National Observatory for Women's Health (Osservatorio per la Salute della Donna) has compiled standards to assess maternity services for deliveries (Osservatorio per la Salute della Donna 2012), but does not propose specific tools for assessing customer satisfaction. In Italy, over 90 per cent of women having a vaginal delivery had their partner in the room during labour and delivery (Ministero della Salute 2013d). No assessment of fathers' satisfaction in maternity services is available in Italy; this kind of assessment is also lacking for other countries in Europe and North America.

In Italy, less than 0.1 per cent of deliveries occur outside hospital (Ministero della Salute 2013d). It is no surprise therefore that there are only four Case Maternità in the country and very few midwives provide delivery care in the home. Although delivering in an SSN hospital is free of charge, delivering at home or in a birth centre may not always be reimbursed by the SSN. Despite evidence that delivering at home may be safe for well-selected women (Cheyney 2014), there is limited interest among professionals, women's advocacy groups and health care providers in supporting the decision of women to deliver at home.

Risk and rights

In Italy, the SSN covers maternity care services for all women, regardless of their economic or citizenship status. However, four intertwined issues prevent women from taking full advantage of the maternity services offered: (1) the north/south divide in health care; (2) the excessive medicalisation of pregnancy; (3) barriers to accessing maternity services among first-generation immigrant women; and (4) an underestimation of the importance of women's empowerment.

Although there is no difference in entitlements, the standard of care across regions varies considerably, with an evident north/south divide. The 2014 report commissioned by the Ministry of Health to assess compliance with the minimum standards of health care and the quality of hospital services documented that southern regions, with the exception of Basilicata, were not fully compliant with the minimum standards of health care and that SSN hospitals in the south of Italy have the poorest performances (Ministero della Salute 2014b), although very positive changes were recorded from the previous report (Ministero della Salute 2012).

As expected, the north/south divide in health care is also reflected in maternity services. Going from north to south, the proportion of smaller birth centres (<500 deliveries per year) and of birth centres based in private hospitals increases, while the proportion of birth centres offering epidural analgesia some of the time (at least during the day on week days) or twenty-four hours a day decreases dramatically. Most concerning of all is the increase in the maternal mortality ratio going from north to south, which peaks at 21.8 maternal deaths per 100,000 deliveries in Sicily, almost twice the national average. The decision of the Ministry of Health to progressively close smaller birth centres (Conferenza Stato Regioni 2010), although based on solid evidence of low cost-efficiency and low safety, is often delayed by the local opposition of those who value the convenience of a short commute over sustainable quality maternity services for all.

Including epidural analgesia among the minimum standards of health care in 2012, i.e. making epidural analgesia an essential level of care provided by all SSN hospitals at no charge, has been controversial, with both the general public and health care professionals supporting either 'natural delivery' or the right of women to request epidural analgesia during labour. Because there is no specific SSN reimbursement for epidural analgesia, hospitals have no financial incentive to provide such a service to women in labour. It is no surprise that the regions with the highest proportion of hospitals offering epidural analgesia are those providing specific dedicated funding. Furthermore, as there is no reporting of epidural analgesia in the CeDAP, nor specific reimbursement, tracking the use of epidural analgesia at the population level is not possible.

A significant medicalisation of pregnancy is documented by the high number of scans during pregnancy (average 5.3 scans) (Ministero della Salute 2013d), the high rate of caesarean deliveries (37.5 per cent in 2010, the highest in Europe) (OECD 2013c) and the high rate of episiotomies (40 per cent – at least twice the rate reported in most European countries) (Istituto Superiore di Sanità 2012; EURO-PERISTAT Project with Surveillance of Cerebral Palsy in Europe (SCPE) and European Surveillance of Congenital Anomalies (EUROCAT) 2013). Medicalisation is the likely consequence of antenatal care being predominantly provided by hospital-based professionals, who specialise in higher risk pregnancies and use a more interventionist approach to care, even in uncomplicated pregnancies and births (Istituto Superiore di Sanità 2012). The north/south divide is also evident in the medicalisation of pregnancy.

The average number of scans during pregnancy is higher in southern Italy, with 41 per cent of women having seven or more scans during pregnancy compared with 20 per cent in northern Italy (Ministero della Salute 2013d). The rate of caesarean deliveries is almost twice that recorded in northern Italy, with a peak in the region of Campania, where over 60 per cent of deliveries occur by caesarean section (Ministero della Salute 2013d). However, the induction of labour is lower in southern Italy, probably as a result of the high rate of caesarean deliveries (Ministero della Salute 2013d). The rate of episiotomy is very high in southern Italy, with 73 per cent of women having this invasive procedure compared with 48 per cent in northern Italy (Grandolfo et al. 2002), although the national rate has been decreasing in the last few years (Istituto Superiore di Sanità

2012). As there is no reporting of episiotomy in the CeDAP, nor specific reimbursement for the procedure, tracking its use at the population level is virtually impossible. Thus, although recipients of maternity care have the right to care at a macro-level, the risks and medicalisation of pregnancy are higher in some areas of Italy.

In 2012 there were 4.8 million foreign residents (7.4 per cent of the population) in Italy, with foreign women having a higher birth rate than Italian women (2.37 and 1.29, respectively) (ISTAT 2013). It is therefore no surprise that, in the last decade, the number of children born to foreign mothers has been progressively increasing (80,000 of newborn babies in 2012 – 15 per cent of all newborn babies) (ISTAT 2014b). A population-based study in the Lazio region documented poorer pregnancy outcomes – including very preterm and preterm birth rates, a low Apgar score, respiratory distress, the need for a neonatal intensive care unit, neonatal death and malformations – among immigrant women compared with Italian women, especially for women from sub-Saharan and West Africa (Cacciani *et al.* 2011).

Although the proportion of women receiving antenatal care is similar among Italian and immigrant women (98.3 and 97.4 per cent, respectively) (Ministero della Salute 2013d), some of the data suggest that access to care may be far from optimal for immigrant women. Compared with Italian women, immigrant women are more likely to initiate prenatal care after the first trimester (13.8 and 2.9 per cent, respectively) (Ministero della Salute 2013d), less likely to attend educational classes on pregnancy, delivery and parenting (41.0 and 63.4 per cent, respectively) or to take folic acid before (8.6 and 23.2 per cent, respectively) and during pregnancy (72.0 and 62.6 per cent, respectively) (Istituto Superiore di Sanità 2012). Immigrant women were more likely to receive antenatal care at an outpatient family services facility than Italian women (61.0 and 11.0 per cent, respectively), less likely to have a caesarean delivery (28.8 and 39.5 per cent, respectively) (Ministero della Salute 2013d) and less likely to have epidural analgesia during labour (6.6 and 19.7 per cent, respectively) (Istituto Superiore di Sanità 2012).

At the micro-level, women have different views about what they want from maternity care. However, some disturbing data suggests that the involvement of women in decisions about their pregnancy and delivery is often limited in Italy and the importance of women's empowerment in relation to childbearing and delivery is still grossly underestimated. A major tool for women's empowerment is childbirth education classes. Although the outpatient family services provide educational classes on pregnancy, delivery and parenting, the offer of such classes is often not tailored to the needs of specific groups of pregnant women (e.g. working women, immigrant women or women living in rural areas), resulting in a low attendance among the women who need these classes the most (Istituto Superiore di Sanità 2012).

Maternity care in Italy is based on the Western medical tradition of physician-attended hospital birth and it is no surprise that women traditionally choose hospital-based professionals for antenatal care. Therefore delivering outside a hospital in Italy is an unlikely option, as there are very few midwifery-led facilities and only a few regions provide partial reimbursement for the expenses of delivering at home or in Casa Maternità.

In the hospital setting support for women in labour is still limited. Epidural analgesia is available in less than half of birth centres, with only 13.3 per cent of facilities providing this option twenty-four hours a day (Pavanello 2012). Increasing the offer of epidural analgesia within SSN facilities will be very challenging with shrinking hospital budgets. It is also interesting to note that no official document listing the hospitals providing epidural analgesia is available from the web site of the Italian Ministry of Health.

Episiotomy is often presented to women in labour as an 'inevitable' or 'emergency' procedure, although the dramatic variations in the proportion of women having an episiotomy among hospitals in the same region (from 5 to 70 per cent of normal deliveries) do not support the view that this procedure is performed according to current guidelines (Assessorato della Sanità Regione Piemonte 2006). Furthermore, many women report not being previously informed in detail about the procedure, the pain involved and the potential short- and long-term side-effects.

Although all delivery rooms in the 1990s were equipped to accommodate the choice of women to take different positions during labour, only a minority of natural births occur where women are free to choose the positions they prefer during labour and delivery (Assessorato della Sanità Regione Piemonte 2006).

Conclusion

In Italy, the SSN offers universal maternity services and is currently engaged in significant efforts to improve access to maternity care for all, despite differences in compliance with the essential levels of care and the excessive medicalisation of pregnancy in different regions. The north/south divide and the growing numbers of foreign women of childbearing age are the greatest future challenges to maternity services in Italy. Acknowledging the importance of women's empowerment will help to reduce the excessive medicalisation of pregnancy in Italy, with positive effects on women and their children and public health in general.

Acknowledgements

A special thanks is given to Gooitske Algera and Philip and Olga Eaton for being lifelong inspirations in women's health and to Nicoletta Dozio MD and Maria Teresa Castiglioni MD for critical review of the manuscript.

References

Assessorato della Sanità Regione Piemonte (2006) *Nascere in Piemonte* (Being born in Pidmont) [in Italian] [online]. Available from: www.regione.piemonte.it/sanita/program_sanita/dip_materno_inf/dwd/nas_piem.pdf. Accessed 24 May 2014.

Assogenerici (2014) La scelta del farmaco branded rispetto al generico "costa" agli italiani 850 mln l'anno (The choice of a brand rather than generic drug is costing Italian citizens 850 million euro every year) [in Italian] [online]. Available from: www.equivalente.it/news/assogenerici/667-assogenerici-la-scelta-del-farmaco-branded-rispetto-al-generico-qcostaq-agli-italiani-850-mln-lanno/. Accessed 27 May 2014.

Bettinelli, M.E., Chapin, E.M. and Cattaneo, A. (2012) 'Establishing the Baby-Friendly Community Initiative in Italy: development, strategy, and implementation', *Journal of Human Lactation*, 28: 297–303.

Cacciani, L., Asole, S., Polo, A., Franco, F., Lucchini, R., De Curtis, M., Di Lallo, D. and Guasticchi, G. (2011) 'Perinatal outcomes among immigrant mothers over two periods in a region of central Italy', *BMC Public Health*, 11: 294–305.

Cheyney, M., Bovbjerg, M., Everson, C., Gordon, W., Hannibal, D. and Vedam, S. (2014) 'Outcomes of care for 16,924 planned home births in the United States: the Midwives Alliance of North America Statistics Project, 2004 to 2009', *Journal of Midwifery and Womens Health*, 59: 17–27.

Conferenza Stato Regioni (2010) 'Linee di indirizzo per la promozione ed il miglioramento della qualità della sicurezza e dell'appropriatezza degli interventi assistenziali nel percorso nascita e per la riduzione del taglio cesareo' (Guidelines for promoting and improving the quality, safety and appropriateness of care in the "Pathway to Birth" and for reducing caesarean section rates) [in Italian], *Gazzetta Ufficiale*, 13: 18 January 2011.

Deneux-Tharaux, C., Carmona, E., Bouvier-Colle, M.H. and Bréart, G. (2006) 'Postpartum maternal mortality and cesarean delivery', *Obstetrics and Gynecology*, 108 (3 Pt 1): 541–548.

Directive 2011/24/EU (2011) 'On the application of patient's rights in cross-border healthcare', *Official Journal of the European Union*, 4 April 2011.

DLgs 151/2001 (2001) 'Testo unico delle disposizioni legislative in materia di tutela e sostegno della maternità e della paternità' (Consolidated act of the legal provisions concerning the safeguard and support of maternity and paternity) [in Italian], *Gazzetta Ufficiale*, 96, 26 April 2001.

DM 24/04/2000 (2000) 'Adozione del progetto obiettivo materno-infantile relativo al "Piano sanitario nazionale per il triennio 1998-2000" (Adopting the mother-and-child focus project within the "National Healthcare Plan for the years 1998-2000") [in Italian]', *Gazzetta Ufficiale* 131 (Suppl. 89), 7 June 2000.

DM 349/2000 (2000) Modificazioni al certificato di assistenza al parto, per la rilevazione dei dati di sanita' pubblica e statistici di base relativi agli eventi di nascita, alla nati-mortalita' ed ai nati affetti da malformazioni (Amendments to the delivery assistance certificate for colleting healthcare and basic statistical data relating to childbirth, stillbirth and newborns with malformations) [in Italian] [online]. Available from: www.trovanorme.salute.gov.it/norme/dettaglioAtto?id=17312. Accessed 24 May 2014.

Donati, S., Senatore, S. and Ronconi, A. (2011) 'Regional maternal mortality working group. Maternal mortality in Italy: a record-linkage study', *British Journal of Obstetrics and Gynecology*, 118: 872–879.

Dossier Ticket 2012 (2014) *Dossier Ticket 2012* [online]. Available from: www.quotidi-anosanita.it/allegati/create_pdf.php?all=3843437.pdf. Accessed 27 May 2014.

DPR 394/99 (1999) 'Regolamento recante norme di attuazione del testo unico delle disposizioni concernenti la disciplina dell'immigrazione e norme sulla condizione dello straniero, a norma dell'articolo 1, comma 6, del decreto legislativo 25 luglio 1998, n. 286' (Procedures for implementing the consolidated act of the provisions on immigration control and regulation of alien status (article 1, paragraph 6 of Law 286/98)) [in Italian], *Gazzetta Ufficiale*, 258, 3 November 1999.

DPR 396/2000 (2000) 'Regolamento per la revisione e la semplificazione dell'ordinamento dello stato civile, a norma dell'articolo 2, comma 12, della legge 15 maggio 1997, n. 127' (Regulations for revision and simplification of the civil status system, according to article 2, paragraph 12, Law 127/1997) [in Italian], *Gazzetta Ufficiale*, 303, 30 December 2000.

Ente Nazionale Previdenza e Assistenza Medici (2012) *Annuario Statistico 2010* (Italian Statistics Yearbook 2010) [in Italian] [online]. Available from: www.enpam.it/la-fondazione/bilancio/annuario-statistico. Accessed 27 May 2014.

Esping-Andersen, G. (1990) *The Three Worlds of Welfare Capitalism*. Cambridge: Polity Press and Princeton: Princeton University Press.

EURO-PERISTAT Project with SCPE and European Surveillance of Congenital Anomalies (EUROCAT) (2013) *European Perinatal Health Report. The Health and Care of Pregnant Women and Babies in Europe in 2010* [online]. Available from: www.europeristat.com. Accessed 30 May 2014.

Ferrera, M. (1996) 'The 'southern model' of welfare in social Europe', *Journal of European Social Policy*, 6: 17–23.

Fortunato, E. (2012) 'Gli infermieri stranieri in Italia: quanti sono, da dove vengono e come sono distribuiti' (Foreign nursing professionals: how many they are, where they come from and where they work) [in Italian], *L'infermiere*, 1: 9–14.

Gonzale, S. (2011) 'The North/South divide in Italy and England: discursive construction of regional inequality', *European Urban and Regional Studies*, 18: 62–76.

Grandolfo, M., Donati, S. and Sereni, A. (2002) *Indagine Conoscitiva sul Percorso Nascita, 2001. Aspetti Metodologici e Risultati Nazionali* (Survey on the 'Pathway to Birth', 2001. Methods and national results) [in Italian] [online]. Available from: www.epicentro.iss.it/problemi/percorso-nascita/ind-pdf/nascita-1.pdf. Accessed 30 May 2014.

Hall, M. and Bewely, S. (1999) 'Maternal mortality and mode of delivery', *Lancet*, 354: 776.

Heritage Foundation (2014) *2014 Index of Economic Freedom* [online] Available from: www.heritage.org/index/. Accessed 20 May 2014.

International Monetary Fund (2013) *World Economic Outlook: Italy*. October 2013 data. [online]. Available from: www.imf.org/external/pubs/ft/weo/2013/02/weodata/weorept.aspx. Accessed 20 May 2014.

ISTAT (2000) *Annuario Statistico Italiano 2000* (Italian Statistics Yearbook 2000) [in Italian] [online]. Available from: www3.istat.it/dati/catalogo/20101119_00/. Accessed 24 May 2014.

ISTAT (2006) *Gravidanza, parto, allattamento al seno, 2004–2005* (Pregnancy, delivery, breastfeeding, 2004-2005) [in Italian] [online]. Available www3.istat.it/salastampa/comunicati/non_calendario/20060605_00/. Accessed 24 May 2014.

ISTAT (2009) *La Vita Quotidiana nel 2009. Analisi multiscopo annuale sulle famiglie "Aspetti della vita quotidiana" Anno 2009* (Daily life in 2009. Annual multipurpose analysis of the Italian families "Aspects of Daily Life" Year 2009) [in Italian] [online]. Available from: www3.istat.it/dati/catalogo/20110121_00/. Accessed 27 May 2014.

ISTAT (2013) *Annuario Statistico Italiano 2013* (Italian Statistics Yearbook 2013) [in Italian] [online]. Available from: www.istat.it/it/archivio/107568. Accessed 24 May 2014.

ISTAT (2014a) Occupati per settore di attività economica (Employed by sector of activity) [in Italian] [online]. Available from: www.istat.it/it/lavoro. Accessed 20 May 2014.

ISTAT (2014b) *Noi Italia, 100 Statistics to Understand the Country We Live In* [online]. Available from: http://noi-italia2014.istat.it/index.php?id=3&L=1. Accessed 28 May 2014.

ISTAT (2014c) Cittadini Stranieri. Popolazione residente per sesso e cittadinanza al 31 dicembre 2012 (Foreign nationals. Resident population by sex and citizenship on 31 December 2012) [in Italian] [online]. Available from: http://demo.istat.it/str2012/index.html. Accessed on 15 October 2014.

Istituto Superiore di Sanità (2012) *Percorso nascita: promozione e valutazione della qualità di modelli operativi. Le indagini del 2008–2009 e del 2010–2011.* Rapporti ISTISAN 12/39 (Pathway to Birth: promoting and assessing the quality of operating models. The 2008-2009 and 2010-2011 surveys. ISTISAN Report 12/39) [in Italian] [online]. Available from: www.iss.it/binary/publ/cont/12_39_web.pdf. Accessed 29 May 2014.

Klein, M.C., Gauthier, R.J., Jorgensen, S.H., Robbins, J.M., Kaczorowski, J., Johnson, B., Corriveau M., Westreich R., Waghorn K., Gelfand M.M. *et al.* (1992) 'Does episiotomy prevent perineal trauma and pelvic floor relaxation?', *Online Journal of Current Clinical Trials*, July: Document No. 20.

Labbok, M.H. (2012) 'Global baby-friendly hospital initiative monitoring data: update and discussion', *Breastfeeding Medicine*, 7: 210–222.

Law 194/78 (1978) 'Norme per la tutela sociale della maternità e sull'interruzione volontaria della gravidanza' (Standards for social maternity safeguards and the voluntary termination of pregnancy) [in Italian], *Gazzetta Ufficiale*, 140, 22 May 1978.

Law 286/98 (1998) 'Testo unico delle disposizioni concernenti la disciplina dell'immigrazione e norme sulla condizione dello straniero' (Consolidated act of the provisions on immigration control and regulation of alien status) [in Italian], *Gazzetta Ufficiale*, 191, 18 August 1998.

Law 40/04 (2004) 'Norme in materia di procreazione medicalmente assistita' (Standards for medically assisted reproduction) [in Italian], *Gazzetta Ufficiale*, 45, 24 February 2004.

Law 405/75 (1975) 'Istituzione dei consultori familiari' (Establishment of the Family Outpatient Services) [in Italian], *Gazzetta Ufficiale*, 227, 27 August 1975.

Law 412/91 (1991) 'Centralità delle regioni nel controllo della spesa sanitaria e unicità del rapporto di lavoro del medico' (The central role of the regions in controlling healthcare expenditure and the exclusiveness of physicians' work contract) [in Italian], *Gazzetta Ufficiale*, 305, 31 December 1991.

Law 833/78 (1978) 'Istituzione del Servizio Sanitario Nazionale' (Establishment of the National Healthcare System) [in Italian], *Gazzetta Ufficiale*, 360, 28 December 1978.

Lo Scalzo, A., Donatini, A., Orzella, L., Cicchetti, A., Profili, S. and Maresso, A. (2009) 'Italy: health system review', *Health Systems in Transition*, 11 (6), 1–216.

Mack Smith, D. (1997) *Modern Italy: a Political History.* Ann Arbor, MI: University of Michigan Press.

Ministero della Salute (2008) *Precisazioni concernenti l'assistenza sanitaria ai cittadini comunitari dimoranti in Italia* (Clarifications on the healthcare provided to European Community citizens who are resident of Italy) [in Italian] [online]. Available from: www.salute.gov.it/imgs/C_17_normativa_1514_allegato.pdf. Accessed 27 May 2014.

Ministero della Salute (2010) *Organizzazione e Attività dei Consultori familiari Pubblici in Italia, Anno 2008* (Organisation and activities of the public outpatient family services in Italy, year 2008) [in Italian] [online]. Available from: www.salute.gov.it/imgs/C_17_pubblicazioni_1406_allegato.pdf. Accessed 29 May 2014.

Ministero della Salute (2012) *Adempimento "mantenimento dell'erogazione dei LEA" attraverso gli indicatori della griglia Lea. Metodologia e Risultati Anno 2010* (Compliance with essential healthcare levels (LEA) assessed through the grid of LEA indicators. Methods and results, year 2010) [in Italian] [online]. Available from: www.salute.gov.it/imgs/c_17_pubblicazioni_1829_allegato.pdf. Accessed 29 May 2014.

Ministero della Salute (2013a) *Personale delle ASL e degli Istituti di cura pubblici* (Personnel of Local Health Units and public hospitals) [in Italian] [online]. Available from: www.salute.gov.it/imgs/C_17_pubblicazioni_1952_allegato.pdf. Accessed 27 May 2014.

Ministero della Salute (2013b) Assistenza primaria – Medici di Medicina Generale e Pediatri di Libera Scelta anno 2011 e trend 2001–2011 (Primary care – general practitioners and family pediatricians, year 2011 and trends for the 2001–2011 period) [in Italian] [online]. Available from: www.salute.gov.it/portale/documentazione/p6_2_8_3_1.jsp?lingua=italiano&id=10. Accessed 27 May 2014.

Ministero della Salute (2013c) Retribuzione dirigenti delle professioni sanitarie (Wages of professionals in the National Healthcare System) [in Italian] [online] Available from: www.salute.gov.it/imgs/C_17_minpag_1061_listaFile_itemName_16_file.pdf. Accessed 30 May 2014.

Ministero della Salute (2013d), *Certificato di assistenza al parto (CeDAP). Analisi dell'evento nascita – Anno 2010* (Delivery Assistance Certificate (CeDAP)). Analysis of childbirth events – year 2010) [in Italian] [online]. Available from: www.salute.gov.it/imgs/C_17_pubblicazioni_2024_allegato.pdf. Accessed 30 May 2014.

Ministero della Salute (2013e) *Relazione del Ministero della Salute sulla attuazione della legge contenente norme sulla tutela sociale della maternità e per l'interruzione volontaria di gravidanza (legge 194/78)* (Ministry of Health report on the implementation of the standards for social maternity safeguards and voluntary termination of pregnancy (Law 194/78)) [in Italian] [online]. Available from: www.salute.gov.it/imgs/C_17_pubblicazioni_2023_allegato.pdf. Accessed 30 May 2014.

Ministero della Salute (2014a) *The National Healthcare System* [in Italian] [online]. Available from: www.salute.gov.it/portale/salute/p1_4.jsp?lingua=italiano&tema=Tu_e_il_Servizio_Sanitario_Nazionale&area=Il_Ssn. Accessed 24 May 2014.

Ministero della Salute (2014b) *Adempimento "mantenimento dell'erogazione dei LEA" attraverso gli indicatori della griglia Lea. Metodologia e Risultati Anno 2012* (Compliance with essential healthcare levels (LEA) assessed through the grid of LEA indicators. Methods and Results, Year 2012) [in Italian] [online]. Available from: www.salastampa.salute.gov.it/imgs/C_17_pubblicazioni_2154_allegato.pdf. Accessed 29 May 2014.

Ministero della Salute News (2011) *Il ruolo delle donne nel Sistema Sanitario Nazionale* (The role of women in the National Healthcare System) [in Italian] [online]. Available from: www.newslettersalute.it/new.php?id=217445. Accessed 27 May 2014.

Ministero della Salute, Sistema Nazionale per le Linee Guida (2011) *Linea Guida 20 – Gravidanza Fisiologica* (Guideline No. 20: the normal pregnancy) [in Italian] [online]. Available from: www.snlg-iss.it/cms/files/LG_Gravidanza.pdf. Accessed 29 May 2014.

Ministero della Salute, Sistema Nazionale per le Linee Guida (2012) *Linea Guida 22 – Taglio Cesareo: una scelta appropriata e consapevole* (Guideline No. 22 – caesarean section: an appropriate and informed choice) [in Italian] [online]. Available from: www.snlg-iss.it/cms/files/LG_Cesareo_finaleL.pdf. Accessed 29 May 2014.

Ministero della Sanità (1994) 'DM Sanità 14/09/1994, n. 739, Regolamento concernente l'individuazione della figura e del relativo profilo professionale dell'infermiere' (Regulations concerning role and professional profile of the nurse professional) [in Italian], *Gazzetta Ufficiale*, 6, 9 January 1995.

Ministero dell'Università e della Ricerca (2012) *Elaborazione su dati MUR – Ufficio di Statistica* (Analysis of the Ministry of University and Research data – Statistical Office) [in Italian] [online]. Available from: http://statistica.miur.it/scripts/IU/vIU0.asp. Accessed 27 May 2014.

National Collaborating Centre for Women's and Children's Health (2008) *Antenatal Care: Routine Care for the Healthy Pregnant Woman*. London: Royal College of Obstetricians and Gynaecologists Press. Available from: www.nice.org.uk/nicemedia/live/11947/40145/40145.pdf. Accessed 22 May 2014.

Niero M. (1996) 'Italy: right turn for the welfare state?'. In: George V. and Taylor-Gooby J. (eds), *European Welfare Policy; Squaring the Circle*. London: Macmillan, pp. 117–135.

OECD (2009) 'Comparing countries' and economies' performances'. In: *PISA 2009 Results*. Paris: OECD Publishing.

OECD (2013a) *OECD Factbook 2013: Economic, Environmental and Social Statistics*. Paris: OECD Publishing.

OECD (2013b) *Economic Surveys: Italy 2013*. Paris: OECD Publishing.

OECD (2013c) *Health at a Glance 2013: OECD Indicators*. Paris: OECD Publishing.

OECD (2014) *OECD Family Database* [online]. Available from: www.oecd.org/social/family/database. Accessed 30 May 2014.

Osservatorio per la Salute della Donna (2012) *Gli standard per la valutazione dei punti nascita* (Standards for the assessment of birth facilities) [in Italian] [online]. Available from: www.ondaosservatorio.it/allegati/Newsdocumenti/articoli%20vari/Manuale%20Punti%20Nascita.pdf. Accessed 30 May 2014.

Palermo C., Montemurro D., Ragazzo F. (2013) *La programmazione del fabbisogno del personale medico nel decennio 2014–2023* (Planning for medical personnel needs for the decade 2014-2023) [in Italian] [online]. Available from: www.anaao.it/amministrazione/tiny_mce/plugins/ajaxfilemanager/uploaded/studio%20programmazione%20fabbisogno_17marzo2014.pdf. Accessed 20 May 2014.

Pavanello S (2012) *Relazione sull'analgesia epidurale durante il travaglio e il parto in Italia* (Report on epidural analgesia during labour and delivery in Italy) [in Italian] [online]. Available from: www.siaarti.it/. Accessed 20 May 2014.

Regione Lombardia Sanità (2012) *Prevalenza, esclusività e durata dell'allattamento al seno in regione Lombardia* (Prevalence, exclusiveness and duration of breastfeeding in

the region of Lombardy) [in Italian] [online]. Available from: www.epicentro.iss.
it/argomenti/allattamento/pdf/report%20allattamento%20rl%202012.pdf.
Accessed 30 May 2014.

UNICEF (2014) *Gli Ospedali Amici dei Bambini in Italia* (Baby-friendly hospitals in
Italy) [in Italian] [online]. Available from: www.unicef.it/doc/152/gli-ospedali-
amici-dei-bambini-in-italia.htm. Accessed 22 May 2014.

United Nations, Department of Economic and Social Affairs (2012) *World Population Prospects: the 2012 Revision* [online]. Available from: esa.un.org/wpp/Excel-
Data/population.htm. Accessed 30 May 2014.

WHO, UNFPA, UNICEF and AMDD (2009) *Monitoring Emergency Obstetric Care*
[online]. Available from: http://unfpa.org/public/publications/pid/3073.
Accessed 30 May 2014.

WHO, UNICEF, UNFPA and the World Bank (2012) *Trends in Maternal Mortality:
1990–2010. WHO, UNICEF, UNFPA and the World Bank Estimates* [online].
Available from: www.who.int/reproductivehealth/publications/monitoring/
9789241503631/en/. Accessed 29 May 2014.

Woolley RJ (1995) 'Benefits and risks of episiotomy: a review of the English-
language literature since 1980. Part I', *Obstetric and Gynecology Surveys*, 50:
806–820.

World Bank (2014) *Mortality Rate, Neonatal (Per 1,000 Live Births)* [online]. Available from: http://data.worldbank.org/indicator/SH.DYN.NMRT. Accessed 6
September 2014.

World Travel and Tourism Council (2014) *Benchmarking of Travel & Tourism in Italy*
[online]. Available from: www.wttc.org/focus/research-for-action/benchmark-
reports/country-results/. Accessed 20 May 2014.

XII Commissione Permanente, Igiene e Sanità (2012) *Indagine conoscitiva sul percorso nascita e sulla situazione dei punti nascita con riguardo all'individuazione di critic-
ità specifiche circa la tutela della salute della donna e del feto e sulle modalità di esercizio
dell'autodeterminazione della donna nella scelta tra parto cesareo o naturale – NASCERE
SICURI* (Survey on the 'Pathway to Birth' programme and birth facilities, specifically focusing on mother-and-child health and women's right to choose between
caesarean section or vaginal delivery – SAFE BIRTH) [in Italian] [online]. Available from: www.senato.it/service/PDF/PDFServer/BGT/688999.pdf. Accessed
29 May 2014.

10 Germany

Nadine Reibling and Monika Mischke

Background

With 81.8 million inhabitants living in sixteen different states, Germany is the most populated country in the European Union. Together with Italy, Germany has the highest share of people aged 65 years and older (Germany/Italy 20.6 per cent, European Union average 17.7 per cent) and is one of the countries with the lowest fertility rates (Statistisches Bundesamt 2013). The historical separation of West Germany (Federal Republic of Germany) and East Germany (German Democratic Republic) is still visible in many areas of social life. In particular, states in the former East Germany are in a less favourable economic position than those in the West, with a lower GDP per capita (West €34,244, East €22,972) and higher unemployment rates (West 4.5 per cent, East 9.0 per cent) (Statistisches Bundesamt 2013). The federal structure of Germany is also important for political decision-making. The state governments participate in federal legislative processes in the second chamber, but also have sole jurisdiction over certain areas, such as the educational system (including childcare).

The majority of migrants in Germany are from European Union member or candidate countries. People from Turkey form the largest single migrant group (Statistisches Bundesamt 2013). In 2012, 68 per cent of women between the ages of fifteen and sixty-four years participated in the labour market. However, 37 per cent of women worked part-time (less than thirty hours) (Statistisches Bundesamt 2013). Women with children in East Germany are more likely to work (East 63 per cent, West 59.3 per cent) and are more likely to work full-time (East 54.7 per cent, West 24.6 per cent) (Keller and Haustein 2012).

Germany as a welfare regime

The German welfare state was founded in 1883 when Otto von Bismarck's law for health insurance for workers was passed in the German Reichstag. Since then, Germany has been identified as the paradigmatic example of the Bismarckian or conservative welfare regime (Esping-Andersen 1990). Social security is primarily organised through insurance, with income-dependent contributions covering the risks of old age, sickness, unemployment and long-term care needs. The organisation of welfare programmes is still relatively fragmented as a result of its historical roots in professional and guild-like security arrangements. In the case of health care, 134 sickness funds currently administer the funding of health care (compared with 1,815 sickness funds in 1970) (Gesetzliche Krankenversicherung Spitzenverband 2013a). The governance of the health care system is based on a corporatist self-regulation system, e.g. prices are negotiated between federal representatives of doctor and hospital associations and the sickness funds in the Federal Joint Committee (Gemeinsamer Bundesausschuss). The federal government steps in only when the corporatist actors cannot come to an agreement.

During its golden age of welfare expansion, Germany built on its existing pre-war social policy arrangements, but greatly expanded both the coverage rates and the benefit levels. Differences between blue-collar and white-collar occupational schemes were widely abolished. As a result of the insurance-based nature of the conservative welfare regime, access to benefits is associated with (previous) employment status, which means that decommodification is lower than in the Nordic welfare states. The insurance-based benefits are still relatively generous compared with other countries worldwide, but, as they are based on earnings-based contributions, they also reproduce existing levels of stratification and income inequality (Esping-Andersen 1990).

From a gender perspective, the German welfare state is characterised by a model of the traditional family ethic with a focus on supporting the male breadwinner, e.g. through income tax splitting (Dingeldey 2001), and with women providing unpaid care work at home (Clasen 2005). Until recently, West German women would often stay at home for several years after childbirth and then return to employment part-time (Rosenfeld *et al.* 2004). Attitudes towards working mothers have become more progressive in recent years, but still lag behind other European countries (Wendt *et al.* 2011). In the past two decades new policies have provided a stronger push towards the participation of women in the labour force and dual-earner families, which was the dominant model in East Germany before reunification (Rosenfeld *et al.* 2004). A total of 15.8 per cent of children in Germany live in poverty or in households that lack basic amenities (Statistisches Bundesamt 2013).

Health care system

In line with its system of welfare provision, health care and sickness benefits are organised as contributions-based health insurance in Germany. However, solidaristic arrangements ensure a quasi-universal coverage of the population. Contributions include coverage for non-working spouses and (non-working) children under twenty-five years of age and the contributions for recipients of unemployment benefits or social assistance are covered by public funds. Self-employed people and those whose income exceeds a defined level can opt out of the statutory insurance and purchase private insurance on the individual insurance market. In 2011, 86 per cent of all employed people were covered by statutory health insurance, 13 per cent had private health insurance and 0.2 per cent were uninsured (Statistisches Bundesamt 2011). Private insurance contributions are risk-based and cover the same benefits as provided in the public system and usually additional services. In addition, there is a smaller supplementary insurance market for dental care, alternative and complementary care, and preferential treatment in hospitals (Busse and Riesberg 2005). The statutory health insurance covers all forms of care (ambulatory, hospital, dental, imaging and drugs), with the exception of long-term care (which is covered by long-term care insurance). Co-payments apply to hospital visits, dental care, medical aids and appliances, and drugs.

In the self-regulatory governance system, the government sets the legal framework for structural changes in the system in consultation with various interest groups. The details of the regulations and their implementation lie with the Federal Joint Committee, which includes representatives of sickness funds as well as doctor and hospital associations; midwives are not represented. Patient organisations are represented, but have no voting powers.

Between 1970 and 2010, total health expenditure in Germany grew from 6 per cent of the GDP to 11.6 per cent. In an OECD comparison, Germany has the third most expensive health care system after the USA (17.7 per cent) and the Netherlands (12.1 per cent) (OECD 2013b).

In 2011, there were 3.84 physicians and 11.37 nurses per 1,000 population, which are both above the OECD average (Table 10.1). Nevertheless, there are urban/rural differences resulting in shortages in rural areas, in particular in the ambulatory sector (Busse and Riesberg 2005). Doctors and midwives who work in private practice are self-employed and primarily

Table 10.1 Human and physical resources in Germany, 2011

Physicians per 1,000 population	3.84
Nurses per 1,000 population	11.37
Medical graduates per 100,000 population	11.76
Nursing graduates per 100,000 population	27.76
Total hospital beds per 1,000 population	8.27
Curative (acute) care beds per 1,000 population	5.33
Obstetricians and gynaecologists per 1,000 population	0.2
Midwives per 1,000 population	0.23

Source: OECD (2013b).

paid on a fee-for-service basis. However, overall spending on physician services is fixed via a global budget. The federal doctor association receives a flat rate per insured person from the sickness funds and reimburses individual doctors for each service provided. This combination of a fixed budget and fee-for-service means that individual doctors do not know the price of their services at the time they provide them because the price is determined by the overall service utilisation in a specific region (Busse and Riesberg 2005).

In 2012, one-third of hospitals were public, one-third were owned by non-profit organisations (e.g. churches) and one-third belonged to private companies (Statistisches Bundesamt 2012a). Statutory insurance covers the costs of services in all three hospital types. Doctors, nurses and midwives working in hospitals receive a salary (Busse and Riesberg 2005). Patients have free access to general practitioners and specialists (no gatekeeping), as well as a free choice of doctor (Reibling 2010; Reibling and Wendt 2012).

The medical degree is the primary requirement for receiving a licence to practise medicine. However, doctors are required to specialise in one of thirty-three fields (including general practice), which requires further education (after their medical degree) of up to five years and another exam (Bundesärztekammer 2003). Only after specialisation can doctors have their own private practice to provide ambulatory care. Doctors who have specialised in gynaecology and obstetrics are, together with midwives, responsible for maternity care.

Licensing for midwives is regulated by federal law (Hebammengesetz 1985). Midwives complete an educational programme over three years at specific midwifery schools (Hebammengesetz 1985). Germany has only recently established midwifery as a college degree and university education still plays only a marginal role in the training of midwives. Midwifery education is based on a standardised curriculum that includes both theoretical education and practical training. Practical training takes place primarily in hospitals (Deutscher Hebammen Verband e.V. 2014a).

Demographic profile

In 2011, life expectancy at birth in Germany was 77.8 years for newborn boys and 82.8 years for newborn girls (Geißler and Meyer 2014). The crude birth rate, i.e. the number of births per 1,000 people, was 8.1 (in 2011) (Statistisches Bundesamt 2012a). As the crude birth rate is hardly comparable across countries, fertility is usually indicated in terms of the total fertility rate, which was 1.36 for Germany in 2011 (OECD 2013a). Germany's fertility rate is relatively low and is far below 2.08 (the rate necessary to ensure the long-term natural replacement of the population) as well as below the OECD average of 1.7 or the EU-21 average of 1.59 (OECD 2013a).

Until 1975, the fertility curves of East and West Germany developed in a similar pattern. Between 1950 and 1965, fertility rose in West Germany from 209 births per 100 women to 248 and in East Germany from 237 births per 100 women to 250 (Geißler and Meyer 2014). This 'baby boom' lasted from the late 1950s until 1965 and is explained by a variety of factors, such as catching up on marriages that were prevented by World War II, decreasing marital age, and economic and social stabilisation. After 1965, fertility rates sharply decreased and reached a low point in the mid-1970s (Geißler and Meyer 2014).

In the following years, however, converse fertility patterns emerged in East and West Germany. In West Germany the mean number of children per 100 women declined from 250 (in 1965) to 128 (in 1985). From 1985 to 1998 fertility rates slightly increased again and since then have fluctuated between 1.3 and 1.4 (Geißler and Meyer 2014).

In East Germany the decline in birth rates between 1965 and 1975 proceeded less dramatically. Population and family policies in the 1970s stimulated a second (albeit more moderate) baby boom between 1975 and 1980, resulting in a fertility rate of 1.94 in 1980 (Rosenfeld *et al.* 2004; Geißler and Meyer 2014). In the subsequent period, fertility declined to 1.6 in 1989. After reunification (November 1989), fertility sharply dropped by 60 per cent and reached a low point of 0.77 in 1994. This 'demographic crisis' can be ascribed to the shock situation at the beginning of the process of reunification (Geißler and Meyer 2014). This process generated enormous social and economic insecurities, as well as new opportunities, and caused many couples to postpone or resign from childbearing (Birg 2001; Geißler and Meyer 2014). Since 1994, fertility has slowly, but constantly, recovered and reached the West German rate of 1.37 in 2007.

In general, childlessness in East Germany increased after reunification. A study from 2008 shows that about 7 per cent of all women born between 1939 and 1963 remained childless, compared with 11 per cent among women born between 1964 and 1968 (Statistisches Bundesamt 2012b). In contrast, in West Germany, 20 per cent of women among the birth cohorts of 1964 to 1968 remained childless (Statistisches Bundesamt 2012b). Regarding the number of children per woman, there is a higher number of one-child families and fewer families with three or more children in East Germany compared with the western part of the country (Geißler and Meyer 2014). In 2008, 33 per cent of East German mothers born between 1959 and 1968 had only one child (26 per cent in West Germany), 44 per cent had two children (in both parts of the country) and 14 per cent had three or more children (21 per cent in West Germany) (Statistisches Bundesamt 2012b). In both parts of the country, women with a higher level of education are more likely to remain childless, have fewer children or have children later in their life (Statistisches Bundesamt 2012b).

In 2011, the average age of mothers giving birth in Germany was 30.6 years. A total of 60 per cent of all newborn babies were born to women aged between 26 and 35 years (Statistisches Bundesamt 2012b). In West Germany, the age at first maternity increased continuously from twenty-four years in 1970 to 29.2 years in 2010; first-time mothers are therefore on average five years older than mothers forty years ago (Statistisches Bundesamt 2012b). In East Germany a higher number of children have been born outside of marriage since the 1960s due to differences in family and social policy entitlements and gender role attitudes (Statistisches Bundesamt 2012b; Rosenfeld *et al.* 2004). After reunification, the age at first maternity had increased to 27.4 years in 2010, which was still about three years lower than in West Germany (Statistisches Bundesamt 2012b) (Table 10.2).

Maternity provision

Gynaecologists[1] and midwives are the main professions responsible for the provision of maternity services. General practitioners or family doctors play no part at any stage (except in very rural settings). Gynaecologists need to provide part of the antenatal care (and can provide all antenatal care), are present at hospital births and perform one postnatal examination of the mother six to eight weeks after birth. Midwives can provide part of the antenatal care, need to be present at every birth (except emergencies) and perform the majority of postnatal care for mother and child (Hebammengesetz 1985).

Germany has 0.2 gynaecologists per 1,000 population (Table 10.2). Most work in private practices in which they provide antenatal and postnatal care to pregnant women and mothers. Moreover, they perform yearly pap smears and prescribe birth control, so many women have a

Table 10.2 Demographic profile of Germany

Population	81.8 million
Women (%)	50.9
Population aged 0–14 years (%)	13.2
Women of childbearing age (15–49 years)[1]	18.4 million (2010)
Population aged 65 years and older (%)	20.6
Population annual growth (%)	0.11
Population density per square kilometre	229
Total fertility rate (births per woman)	1.36
Crude birth rate per 1,000 people	8.1
Crude death rate per 1,000 people	10.4
Urban population (%)	35.4
Ethnic groups (breakdown)	9.1% residents with foreign nationality; 79.4% from European countries. The largest migrant group is from Turkey – 21.8% of all residents with foreign nationality (2012)

Sources: Statistisches Bundesamt (2013); 1 Statistisches Bundesamt (2012b).

regular gynaecologist before their first pregnancy. An appointment with their regular gynaecologist usually represents the first contact with the health care system for pregnant women. Gynaecologists in private practice are usually not involved in childbirth, although some have private beds in hospitals where they can deliver their patients' babies.

In 98 per cent of cases childbirth takes place in a hospital setting (Braun 2006). In 2012, Germany had 2017 hospitals with 8537 beds in obstetrics located in 430 obstetric departments (Statistisches Bundesamt 2012a). Only specific perinatal hospitals are licensed to deliver and care for preterm babies with birth weights of 1,500 g or less. Hospitals generally have anaesthetists on-site or on-call for epidural anaesthesia and caesarean sections. Following the WHO/UNICEF Baby-Friendly Hospital Initiative, hospitals can apply for the certification 'Baby-Friendly'. This is currently held by eighty-two hospitals in Germany (Babyfreundliches Krankenhaus e.V. 2014). Compared with other OECD countries, Germany has a high average number of hospital days after the birth (2011: Germany 4.4, OECD average 3.9) (OECD 2013b). However, the number of postnatal days in hospital has been declining steadily since 2000.

Midwives perform different roles in maternity care and work in different settings. Self-employed midwives can manage births with full responsibility at home, in birth centres or in hospitals (Braun 2006). In 2011, Germany had 0.23 midwives per 1,000 population, which is below the OECD average of 0.37. As Germany has a relatively elderly population and a low fertility rate, a better comparison may be the number of midwives per 1,000 live births. With 28.66 midwives per 1,000 live births, Germany is only slightly below the OECD average of 30.89.

A survey of 3603 midwives in Germany indicates that 4 per cent work only as (hospital) employees, 28 per cent work in hospitals and are also self-employed, 61 per cent are exclusively self-employed and 7 per cent are not professionally active (Albrecht *et al.* 2012). About 62 per cent of all self-employed midwives do not offer deliveries, but rather specialise in pre-natal and antenatal care (Albrecht *et al.* 2012).

There are several options for mothers to deliver their children with midwives only: as home births, in birth centres or in midwifery-led delivery wards (Hebammenkreißsaal). Birth centres are independent institutions owned and managed by self-employed midwives with delivery rooms and limited technical equipment, e.g. cardiotocographs. There are around 130 birth centres in Germany (Deutscher Hebammen Verband e.V. 2014b). Midwifery-led delivery wards (Hebammenkreißsäle) are delivery wards in hospitals where midwives are solely responsible for births without the presence of doctors. These wards are a relatively new development. There were only fourteen in all of Germany in 2013 (Deutscher Hebammen Verband e.V. 2014c).

Even though home births and birth centres have become more popular over the last two decades (1991, 0.46 per cent of all births; 2010, 1.68 per cent), they are still rare, representing less than 2 per cent of all births

(Albrecht *et al.* 2012; Gesellschaft für Qualität in der außerklinischen Geburtshilfe e.V. 2014). Two-thirds of births outside hospital take place in birth centres and one-third take place at home. As midwives who attend births outside hospital are encouraged, but not required, to document these births, these statistics rely to some extent on estimations (Gesellschaft für Qualität in der außerklinischen Geburtshilfe e.V. 2014).

Since 2010 the remuneration of midwives has been an ongoing issue of political and media debate (Deutscher Bundestag 2014). The National Midwifery Association advocates for changes in the remuneration for out-of-hospital births. Self-employed midwives who perform deliveries are required to have liability insurance, which covers claims from complications and deaths. Only two or three insurance companies offer such insurance and premiums increased from €404 in 2000 to €5,091 in 2014 (Deutscher HebammenVerband e.V. 2014b). The National Midwifery Association argues that many midwives have difficulty in paying the insurance premium based on the remuneration they receive for the deliveries. Midwives who do have insurance claims have later difficulties with taking out insurance. Even though reliable statistics do not exist, survey data indicate that 10–25 per cent of self-employed midwives have stopped performing deliveries, which has reduced the availability of choice in the place of birth (Albrecht *et al.* 2012). The health minister has recently announced that sickness funds will increase the remuneration for midwives to cover the increase in premiums. The ministry also negotiates with private insurance companies with the aim of extending the liability coverage of midwives in the future (Ärztezeitung 2014).

Maternity entitlements

Maternity leave was first introduced in 1952. The current duration of maternity leave is fourteen weeks, of which six weeks should be taken before the birth and eight weeks following confinement. The latter eight weeks are obligatory for reasons of health protection for the child and the mother. Before birth, women may continue to work until the birth only if they explicitly declare that it is their personal decision to do so (Blum and Erler 2013).

The payment of maternity leave is 100 per cent of earnings, with no ceiling on payments. Benefits are covered by the mother's health insurance, which pays €13 per day, and her employer, who pays the remainder. In most cases, the employer bears the bulk of the costs of maternity leave benefits. Mothers with an income below €390 per month are paid solely by their health insurance. Unemployed mothers who are registered as such, and thus receive unemployment benefit, also receive maternity leave benefit from their health insurance, which is equal to their unemployment benefit. Self-employed women and women not involved in the labour market have no statutory right to maternity leave benefits (Blum and Erler 2013).

Paternity leave, defined as a short period of leave immediately following the birth of a child and only available to the father (either paid or unpaid), does not exist in Germany (Blum and Erler 2013).

From 1979 until the introduction of parental leave in West Germany in 1986, mothers were entitled to stay at home for four months after childbirth as part of maternity protection regulations. In 1986 a separate law regulating parental leave came into effect that entitled both mothers and fathers to take parental leave for a period of up to three years. A flat-rate and means-tested childrearing benefit was paid for up to two years (Deven and Moss 2005). In practice, almost only mothers took advantage of the parental leave entitlement and many West German women took advantage of a long, mostly unpaid, leave period followed by part-time work as long as their children were young (Rosenfeld *et al.* 2004). In contrast, East German mothers mostly returned to full-time employment after the 'birth year' (one year of paid leave for mothers after giving birth), which was introduced in 1976 (Rosenfeld *et al.* 2004; Trappe 1995). Parental leave was reformed in 2007. The formerly means-tested and flat-rate benefit was replaced by an unconditional wage replacement of about 67 per cent of the former mean income of the parent taking the leave. Parental leave is still a family benefit, thus both parents are equally entitled to take it. The actual wage replacement rate of the benefit is slightly graded according to income.[2] The maximum payment is €1,800 a month; the minimum payment is €300 a month, which is also granted to parents without any prior income, e.g. for students or those not actively involved in the labour market. Since 2011, the long-term unemployed are no longer eligible for this minimum payment because benefits are now credited against social assistance payments. Parents who are unemployed long term thus receive social assistance payments only and do not also receive the minimum parental leave benefit of €300 (Bundesministerium für Familie, Senioren, Frauen und Jugend 2012; Blum and Erler 2013).

The maximum duration of benefit is fourteen months, including two non-transferable months for the partner who takes less leave (usually the father). The parental benefit, as well as the non-transferable months reserved for the partner, may also be spread over a period twice as long, i.e. over a maximum of twenty-eight months. Benefits are then reduced by 50 per cent so that the total amount remains the same. Recipients of the parental benefit are allowed to work for up to thirty hours a week. If they do so, however, the amount of parental benefit is calculated as a percentage of the 'lost income', i.e. the margin between the present income from part-time work and the former income.

In addition to the parental leave period of up to fourteen months, parents can take unpaid childcare leave until the child's third birthday. During this period, job security is guaranteed.

The parental leave reform in 2007 aimed to increase the take-up of leave by fathers. Data from the Federal Office of Statistics show that the proportion of fathers taking parental leave rose from 3.3 per cent in 2006 to 27.8 per cent in 2011 (Blum and Erler 2013).

Childbirth in Germany

Antenatal care

Pregnant mothers are expected to receive regular antenatal care. Antenatal care usually starts with a mother's visit to her regular gynaecologist, who determines whether or not she is pregnant. During this visit the doctor performs an assessment of the medical history of the woman, her family and her previous pregnancies, as well as an assessment of her social and work situation (Gemeinsamer Bundesausschuss 2013). This information is listed in a booklet called mother passport (Mutterpass), which the woman is encouraged to carry with her throughout her pregnancy. Further antenatal visits are recorded in the booklet so that the hospital and the different providers who may be involved in antenatal care (e.g. the midwife) are informed about the current medical status and the development of the pregnancy. National data from 2008[3] reveal that 0.3 per cent of women who delivered their babies in hospitals had no mother passport, which indicates that almost 99 per cent of pregnant women have at least one antenatal care visit (Bundesgeschäftsstelle Qualitätssicherung 2009). A total of 45.6 per cent of pregnant women had their first visit before the ninth week of their pregnancy, 37.8 per cent had their first visit between weeks nine and twelve, and 9.7 per cent had their first antenatal visit after the first trimester (Bundesgeschäftsstelle Qualitätssicherung 2009).

One of the entries in the mother passport is a determination of whether the woman has a high-risk pregnancy. Several factors can lead to this status being assigned, including existing chronic conditions (e.g. diabetes), previous pregnancy complications, as well as whether the first-time mother is younger than eighteen or older than thirty-five years (Gemeinsamer Bundesausschuss 2013). Data from 2008 indicate that 28.4 per cent of pregnant women are assigned the high-risk pregnancy status, but 64.6 per cent have at least one documented pregnancy risk (Bundesgeschäftsstelle Qualitätssicherung 2009). Women with a high-risk pregnancy status are entitled to more frequent antenatal care visits (including ultrasound scans) and to prenatal diagnoses (including amniocentesis). Prenatal diagnostic tests for women with 'normal' pregnancies are usually not covered by sickness funds (Gemeinsamer Bundesausschuss 2013). Only 4.2 per cent of pregnant mothers had an amniocentesis (Bundesgeschäftsstelle Qualitätssicherung 2009).

Further antenatal care includes once-off serological tests (rubella, HIV, hepatitis B, Chlamydia trachomatis) and monthly examinations (weight checks, blood pressure checks and urine tests) until the last two months of pregnancy, when examinations are performed fortnightly (Gemeinsamer Bundesausschuss 2013). In 2008, 6.2 per cent of pregnant women had seven or less antenatal care visits, 43.5 per cent had eight to eleven visits and 42.1 per cent had twelve or more (no information for 8.6 per cent) (Bundesgeschäftsstelle Qualitätssicherung 2009).

The public insurance system covers three ultrasound scans in antenatal care. The ultrasound scan in the second trimester often includes an extended sonographic examination with biometry and a systematic examination of foetal morphologies. Only doctors with specific qualifications are allowed to perform this examination, which requires pregnant women to visit a hospital or specialised practice (Gemeinsamer Bundesausschuss 2013). In 2008, 4 per cent of pregnant mothers had less than the three recommended ultrasound scans, 65.5 per cent had three or four scans and 22.1 per cent had five or more ultrasound scans during their pregnancy (Bundesgeschäftsstelle Qualitätssicherung 2009). Women are also encouraged to be tested for gestational diabetes between the twenty-fourth and the twenty-seventh week of their pregnancy (Gemeinsamer Bundesausschuss 2013).

Midwives can perform all antenatal tests except ultrasound scans if the doctor has no concerns about the development of the pregnancy (Gemeinsamer Bundesausschuss 2013). In practice, women who have chosen a midwife often alternate between seeing their doctor and a midwife for their monthly check-ups. Women with public health insurance are also entitled to attend antenatal classes, which are usually held by midwives in hospitals, birth centres or at their private practice (Bundeszentrale für gesundheitliche Aufklärung 2014a).

Women are encouraged to register with their chosen hospital or birth centre several weeks before their delivery (Gemeinsamer Bundesausschuss 2013). Pregnant women generally have a free choice of hospital, even though there may, in practice, be no choice in rural areas. Maternity units regularly offer evenings at which they inform pregnant mothers and their partners about the ward (e.g. whether it offers water births) and show them their facilities.

Intrapartum care

Childbirth in Germany is widely medicalised and 98 per cent of births occur in a hospital setting (Gesellschaft für Qualität in der außerklinischen Geburtshilfe e.V. 2014). However, midwives have a strong legal position in the birth process. Their presence at a birth is obligatory and, even in hospitals, midwives support the pregnant woman for most of the delivery (Hebammengesetz 1985). Midwives have the legal right to perform deliveries without doctors, but doctors are required to be accompanied by midwives (except in emergencies) (Hebammengesetz 1985). In the hospital setting, however, there is often a hierarchy in which doctors give orders once they are present. In practice, this can also vary depending on the relative experience of the attendant doctor and the midwife (Braun 2006).

Women legally have a free choice of place of birth, but, in practice, it may be difficult to have a home birth or a delivery in a birth centre as birth centres are not available nationwide and only 29 per cent of all self-employed midwives offer delivery services (Gesetzliche Krankenversicherung Spitzenverband 2013). Although sickness funds cover the costs of childbirth in all settings, only certain funds cover midwives' on-call fee, so out-of-hospital births can lead to out-of-pocket costs for the family (Albrecht *et al.* 2012).

Medical intervention in the birth process is a matter of controversy in scientific and professional debates and a central focus of the natural birth movement. A general trend can be observed towards more flexible criteria for the justification of medical interventions, such as caesarean sections or induced births (Hickl 2002). Clear medical indications, such as the imminent danger of the mother's or baby's life, account for only a small number of medical interventions (Hickl 2002). The majority of decisions about medical interventions occur in situations in which medical information, the mother's preferences, the doctor's judgement and organisational considerations may all determine the likelihood of intervention (Hickl 2002). On the one hand, there is a concern about the increasing rates of interventions and doctors are seen as causing these interventions through high levels of risk aversion and unnecessary preventive interventions (Hickl 2002). On the other hand, doctors may have become more sensitive towards patient preferences and many women express a high desire for safety in childbirth (Hickl 2002). There is no general rule for who has the decision-making power about interventions in the birth process. Mothers generally need to agree to all medical interventions unless there is an immediate threat to the mother or baby, but, in practice, if doctors or midwives make suggestions for interventions, pregnant mothers often agree (particularly if it is their first birth).

The global rate of caesarean sections has increased dramatically in recent years. In OECD countries, caesarean sections have almost doubled from 14 per cent of all births in 1991 to 26 per cent in 2009 (OECD 2011). With 30 per cent of births by caesarean section in 2009, Germany is above the OECD average. Despite the uniform rise in all countries, there is a substantial variation from 14 per cent in the Netherlands to 43 per cent in Turkey. An explanation for the rise in caesarean section rates in Germany has proved difficult. Caesarean sections are more likely to occur with first births. A total of 63 per cent of caesarean sections are for first-time mothers, compared with 54 per cent of vaginal deliveries (Kolip 2012). The age of mothers is significantly higher (31.5 years) for caesarean sections than for vaginal deliveries (30.4 years) (Kolip 2012). Caesarean

sections increase the likelihood of a caesarean section in subsequent pregnancies: 66.5 per cent of caesarean sections for subsequent deliveries are
for mothers who had a previous caesarean section, compared with 9.7 per
cent of those who had a previous vaginal delivery (Kolip 2012). Clearly
caesarean sections by choice are not the main driver for this growing rate
because they account for only about 2 per cent of all births (Haller *et al.*
2002). However, 58 per cent of caesarean sections were planned before
contractions started (Kolip 2012). Not only the characteristics of the pregnant woman, but also organisational factors may determine intervention
rates. As regions vary between 17 and 51 per cent in their caesarean
section rates (Bertelsmann Stiftung 2010), it seems likely that organisational factors play a part in these decisions. Hospitals in Germany are
remunerated via diagnosis-related groups, which means that they receive a
flat rate by patient with a specific diagnosis (and potentially extra payments when there are complications). Even though caesarean sections
have a higher diagnosis-related group rate, it is difficult to say how the
payment compares with the real costs for the hospital (Haller *et al.* 2002).
As there is no time limit for labour in Germany, planned caesarean sections have the advantage of being easy to manage within the hospital
routine. Nevertheless, most births do not take longer than twelve hours
(10 per cent, one to three hours; 29 per cent, three to six hours; 30 per
cent, six to twelve hours; 6 per cent, twelve to eighteen hours; 2 per cent,
eighteen hours and over; 22 per cent, unclear) (Bundesgeschäftsstelle
Qualitätssicherung 2009).

Even though many hospitals offer delivery rooms with options for different birth positions and they may generally support a natural birth,
medical interventions and the use of technology are the rule rather than
the exception. In 2008 (most recent data), 25 per cent of births were
induced and 62 per cent of all births included some form of anaesthesia
(Bundesgeschäftsstelle Qualitätssicherung 2009). In 95 per cent of all
births, cardiotocographs were used for monitoring and 50 per cent of all
pregnant women were attached to a cardiotocograph continuously
throughout labour (Bundesgeschäftsstelle Qualitätssicherung 2009). One
medical intervention on the decline in Germany is episiotomy. In 2002, 41
per cent of all births involved an episiotomy compared with 30 per cent in
2008. Compared with other European countries, Germany holds a
medium position in episiotomy rates (Zeitlin *et al.* 2010).

Postnatal care

Postnatally, women are entitled to care from midwives for eight weeks,
including daily home visits for the first ten days after delivery (Bundeszentrale für gesundheitliche Aufklärung 2014b). Postnatal care by midwives
includes care for the mother (monitoring the health of the mother, in
particular the lochia and the remission of the uterus, as well as the healing

of birth wounds) and the baby (health and general development, e.g. weight, food intake and excretion) (Bundeszentrale für gesundheitliche Aufklärung 2014b). Midwives also support new mothers with various practical and personal problems that may arise in the first few weeks after birth (Bundeszentrale für gesundheitliche Aufklärung 2014b). Midwives do not automatically visit new mothers after birth. Instead, pregnant women actively search for a midwife in their area before birth. Pregnant women from lower social classes may not always be aware of their rights and may take less advantage of these services; however, they often have additional challenges and require extra support. The use of 'family midwives' who visit families with social challenges (e.g. poverty or a low level of education) is seen as a strategy for early intervention. Until recently, only a limited number of family midwives were available in communities with pilot projects. In 2012 the federal government began to provide states and municipalities with funding to implement a nationwide network of family midwives for underprivileged families (Bundeskinderschutzgesetz 2011).

The National Breastfeeding Committee in Germany recommends exclusive breastfeeding for the first six months and continued breastfeeding with complementary food after the six-month period (National Breastfeeding Committee 2013). The committee makes no recommendation for the overall length of breastfeeding 'since this should be an individual decision of mothers and their babies' (National Breastfeeding Committee 2013).

Data on breastfeeding in Germany are patchy and there is no national prospective study of mothers' breastfeeding behaviour. However, all available data sources indicate that breastfeeding behaviour does not meet the recommendations of the National Breastfeeding Committee and international organisations such as the WHO (Dulon *et al.* 2001; Kohlhuber *et al.* 2008; Lange *et al.* 2007; Peters *et al.* 2006; Yngve and Sjöström 2001). A prospective study from 1997–1998 indicates that, although 90 per cent of German mothers started to breastfeed after birth, only 70 per cent continued to breastfeed two months after birth and 45 per cent breastfed exclusively at that time. After six months, about half of mothers continue to breastfeed (Dulon *et al.* 2001; Kohlhuber *et al.* 2008). Nevertheless, this situation represents an improvement on the situation in the 1980s and 1990s. A retrospective analysis of breastfeeding of birth cohorts indicates that exclusive breastfeeding for six months increased from 20 per cent in 1988 to 48 per cent in 1999 and declined afterwards to 35 per cent in 2005. Despite the downturn in exclusive breastfeeding, breastfeeding rates in general are at a peak since the first data point in 1986.

Finally, a comparison of breastfeeding in East and West Germany in 1997–1998 points to breastfeeding as an issue related to both maternal and child health as well as women's labour force participation. Even though the reunification of Germany occurred two decades ago, breastfeeding rates differ between the two parts of the country. Although East

German women are more likely to breastfeed immediately after birth (East 97.1 per cent, West 88.7 per cent), West German women breastfeed their children for longer: 48.5 per cent of West German women breastfed their children exclusively for four months after birth compared with 32.5 per cent in East Germany (Dulon *et al.* 2001). East German women are more likely to indicate that they stopped breastfeeding because they returned to work (Dulon *et al.* 2001). In East Germany, a fast return to the labour market was the societal norm, whereas in West Germany most women stayed at home for several years. Germany still has relatively generous leave regulations (with one year of paid parental leave and a guarantee of return to a job for three years), so women can dedicate time to caring for their child (including breastfeeding). Against the background of evidence which indicates that periods of leave have a detrimental effect on women's occupational success and earnings (Rippeyoung and Noonan 2012), recent social policy in Germany and changing societal values are promoting earlier labour market re-entry for women in the western part of the country. How changes in labour market participation will affect breast-feeding patterns in the future is uncertain.[4]

Low birthweight is measured as the proportion of babies with a birth-weight below 2.5 kilograms as a percentage of the total number of live births. In Germany, 6.9 per cent of babies were born with a low birth-weight in 2010. This number is the same as the OECD average.

In Europe, the preterm birth rate (measured as a percentage of the total number of live births) varies roughly between 5 and 10 per cent, with a rate of about 8 per cent in Germany. Most problematic in terms of short- and long-term health outcomes are preterm births before the thirty-second week of gestation, which account for about 1 per cent of all births in Germany as well as in other countries (Bergmann and Dudenhausen 2003; Zeitlin *et al.* 2010).

The maternal mortality rate indicates the number of all maternal deaths from direct or indirect obstetric causes per 100,000 live births (Zeitlin *et al.* 2010; Bundesinstitut für Bevölkerungsforschung 2013). As in most parts of Europe, maternal mortality in Germany has continuously dropped to a very low level. In 1980, the maternal mortality rate was 19.8 and decreased rapidly to a low rate of 4.6 maternal deaths per 100,000 live births in 2012 (Bundesinstitut für Bevölkerungsforschung 2013). World-wide, Germany has one of the lowest maternal mortality rates (Bundesinstitut für Bevölkerungsforschung 2013).

German data on perinatal mortality includes stillbirths (or foetal deaths) with a birthweight of at least 500 g at or after 22 weeks of gestation as well as early neonatal deaths, i.e. deaths during the first seven days after a live birth (Bundesinstitut für Bevölkerungsforschung 2013). The peri-natal mortality rate is calculated by dividing the number of babies who died by the total number of births (including stillbirths and live births). The rates differ slightly between male and female babies. In 2011, the perinatal death rate per 1,000 births (including stillbirths and live births) was 5.7 for male and 5.3 for female babies (Bundesinstitut für Bevölkerungsforschung 2013). International comparisons of perinatal and infant mortality rates are limited as a result of differences in definitions and registration practices (Bundesinstitut für Bevölkerungsforschung 2013). Using the foetal mortality rate (deaths at or after 28 weeks of gestation), perinatal mortality in 2010 ranged from 1.5 per 1,000 births in the Czech Republic to 4.3 in France. Germany recorded a rate of 2.3 per 1,000 births (Zeitlin *et al.* 2010).

Infant mortality is calculated as the number of babies who die during the first year after birth per 1,000 live births (Bundesinstitut für Bevölkerungsforschung 2013). Between 1970 and 2010, infant mortality decreased from 22.5 infant deaths in 1970 to 3.4 infant deaths per 1,000 live births in 2010 (Table 10.3) (OECD 2013b). During this period of time the sharpest decrease in infant mortality took place during the 1980s, with a reduction of 45 per cent between 1970 and 1980 (i.e. from 22.5 infant deaths per 1,000 live births in 1970 to 12.4 infant deaths in 1980). With 3.6 infant deaths per 1,000 live births in 2011, Germany had a middle position compared with other European countries, in which mortality rates ranged from 2.1 in Sweden to 9.4 in Romania (Bundesinstitut für Bevölkerungsforschung 2013).

Consumer involvement

Evidence from Denmark indicates that women are more satisfied when they deliver in midwifery units than in obstetric units (Overgaard *et al.* 2012). Part of the explanation seems to be the importance of emotional support, listening and retaining a sense of control during labour (Waldenström *et al.* 2004).

In Germany, there is hardly any scientific research available on consumer involvement, preferences or satisfaction. A recent German study conducted by the Bertelsmann Foundation in spring 2012[5] analysed the attitudes of 1504 mothers who recently delivered towards different methods of delivery. The majority of women were satisfied with the care provided (Kolip 2012). The results showed that most women see vaginal birth as preferable, but, at the same time, strongly support women's choice to opt for a caesarean section (Kolip 2012). More than 80 per cent of the women surveyed indicated that technological equipment makes them feel safer and only a minority argued for less technology and fewer doctor's visits to increase women's confidence in giving birth using her own strength (Kolip 2012). However, the same survey also shows that women's attitudes are strongly dependent on their type of delivery. Women who had a vaginal birth are significantly less supportive of caesarean sections, assess them as less safe and believe more strongly that a normal delivery strengthens the bond between mother and child (Kolip 2012).

Table 10.3 Birth interventions and outcomes for selected years in Germany

	1970	1980	1990	2000	2010
Maternal mortality[1]	51.8	20.6	9.1	5.6	5.2
Perinatal mortality per 1,000 live and stillbirths[2]	25.3	12.1	6.3	6.1	5.4
Neonatal mortality per 1,000 live births[2]	17.2	8.1	3.7	2.7	2.3
Infant mortality per 1,000 live births[2]	22.5	12.4	7.0	4.4	3.4
Induction (% of all births)[3]	–	–	–	23.7 (2001)	25.3 (2008)
Forceps (% of all births)[4]	–	–	2.3 (1994)	1.6	0.6
Vacuum (% of all births)[4]	–	–	5.7 (1994)	4.8	5.3
Caesarean section per 1,000 live births[4]	–	–	157	208.8	302.9 (2009)
Episiotomy (% of all vaginal births)[3]	–	–	–	41.2 (2001)	29.6 (2008)
Anaesthesia[3]	–	–	–	55.8 (2001)	62.4 (2008)

Sources: 1 WHO (2012); 2 OECD (2013b); 3 Bundesgeschäftsstelle Qualitätssicherung (2009); 4 Gesundheitsberichterstattung des Bundes (www.gbe-bund.de).

To enable citizens to make informed decisions regarding their pregnancy and delivery, several internet sites offer extensive information and advice. Among the providers is the Institute for Quality and Efficiency in Healthcare, an independent scientific institution that was established to support evidence-based decision-making in the German health care system. The private Bertelsmann Foundation, which conducts research on health-related topics, provides an internet site with information related to childbirth with a focus on caesarean sections. The Federal Centre for Health Education (Bundeszentrale für gesundheitliche Aufklärung), which was established in 1967 to reduce health risks and encourage health-promoting lifestyles, also maintains several internet sites for women and (future) parents. A health site for women provides information on women's health and a family site provides information about contraception, family planning, pregnancy and childbirth.

The internet site White List (Weiße Liste) provides an online database for searching and comparing hospitals and doctors. It is funded by the Bertelsmann Foundation in co-operation with a number of other non-profit organisations, such as self-help organisations and sickness funds. With regard to childbirth, the database provides hospital-specific statistics on the quality and availability of facilities, services and personnel, as well as patients' experiences in general (not differentiated by diagnosis). Among other items, hospitals can be compared with regard to the frequency of normal births, caesarean sections and perineal ruptures, the number and formal qualification of doctors, and the type of birth-related medical and non-medical services provided. However, the figures provided are not always complete and are difficult to interpret without additional knowledge of the hospital and expertise in the relevant indicators.

Finally, there are 1,200 'pro familia' agencies, the leading non-governmental service and consumer organisation for sexual and reproductive health and rights in Germany, which offer counselling on pregnancy, abortion and sterilisation.

Risk and rights

Pregnant women in Germany have extensive rights to maternity care and free choice of birth place, hospital, doctor and midwife.[6] However, this choice is often restricted by limited availability, especially in rural areas. The health care system acknowledges that birth involves many personal and social changes for the mother and her family and supports families through generous midwifery care before and after birth. Midwives report that they increasingly take over responsibilities that used to lie with the extended family (e.g. instructions on infant care and cooking) (Schmidt 2014). Despite this notion of childbirth as a major life event and women as deserving of personalised support via midwives, maternity care in Germany is strongly medicalised and organised around risks.

At the micro-level, most women seem to be risk-averse and prefer hospital births despite the free choice of birth place. Nevertheless, this preference of hospitals and technology also needs to be interpreted in the context of current practice. In a country where almost all births occur in hospitals and obstetric guidelines suggest 'warning' women of the risks of out-of-hospital births (Deutsche Gesellschaft für Gynäkologie und Geburtshilfe e.V. 2012), a decision for a home birth or a delivery in a birth centre indicates a deviation from the 'normal' method of childbirth. Risk is an important category in maternity care. The initial visit during which pregnancy is determined involves an extensive risk assessment and documentation in the Mother Passport. Although this risk assessment and the category of high-risk pregnancies involves additional entitlements and supports the exchange of information among providers, it also communicates to pregnant women that their pregnancy may be 'risky' and not 'normal'.

At the meso-level, midwives and doctors share the responsibility for maternity care, but often have different perceptions of risk and the appropriate place of birth. While doctors' associations prioritise (potential) risk avoidance, midwives argue that women's experience of the delivery should also be an important criterion in assessing the relative value of hospital and home or birth centre births. Although empirical evidence clearly shows that all forms of delivery in Germany are 'safe'[7] and differences (if any) are small (Gesellschaft für Qualität in der außerklinischen Geburtshilfe e.V. 2011a), evidence on how 'small' the differences are is both limited and ambiguous (David *et al.* 2004; Birthplace in England Collaborative Group 2011; Gesellschaft für Qualität in der außerklinischen Geburtshilfe e.V. 2011b). Until the evidence reaches a consensus on the relative risks associated with different places of birth, the decision about how to deal with (potential) risk will remain with the pregnant woman. Different interpretations of risk by both professional groups are unlikely to be objective, but are instead used to support their respective professional interests.

These professional interests are also important for developments at the macro-level as doctors' associations and hospital associations (but not midwives) are members of the Federal Joint Committee (Gemeinsamer Bundesausschuss), which consults about structural reform and works out the details of the implementation of political decisions. In 2001, the Gemeinsamer Bundesausschuss commissioned national quality reports in obstetrics (Bundesgeschäftsstelle Qualitätssicherung 2009). The selected quality indicators focused on dramatic and rare outcomes (e.g. maternal mortality, acidosis) rather than on quality indicators for 'normal' childbirth (the psychological health of the mother, breastfeeding). As these are the only indicators available for women for a standardised comparison of hospitals, risk is reinforced as the major criterion for decision-making.

In Germany, gynaecologists and midwives share the right to provide care for pregnant women and attend deliveries. In general, specialists play an important part in the German health care system, which explains why general practitioners are not involved in maternity care. Although all the professions accept that midwives are present at childbirth, participate in pre-natal care and have a dominant role in postnatal care (Bund Deutscher Hebammen e.V. 2001; Deutsche Gesellschaft für Gynäkologie und Geburts-hilfe e.V. 2012), there are professional disputes about their role and their relationship with doctors. First, if and when doctors need to be present is not clearly defined. The National Midwifery Association argues that doctors do not need to be present at 'normal' births (Bund Deutscher Hebammen e.V. 2001) and there are arrangements (such as midwifery-led delivery wards in hospitals) in which doctors are only called in when complications arise. The German Association for Gynaecology and Obstetrics, on the other hand, argues that doctors should be present at hospital births at the start of bearing-down pains (Deutsche Gesellschaft für Gynäkologie und Geburts-hilfe e.V. 2012), which is the usual practice in most hospitals. Second, it is contested whether midwives should work under the authority of doctors when they are present (Bund Deutscher Hebammen e.V. 2001; Deutsche Gesellschaft für Gynäkologie und Geburtshilfe e.V. 2012). This may be regu-lated differently across hospitals and may also vary in practice depending on the relative experience of the doctor and midwife (Braun 2006). Neverthe-less, midwives always retain the right to inform doctors when they see an ordered course of action as a risk to the mother or child and can refuse such orders (Hebammengesetz 1985). Third, doctors challenge births outside hospitals for safety reasons (Le Ker 2012). The German Association for Gynaecology and Obstetrics recommends that doctors should inform preg-nant women of the higher risk of births outside hospital (Deutsche Gesell-schaft für Gynäkologie und Geburtshilfe e.V. 2012), while the National Midwifery Association claims there are no differences in birth outcomes for normal births outside hospitals (Bund Deutscher Hebammen e.V. 2001).

A German study that compared mother and infant health for births in birth centres and hospitals (adjustment of clinical birth population to birth centre risks) indicates that hospitals and birth centres have signi-ficant advantages and disadvantages for different outcomes (David *et al.* 2004). Among the birth centre births, the risk of postpartum bleeding was higher, as were low five-minute Apgar scores among babies of first-time mothers (David *et al.* 2004). Birth centre births also had significantly more neonatal interventions (David *et al.* 2004). Hospital births had more surgery (including episiotomies) and more DR III and IV perineal rup-tures as well as more transfers of babies to paediatric departments. Infant and maternal mortality seem to be similar in both settings, but are difficult to study as they are rare events (David *et al.* 2004). Infant mortality among births outside hospitals was 1.1 per 1,000 births in 2011, but this statistic is based on only eleven cases of babies who died because the absolute number of out-of-hospital births is so small (Gesellschaft für Qualität in der außerklinischen Geburtshilfe e.V. 2011a).

Technology plays an important part both in antenatal and intrapartum care in Germany. In particular, the use of ultrasonography and cardiotocographs exceeds the German recommendations (Gemeinsamer Bundesausschuss 2013). Although three ultrasound scans are recommended in Germany, 22 per cent of pregnant women have five or more ultrasound scans (Bundesgeschäftsstelle Qualitätssicherung 2009). The use of cardiotocographs is only recommended with medical indications (Gemeinsamer Bundesausschuss 2013), but is regularly used both for antenatal care in the last trimester and during labour (Braun 2006; Bundesgeschäftsstelle Qualitätssicherung 2009). Although the use of technology is not always backed up by clinical evidence, most pregnant women appreciate technology, particularly in antenatal care. In a 2012 study of 1,504 recent mothers, more than 80 per cent indicated that technological equipment makes them feel safer and only a minority argued for less technology and fewer doctor's visits to increase women's confidence to give birth using their own strength (Kolip 2012).

Conclusion

The traditional family model, which supports a male breadwinner and a female care-giver, is slowly evolving into a dual-earner family model. Fathers are encouraged to take parental leave and women are expected to return to the labour market sooner. However, there is still a huge lack of childcare facilities that are necessary to achieve a better work–life balance for dual-earner couples. Moreover, there continues to be a strong normative opposition towards this model in conservative parts of society, especially in West Germany.

Pregnancy and childbirth are strongly medicalised and make heavy use of technology. Ninety-eight per cent of births occur in a hospital setting, which is supported by both doctors and the majority of women, who aim to minimise risk and appreciate the availability of technology and anaesthesia. Almost all women favour a vaginal delivery; however, every third child is born via a caesarean section. The number of birth centres and home births is increasing, but both options remain marginal phenomena.

There is little indication that the German maternity care system will undergo dramatic reforms in the near future. Two opposing trends will affect the manner in which children are born in Germany. On the one hand, we observe a new emphasis on natural births and midwifery care. The number of out-of-hospital births has grown slowly, but steadily. New care arrangements (such as midwifery-led maternity wards) are increasing and hospitals that compete for the decreasing number of pregnant women are responding to women's preferences by offering homeopathic treatments, water births and more individualised care. On the other hand, the age at first pregnancy and the number of pregnancies defined as 'risky' are increasing. Anaesthesia and caesarean sections are becoming less risky and are therefore likely to increase as they are seen as a safe alternative to natural childbirth. Finally, the high rate of caesarean section itself leads to a growth in further caesarean sections. At this point in time, Germany largely lacks a women's voice regarding maternity care. This may, in part, be the result of a maternity care system that supports techno-logical, specialised care by doctors and personal support by midwives as well as free choice for pregnant women.

Notes

1 Doctors receive a specialisation in 'gynaecology and obstetrics'. They are not separate specialty fields. Gynaecologist is the term commonly used in the German setting.
2 For incomes below €1,000, the replacement rate gradually goes up to 100 per cent, i.e. by 0.1 percentage points per every €2 of the margin between the income and €1,000. For higher incomes the rate gradually decreases to 65 per cent. Couples with an annual income of more than €500,000 (€250,000 for single parents) are not entitled to parental leave benefits (Blum and Erler 2013).
3 2008 is the year from which the most recent data for obstetric parameters are available at the national level.
4 The legal protection of working mothers grants breastfeeding times of one hour a day (or half an hour twice a day) (Mutterschutzgesetz §7, Abs.1).
5 The study was part of the 2012 Gesundheitsmonitor (Health Care Monitor), which is conducted regularly by the Bertelsmann Foundation and BARMER GEK (a public health insurance company) to monitor public opinion towards the health care system in Germany.
6 Choice of doctor and midwife denotes mostly outpatient care. Although there are arrangements in which a woman can choose a doctor or midwife who accom-panies her during the delivery, the standard hospital birth includes no provider choice because doctors and midwives work in shifts.
7 'Safe' in this context means that birth outcomes (including mortality) are in the range of (richer) OECD countries and low in both historical and international comparison.

Useful web sites

Bundeszentrale für gesundheitliche Aufklärung	www.bzga.de/home/ www.frauengesundheitsportal.de www.schwanger-info.de www.familienplanung.de
White List	www.weisse-liste.de
Pro-Family	www.profamilia.de

References

Albrecht, M., Loos, S., Sander, M. Schliwen, A. and Wolfschütz, A. (2012) *Ver-sorgungs- und Vergütungssituation in der außerklinischen Hebammenhilfe: Ergebnis-bericht für das Bundeministerium für Gesundheit* (Supply and payment situation in out-of-hospital midwife care: report for the Federal Ministry of Health) [in German]. Berlin: IGES Institut.

Ärztezeitung (2014) 'Haftpflicht: Gröhe gibt bei Hebammen Gas' (Liability insurance: Gröhe is hitting the gas with midwives) [in German], *Ärztezeitung*, 8 May [online]. Available from: www.aerztezeitung.de/politik_gesellschaft/article/860402/haftpflicht-groehe-gibt-hebammen-gas.html?sh=1&h=878090519. Accessed 13 May 2014.

Babyfreundliches Krankenhaus e.V. (2014) *Ausgezeichnete Mitglieder* (Awarded Members) [in German] [online]. Available from: www.babyfreundlich.org/fachkraefte/initiative-babyfreundlich/ausgezeichnete-mitglieder.html#tab-484–1. Accessed 2 April 2014.

Bergmann, R.L. and Dudenhausen, J.W. (2003) 'Prediction and prevention of preterm birth', *Gynäkologe*, 36 (5): 391–402.

Bertelsmann Stiftung (2010) *Regionale Unterschiede in der Gesundheitsversorgung: Kaiserschnittrate nach Kreisen 2010* (Regional differences in the provision of healthcare: caesarean rate by district) [in German] [online]. Available from: www.faktencheck-kaiserschnitt.de. Accessed 14 April 2014.

Bundesinstitut für Bevölkerungsforschung (2013) *Bundesinstitut für Bevölkerungsforschung* (Federal Institute for Population Research) [in German] [online]. Available from: www.bib-demografie.de/DE/Home/home_node.html. Accessed 8 April 2014.

Birg, H. (2001) *Die demographische Zeitenwende: der Bevölkerungsrückgang in Deutschland und Europa ; [mit 25 Tabellen]* (Demographic change: population decrease in Germany and Europe) [in German]. Munich: Beck.

Birthplace in England Collaborative Group (2011) 'Perinatal and maternal outcomes by planned place of birth for healthy women with low risk pregnancies: the Birthplace in England National Prospective Cohort Study', *BMJ*, 343 (4): d7400.

Blum, S. and Erler, D. (2013) 'Germany country note'. In: Moss, P. (ed.), *International Review of Leave Policies and Research 2013* [online]. Available from: www.leavenetwork.org/lp_and_r_reports/. Accessed 13 January 2014.

Braun, B. (2006) *Geburten und Geburtshilfe in Deutschland* (Births and obstetrics in Germany) [in German], GEK Schriftenreihe zur Gesundheitsanalyse, 43. St Augustin: Asgard-Verlag.

Bund Deutscher Hebammen e.V. (2001) *Empfehlungen zur Zusammenarbeit von Hebamme und Ärztin/Arzt in der Geburtshilfe* (Recommendations for the collaboration between midwives and obstetricians) [in German] [online]. Available from: www.hebammenverband.de/aktuell/standpunkte/empfehlungen/. Accessed 17 April 2014.

Bundesärztekammer (2003) *(Muster-)Weiterbildungsordnung 2003* ((Exemplary) regulation on further education) [in German] [online]. Available from: www.bundesaerztekammer.de/downloads/20130628-MWBO_V6.pdf. Accessed 2 April 2014.

Bundesgeschäftsstelle Qualitätssicherung GmbH (2009) *Bundesauswertung 2008 Geburtshilfe* (National results 2008: obstetrics) [in German] [online]. Available from: www.bqs-outcome.de. Accessed 3 April 2014.

Bundeskinderschutzgesetz (2011) 'Gesetz zur Stärkung eines aktiven Schutzes von Kindern und Jugendlichen' (Law for the improvement of a (pro)active protection of children and adolescents) [in German], *Bundesgesetzblatt*, I (70): 2975–2982.

Bundesministerium für Familie, Senioren, Frauen und Jugend (ed.) (2012) *Elterngeld und Elternzeit. Das Bundeselterngeld- und Elternzeitgesetz* (Parental benefit and parental leave. The federal law for parental leave) [in German], 11th edn. Berlin: BMFSFJ.

Bundeszentrale für gesundheitliche Aufklärung (2014a) *Kurse zur Geburtsvorbereitung* (Antenatal classes) [in German] [online]. Available from: www.familienplanung.de/schwangerschaft/geburtsvorbereitung/geburtsvorbereitungskurs/. Accessed 3 April 2014.

Bundeszentrale für gesundheitliche Aufklärung (2014b) *Wochenbett-Betreuung* (Postnatal care) [in German] [online]. Available from: www.familienplanung.de/schwangerschaft/nach-der-geburt/wochenbett-betreuung/. Accessed 3 April 2014.

Busse, R. and Riesberg, A. (2005) *Health Care Systems in Transition: Germany*. Copenhagen: European Observatory on Health Systems and Policies.

Clasen, J. (2005) *Reforming European Welfare States*. Oxford: Oxford University Press.

David, M., Pachaly, J., Vetter, K. and Kentenich, H. (2004) 'Geburtsort Geburtshaus – Perinataldaten im Vergleich zu Klinikentbindungen in Bayern und Berlin' (Birthplace birth centre – perinatal outcomes in comparison with hospital births in Bavaria and Berlin) [in German], *Zeitschrift für Geburtshilfe und Neonatologie*, 208 (3): 110–117.

Deutsche Gesellschaft für Gynäkologie und Geburtshilfe e.V. (2012) 'Empfehlungen zur Zusammenarbeit von Arzt und Hebamme in der Geburtshilfe – Aus ärztlicher Sicht' (Recommendations for the cooperation of doctor and midwife in obstetrics – a medical perspective) [in German], *Arbeitsgemeinschaft der Wissenschaftlichen Medizinischen Fachgesellschaften (AMWF) e.V Online*, 015/030 [online]. Available from: www.awmf.org/uploads/tx_szleitlinien/015–030l_S1_Zusammenarbeit_Arzt_Hebamme_2013–05.pdf. Accessed 12 May 2014.

Deutscher Bundestag (2014) *Sorge um flächendeckende Geburtshilfe* (Worries about comprehensive coverage with obstetric care services) [in German] [online]. Available from: www.bundestag.de/mobil/aktuell/textarchiv/2014/49969914_kw12_de_hebammen/index.html. Accessed 2 April 2014.

Deutscher Hebammen Verband e.V. (2014a) *Deutscher Hebammen Verband e.V.: Ausbildung* (Vocational training for midwives) [in German] [online]. Available from: www.hebammenverband.de/beruf-hebamme/ausbildung/. Accessed 1 April 2014.

Deutscher Hebammen Verband e.V. (2014b) *Haftpflichtvertrag für ein Jahr unterschrieben, weiterhin keine langfristige Lösung in Sicht* (Liability insurance contracts signed for one year, still no long-term solution in sight) [online]. Available from: www. hebammenverband.de/aktuell/nachricht-detail/datum/2014/03/28/artikel/haftpflichtvertrag-fuer-ein-jahr-unterschrieben-weiterhin-keine-langfristige-loesung-in-sicht/. Accessed 2 April 2014.

Deutscher Hebammen Verband e.V. (2014c) *Hebammenkreißsäle in Deutschland* (Midwife-led delivery wards in Germany) [in German] [online]. Available from: www.hebammenverband.de/familie/hebammen-kreisssaele/. Accessed 2 April 2014.

Deven, F. and Moss, P. (2005) *Leave Policies and Research. Reviews and Country Notes* [online]. Available from: www.leavenetwork.org/fileadmin/Leavenetwork/Annual_reviews/2005_annual_report.pdf. Accessed 13 January 2014.

Dingeldey, I. (2001) 'European tax systems and their impact on family employment patterns', *Journal of Social Policy*, 30 (4): 653–672.

Dulon, M., Kersting, M. and Schach, S. (2001) 'Duration of breastfeeding and associated factors in Western and Eastern Germany', *Acta Paediatrica*, 90 (8): 931–935.

Esping-Andersen, G. (1990) *The Three Worlds of Welfare Capitalism.* Cambridge: Polity Press.

Geißler, R. and Meyer, T. (2014) 'Struktur und Entwicklung der Bevölkerung' (Population structure and development) [in German]. In: R. Geißler (ed.), *Die Sozialstruktur Deutschlands.* Wiesbaden: Springer Fachmedien, pp. 27–58. Available from: http://link.springer.com/chapter/10.1007/978–3–531–19151–5_3. Accessed 3 April 2014.

Gemeinsamer Bundesausschuss (2013) 'Richtlinien des Gemeinsamen Bundesausschusses über die ärztliche Betreuung während der Schwangerschaft und nach der Entbindung ("Mutterschafts-Richtlinien") (Guidelines of the Federal Joint Committee on the medical assistance during pregnancy and after birth ("Maternity guidelines")) [in German], *Bundesanzeiger,* AT (B2).

Gesellschaft für Qualität in der außerklinischen Geburtshilfe e.V. (2011a) *Außerklinische Geburtshilfe in Deutschland – Qualitätsbericht 2011* (Out-of-hospital childbirth in Germany – quality report 2011) [in German]. Auerbach: Verlag Wissenschaftliche Scripten.

Gesellschaft für Qualität in der außerklinischen Geburtshilfe e.V. (2011b) *Pilotprojekt zum Vergleich klinischer Geburten im Bundesland Hessen mit außerklinischen Geburten in von Hebammen geleiteten Einrichtungen bundesweit* (Pilot project for the comparison of hospital births with out-of-hospital births in midwife-led facilities in the state of Hessen) [in German] [online]. Available from: www.quag.de/downloads/VergleichGeburtenGKV-SV.pdf. Accessed 17 April 2014.

Gesellschaft für Qualität in der außerklinischen Geburtshilfe e.V. (QUAG) (2014) *QUAG – Geburtenzahlen in Deutschland* (QUAG – birth figures in Germany) [in German] [online]. Available from: www.quag.de/quag/geburtenzahlen.htm.

Gesetzliche Krankenversicherung Spitzenverband (2013) *Vertragspartnerliste Hebammen* (List of contracted midwives) [in German] [online]. Available from: www.gkv-spitzenverband.de/presse/zahlen_und_grafiken/gkv_kennzahlen_hebammen/gkv_kennzahlen_hebammen_1.jsp. Accessed 3 April 2014.

Haller, U., Hepp, H. and Winter, R. (2002) 'Section nach Wunsch oder elektive Section: Aufforderung zum Umdenken' (Section on demand or elective section: a call for a reconsideration) [in German], *Gynäkologisch-geburtshilfliche Rundschau,* 42: 1–3.

Hebammengesetz (1985) Gesetz über den Beruf der Hebamme und des Entbindungspflegers (Hebammengesetz – HebG) (Law on the profession of midwives) [in German]. BGB I. I S.209.

Hickl, E.-J. (2002) 'Wandlungen in der Kaiserschnittindikation' (Changing indications for caesarean sections) [in German], *Gynäkologisch-geburtshilfliche Rundschau,* 42 (1): 15–18.

Keller, M. and Haustein, T. (2012) 'Vereinbarkeit von Familie und Beruf: Ergebnisse des Mikrozensus 2010' (Reconciliation of work and family life: results from the census 2010) [in German], *Wirtschaft und Statistik,* January: 30–51.

Kohlhuber, M., Rebhan, B., Schwegler, U., Koletzko, B. and Fromme, H. (2008) 'Breastfeeding rates and duration in Germany: a Bavarian cohort study', *The British Journal of Nutrition,* 99 (5): 1127–1132.

Kolip, P. (2012) 'Einflussfaktoren auf den Geburtsmodus: Kaiserschnitt versus Spontangeburt' (Influencing factors on the mode of birth: caesarean section versus vaginal delivery) [in German], *Gesundheitsmonitor,* 3/2012.

Lange, D.C., Schenk, L. and Bergmann, R. (2007) 'Verbreitung, Dauer und zeitlicher Trend des Stillens in Deutschland' (Breastfeeding in Germany: prevalence, duration and trends) [in German], *Bundesgesundheitsblatt – Gesundheitsforschung – Gesundheitsschutz*, 50 (5–6): 624–633.

Le Ker, H. (2012) 'Streit um Hausgeburten: Kuschelatmosphäre plus High-Tech-Medizin' (Controversy around home births: cosy atmosphere plus high-tech medicine) [in German], *SPIEGEL Online* [online]. Available from: www.spiegel.de/#action=404&ref=hpinject404. Accessed 2 April 2014.

National Breastfeeding Committee (2013) *Information on Breastfeeding for Expectant Mothers* [online]. Available from: www.bfr.bund.de/cm/350/stillempfehlungen_fuer_schwangere_englisch.pdf. Accessed 2 April 2014.

OECD (2011) *Health at a Glance 2011: OECD Indicators* [online]. Available from: www.oecd-ilibrary.org/social-issues-migration-health/health-at-a-glance-2011/caesarean-sections_health_glance-2011-37-en. Accessed 13 May 2014.

OECD (2013a) *OECD Family Database: Child Well-being Module* [online]. Available from: www.oecd.org/social/soc/oecdfamilydatabasechildwell-beingmodule.htm. Accessed 20 November 2013.

OECD (2013b) *OECD Health Data 2013* [online]. Available from: www.oecd.org/health/healthdata. Accessed 4 March 2014.

Overgaard, C., Fenger-Gron, M. and Sandall, J. (2012) 'The impact of birthplace on women's birth experiences and perceptions of care', *Social Science & Medicine*, 74 (7): 973–981.

Peters, E., Wehkamp, K.-H., Felberbaum, R.E., Krüger, D. and Linder, R. (2006) 'Breastfeeding duration is determined by only a few factors', *The European Journal of Public Health*, 16 (2): 162–167.

Reibling, N. (2010) 'Healthcare systems in Europe: towards an incorporation of patient access', *Journal of European Social Policy*, 20 (1): 5–18.

Reibling, N. and Wendt, C. (2012) 'Gatekeeping and provider choice in OECD healthcare systems', *Current Sociology*, 60 (4): 489–505.

Rippeyoung, P.L.F. and Noonan, M.C. (2012) 'Is breastfeeding truly cost free? Income consequences of breastfeeding for women', *American Sociological Review*, 77 (2): 244–267.

Rosenfeld, R.A., Trappe, H. and Gornick, J.C. (2004) 'Gender and work in Germany: before and after reunification', *Annual Review of Sociology*, 30: 103–124.

Schmidt, L. (2014) 'Ich bin beste Freundin und Therapeutin in einem' (I am best friend and therapist at the same time) [in German], *Frankfurter Allgemeine Zeitung (FAZ)* [online]. Available from: www.faz.net/aktuell/gesellschaft/gesundheit/hebammen-ich-bin-bes. Accessed 17 April 2014.

Statistisches Bundesamt (2011) *Sozialleistungen: Angaben zur Krankenversicherung* (Social security benefits: data on health insurance) [in German]. Wiesbaden (Fachserie 13) [online]. Available from: www.destatis.de/DE/Publikationen/Thematisch/Bevoelkerung/HaushalteMikrozensus/KrankenversicherungMikrozensus2130110119004.pdf?__blob=publicationFile. Accessed 15 April 2014.

Statistisches Bundesamt (2012a) 'Grunddaten der Krankenhäuser' (Basic hospital data) [in German], *Fachserie Gesundheit*, 12 (6.1.1) [online]. Available from: www.destatis.de/DE/Publikationen/Thematisch/Gesundheit/Krankenhaeuser/GrunddatenKrankenhaeuser2120611127004.pdf?__blob=publicationFile. Accessed 2 April 2014.

Statistisches Bundesamt (2012b) *Geburten in Deutschland*, 2012 (Births in Germany, 2012) [in German]. Wiesbaden: Statistisches Bundesamt.

Statistisches Bundesamt (2013) *Statistisches Jahrbuch Deutschland 2013* (Statistical Yearbook Germany 2013) [in German]. Wiesbaden: Statistisches Bundesamt.

Trappe, H. (1995) *Emanzipation oder Zwang?: Frauen in der DDR zwischen Beruf, Familie und Sozialpolitik* (Emancipation or coercion: Women in the GDR between job, family and social policy) [in German]. Berlin: Akademie-Verlag.

Waldenström, U., Hildingsson, I., Rubertsson, C. and Rádestad, I. (2004) 'A negative birth experience: prevalence and risk factors in a national sample', *Birth: Issues in Perinatal Care*, 31 (1): 17–27.

Wendt, C., Mischke, M. and Pfeifer, M. (2011) *Welfare States and Public Opinion: Perceptions of Healthcare Systems, Family Policy and Benefits for the Unemployed and Poor in Europe*. Cheltenham: Edward Elgar.

World Health Organization (2012) *Trends in Maternal Mortality: 1990 to 2010. WHO, UNICEF, UNFPA and The World Bank Estimates* [online]. Available from: http://whqlibdoc.who.int/publications/2012/9789241503631_eng.pdf?ua=1. Accessed 13 January 2014.

Yngve, A. and Sjöström, M. (2001) 'Breastfeeding in countries of the European Union and EFTA: current and proposed recommendations, rationale, prevalence, duration and trends', *Public Health Nutrition*, 4 (2B): 631–645.

Zeitlin, J., Mohangoo, A. and Delnord, M. (eds) (2010) *European Perinatal Health Report. Health and Care of Pregnant Women and Babies in Europe 2010*. Paris: EUROPERISTAT.

11 The Netherlands

Monika Ewa Kaminska

Background

The Netherlands is a decentralised unitary state in Western Europe consisting of twelve provinces. It is a constitutional monarchy, with a king or queen as the formal head of state, and a parliamentary representative democracy. The Netherlands has been described as a consociational state due to the practice of striving for a broad consensus on significant issues within the political realm and society alike (Visser and Hemerijk 1997), with different segments of society enjoying a large degree of autonomy (Andeweg and Irwin 2005).

The Dutch economy is among the world's top twenty in terms of total GDP. Financial and commercial services are the main drivers of the economy, with business services being the dominant sector. Industrial activity is concentrated in food processing, chemicals and petroleum refining, and electrical and electronic machinery (Schäfer *et al.* 2010: 1). In 2011, the GDP per capita (current prices, adjusted for purchasing power parity) was US$43,000, the second highest in the European Union, and the fifth highest in the OECD. After high growth rates of the GDP in the 1990s (4.7 per cent in 1999), the Dutch economy slumped, then accelerated in 2004 and grew until 2007. It was then hit by the current economic crisis and registered negative GDP growth in 2009, 2012 and 2013 (OECD 2013a; European Commission 2014).

The Netherlands as a welfare regime

The Dutch welfare state is difficult to classify into one of the established families of welfare state systems. Its social security system displays characteristics of both the 'Bismarckian-type social insurance for workers' and 'universal, so-called people's insurances that cover all citizens' (van Oorschot 2009: 366). This has allowed it to be classified as a social democratic, conservative/continental, liberal or hybrid type (Arts and Gelissen 2010).

Esping-Andersen assigned the Netherlands to the social democratic type of welfare regime based on its superior performance on decommodification and stratification effects and the strong manifestation of socialist regime attributes. However, based on the functioning of its labour market, the Netherlands appeared in the continental cluster which strongly nourishes exit and reduced labour supply (Esping-Andersen 1990). In Esping-Andersen's later work, although 'important elements of [the Dutch] income maintenance system are closer to the Nordic universalistic model' (Esping-Andersen 1996: 84), the Netherlands features in the group of continental/conservative welfare states, where 'the Christian democratic "subsidiarity principle" has institutionalised familialism' by 'supporting the male-breadwinner/female-carer model with transfers'[1] (Esping-Andersen 1996: 66) and complementing it with 'underdeveloped social care services' (Esping-Andersen 1996: 71).

The Dutch welfare system can be characterised by a high degree of corporatism and comprehensiveness (van Oorschot 2009: 365), although over the past few decades the emphasis has shifted from inclusive solidarity towards exclusive selectivity and from collective responsibility towards individual responsibility (van Oorschot 2009: 374), a change also affecting the health care system. Meulders and O'Dorchai (2007) indicate that '[h]istorically, the process of "democratic pacification" (via pillarisation) in the Netherlands has led, on the one hand, to tolerance and accommodation, mainly in the public sphere, and to basic income policies, and, on the other, to a strengthened idea of family privacy and women homemakers' (Meulders and O'Dorchai 2007: 8). Traditionally, a nuclear Dutch family leads an autonomous and self-determining life 'free from government interference' (van Daalen 2007: 621).

Between 1849 and 1990, the labour market participation of (especially married) women in the Netherlands was much lower than in Belgium, Denmark, France, Germany, Sweden or the UK (van Daalen 2007: 621). In the early 1990s, the female participation rates of 40–45 per cent were among the lowest within the OECD (OECD 1993). Since then, 'social policies have increasingly focused on facilitating the work/life balance for Dutch mothers' (Meulders and O'Dorchai 2007: 8), although the familialistic bias persists. Overall, 'the female employment rate increased from 30 per cent in 1975 to almost 70 per cent in 2011 (above the OECD average of 60 per cent)' (OECD 2013c). However, 76.7 per cent of all employed women work part-time, including 75 per cent of women with dependent children (OECD 2013c), which adversely affects women's earnings and career profiles compared with men (a high gender pay gap mainly due to differences in working hours, a low share of female supervisory staff and a large gender-based pension gap) (OECD 2013c). The labour market outcomes cannot be considered separately from the duration and generosity of maternity entitlements, and the availability of childcare facilities.

Health care system

The Dutch health care system, in a similar way to the welfare state within which it is embedded, defies classification. It can be described as 'rooted in the "Bismarckian" social insurance tradition' (Schäfer *et al.* 2010: 13), but displays characteristics of different types of health care system. Until the mid-1970s it was very compound and consisted of 'several separate sub-schemes', each representing the 'ideational and organisational character-istics of three health care system types: the National Health Service, the social health insurance, and the private health insurance system' (Götze 2010: 1, 37). In the following decades several structural reforms culmin-ated in the 2006 Health Insurance Act, which introduced a universal health insurance scheme for the whole population as a 'further innovation of the old Bismarckian system' (Schäfer *et al.* 2010: 13, 167). The reforms have produced a unitary, but hybrid, health care system: it is regulated by the state, but financed mainly by social insurance contributions, with pro-vision delegated to private entities (Böhm *et al.* 2013).

The 2006 reforms reinforced the role of market mechanisms (OECD 2012a). Consequently, health care in the Netherlands can be character-ised by 'a shift from supply towards a needs-based health care' (Den Exter 2010: 1031). Despite cost-containment reforms, health care spending in the Netherlands has grown in recent years following a sharp increase in the volume of care and in the already high incomes of doctors; however, generic drug prices decreased significantly (OECD 2012a: 107, 109, 113). The total health expenditure as a share of GDP reached 11.9 per cent in 2011. It tops the European Union charts and comes second within the OECD. Health spending per capita (US$5,099 in 2011, adjusted for pur-chasing power parity) is the fourth highest within the OECD (OECD 2013b). Public funding covers 85.6 per cent of current health spending (above the OECD average of 72.2 per cent) (OECD 2013a).

Primary, secondary and long-term care are mainly provided by private providers, while preventive care is primarily provided by the public health services. Although unusual for a social health insurance system, the Nether-lands belongs to 'strong gatekeeping and low supply states', characterised by 'extensive gatekeeping arrangements regulating access to specialist care and a very low number of health care providers (except for nurses) and medical technology' (Reibling 2010: 15). Primary care has historically been a strong foundation of the Dutch health care system and, crucially for the develop-ment of Dutch maternity care, it is considered to prevent the unnecessary use of costly secondary care and remains a policy priority (Schäfer *et al.* 2010: 13, xx). Primary care providers include general practitioners and midwives, who function as gate-keepers: any specialist and hospital care, including paediatric and gynaecological care, with the exception of emergency cases, is available exclusively on referral (Schäfer *et al.* 2010: xxv). Secondary care is offered within hospitals and mental health care institutions by medical specialists who traditionally work within hospital structures in both inpatient and outpatient care (Schäfer *et al.* 2010: 18). In recent years, a growing number of specialists have participated in independent treatment centres. Hospitals have inpatient and outpatient units and twenty-four-hour emergency wards. Patients whose conditions are not life-threatening are supposed to consult a general practitioner for out-of-hours care. Well-developed long-term care is offered against long-term care insurance and is provided in nursing homes or in the patient's home (OECD 2012a: 117).

Access to (primary) care is facilitated by the comprehensive basic mandatory health insurance scheme based on the principles of equal access and solidarity (Den Exter 2010). Few people in the Netherlands give up medical visits for financial reasons (Westert *et al.* 2010). The dispersion in the age of death, a measure of inequality in health status, is among the lowest within the OECD (Joumard *et al.* 2010). The supply side of the Dutch health care system is more constrained than in many other OECD countries (Table 11.1) and the volume of health care services (doctor consultations, inpatient discharge rates and average length of stay in acute care) is low compared with the OECD average (OECD 2012a: 103).

The Dutch Ministry of Health, Welfare and Sport (Ministerie van Volksgezondheid, Welzijn en Sport) is responsible for public health and health care, welfare and socio-cultural work, and sport. Autonomous agencies operating under the Ministry of Health, Welfare and Sport include the National Institute for Public Health and Environment (Rijksinstituut voor Volksgezondheid en Milieu). The supervision and management of the health care system are delegated to independent bodies – for example, the Healthcare Inspectorate (Inspectie voor de Gezondheidszorg) and the National Healthcare Institute (Zorginstituut Nederland). Following the introduction (in 2006) of managed competition as the central regulatory mechanism in the health care arena, the role of the government has 'changed from direct control of volumes, prices and productive capacity to setting the "rules of the game"

Table 11.1 Human and physical resources in the Netherlands

Physicians per 1,000 population	3 (2010)
Nurses per 1,000 population	11.8 (2010)
Medical graduates per 100,000 population	14.5 (2011)
Nursing graduates per 100,000 population	38.6 (2011)
Total hospital beds per 1,000 population	4.7 (2009)
Curative (acute) care beds per 1,000 population	3.3 (2011)
Gynaecologists, total	973 (2014)[a]
Midwives	2.692, 1.5% of them being men (2012)[b]

Sources: OECD (2013a); a NVOG (2014); b NIVEL (2013).

and overseeing whether markets are working properly' (Schäfer *et al.* 2010: 21–22). However, the Ministry of Health, Welfare and Sport (supported by the National Healthcare Institute) continues to define the benefits package.

Demographic profile

The Netherlands is the most densely populated country in the European Union (Table 11.2). Annual population growth rates have fallen since the 1970s to 0.21 per cent in 2007 (OECD 2013a). In 2012 the estimated net migration was 50,000 (World Bank 2013). Between 1970 and 2011, life expectancy at birth in the Netherlands has increased from 73.6 to 81.3 years (OECD 2013b).

Since 1973, Dutch fertility rates have been below the replacement level. After a significant drop between 1970 (2.57) and 1983 (1.47), fertility rates increased at an irregular pace to reach 1.8 in 2010 (OECD 2013a). For decades, mothers in the Netherlands were among the oldest in Europe (Garssen and Nicolaas 2008), but, in 2010, seven other European countries had higher rates of mothers aged thirty-five years and older (European Perinatal Health Report 2013). Non-Western women (mainly Surinamese, Turkish and Moroccan) play an increasing part in the fertility trends. In 2008, they constituted 13.5 per cent of all women of fertile age in the Netherlands (Garssen and Nicolaas 2008).

Maternity care provision

Dutch maternity care is based on the midwifery model. It differs significantly from that encountered in other industrialised countries in its

Table 11.2 Demographic profile of the Netherlands, 2012

Population	16,754,960
Women (%)	50.5
Population aged 0–14 years (%)	17.2
Women of childbearing age (15–44 years) (%)	19
Population aged 65 years or older (%)	16.5
Population annual growth (%)	0.21 (2007)
Population density per square kilometre	403.3
Total fertility rate (births per woman)	1.8 (2010)
Crude birth rate per 1,000 people	10.8[a]
Crude death rate per 1,000 people	8.4[a]
Urban population (%)	84[a]
Ethnic groups (breakdown)	79.1% ethnic Dutch; 9.3% Western origin; 2.4% Turkish; 2.2% Moroccan; 2% Surinamese; 0.9% Antillan/Aruban; 4.1% other non-Western[b]

Sources: OECD (2013a); a WHO (2014); b Statistics Netherlands (2014).

ideology, organisation and practice; these are embedded in specific social structures and the cultural context that generated and sustains those structures (De Vries and Lemmens 2006; Christiaens and Bracke 2007). The cultural context includes the importance of home and the nuclear family, specific ideas about the role of women as home-makers, thriftiness in the use of medicine and the social norms of 'not behaving differently from others' and 'not sticking out one's head' (De Vries 2005: 138–179; De Vries *et al.* 2013).

Ideologically, pregnancy, labour and the puerperium in the Netherlands are regarded as physiological rather than medical events (De Vries and Buitendijk 2012). Home delivery is seen as safe and is expected to proceed normally (Ziekenfondsraad 1987), while 'a desire of an obstetrician-supervised pregnancy and hospital delivery is seen as a challenge to the "physiological" norm' (Christiaens and Bracke 2007: e12). Many Dutch women never see a physician or make a hospital visit throughout their reproductive lifetime of pregnancies and births (Katz Rothman 2001: 183). An expectative approach prevails and any medical intervention should be minimised, as it does not belong to the cultural definition of normal deliveries (Abraham-van der Mark 1996: 3–4). Consequently, '[p]regnant women are not regarded as ill patients, unless something goes actually wrong or unless the delivery is expected to be difficult for previously assessed reasons' (van Teijlingen 2004: 163–164). Indeed, the Dutch literature and Dutch midwives in their practice refer to pregnant women as clients, not patients.

Organisationally, the most distinguished feature of Dutch maternity care is the strict division between primary care (provided by autonomous community midwives) for women with low-risk ('normal') pregnancies and secondary care (provided by gynaecologists and clinical midwives in general hospitals) for women with high-risk ('complicated') pregnancies. In the case of major complications, tertiary care is provided by gynaecologists in academic hospitals. Thus the system distinguishes between two groups of pregnant women who are cared for by different tiers, different professions and different organisations (Pieters 2013: 71). The financial structure and compensation for the two groups are different and data on perinatal care are collected at the different levels and are not assembled for the individuals attending different echelons (Pieters 2013: 73).

Primary care midwives operate as autonomous medical practitioners (Smeenk and Ten Have 2003: 155). They are usually self-employed and work without the guidance or control of an obstetrician. The state has supported the position of midwives through the promotion of the professionalisation of midwifery and the normality of childbirth by means of legislation and insurance (Christiaens *et al.* 2013: e5). Midwives' authority in the 'uncomplicated natural course of labour' without the use of obstetrical instruments was established by the first Dutch Law of Medical Practice in 1865 (Amelink-Verburg and Buitendijk 2010). The sickness insurance system introduced in 1941 established the monopoly (*primaat*) of midwives over normal deliveries. Midwives became exclusively responsible for delivering services in home births to pregnant members of sickness funds (van Teijlingen 2004).[2] Hospitalisation was only covered by insurance in the case of medical issues (Abraham-van der Mark 1996). In 1974, a restructuring of the health care system strengthened care levels with gate-keeping functions (Structuurnota Gezondheidszorg 1974). This corroborated the idea that low-risk pregnant women should be served by midwifery practices, with only high-risk pregnancies being addressed by gynaecologists in the hospital setting (Pieters 2013: 71).

Risk selection and the resulting assignment to primary or secondary care is based on the List of Obstetric Indications (Verloskundige Indicatielijst), which specifies referral criteria. The official List of Obstetric Indications, published in 1973, has been revised three times – in 1987, 1999 and 2003 – by the Royal Dutch Organisation of Midwives (Koninklijke Nederlandse Organisatie van Verloskundigen) and the Dutch Association for Obstetrics and Gynaecology (Nederlandse Vereiniging voor Obstetrie en Gynaecologie) (Amelink-Verburg and Buitendijk 2010). Since the 1987 revision, primary care midwives have been responsible for assessing the risk and deciding about the need to refer a woman to secondary care (Smeenk and Ten Have 2003: 155). Following the 2006 health care system reform, the government has favoured a more market-oriented approach towards care, which led to the disappearance of the protective regulations of midwifery-led care (*primaat*) (Christiaens *et al.* 2013).

Midwives in the Netherlands are educated in a four-year bachelor programme in one of the four midwifery colleges. In addition, they can follow a midwifery master's programme (Manniën *et al.* 2012). In 2012, almost 60 per cent of practising midwives worked in primary care, which is one per 1586 women of fertile age (15–39 years). About 50 per cent of all midwives (co-)owned their own practice. In total, there were 511 practices. Almost 28 per cent of all midwives worked as clinical midwives in hospitals under the supervision of an obstetrician. Others were employed at health centres or midwifery practices. Most (54 per cent) midwives worked part-time. An average annual caseload of a full-time primary care midwife consists of the antenatal, intrapartum and postnatal care of about 105 women (Nederlands Instituut voor Onderzoek van de Gezondheidszorg 2013). The professional profile of the midwife, developed by the Royal Dutch Organisation of Midwives, emphasises the prevention of unnecessary medical intervention in low-risk pregnancies (Smeenk and Ten Have 2003) and the unity of the midwifery profession (including independent midwives and hospital-based clinical midwives) based on the physiological paradigm (Christiaens *et al.* 2013).

To become a gynaecologist, twelve years of education and training are required: six years of studying medicine at an academic level and another six years of specialisation in gynaecology/obstetrics. Gynaecologists are trained in risk reduction and prefer to have events unfold in the hospital setting (Pieters 2013: 74). They work exclusively in hospitals. Residents are employed in academic hospitals and are responsible for consultations; they are present in the delivery rooms. Residents have vast autonomy and obstetricians only intervene when major complications arise.

Midwives and gynaecologists have to register in a publicly available register to be able to practice. To maintain their registered status, midwives have to document a minimum of 2080 working hours in five years.

The collaboration between the Royal Dutch Organisation of Midwives and the Dutch Association for Obstetrics and Gynaecology involves the elaboration of the List of Obstetric Indications. In some regions, midwifery practices and hospital obstetric departments work together in maternity collaboratives to define policy at the regional level and to identify and address problems. The co-operation is not always adequate, partly due to the professional competition of the two groups (Pieters 2013: 74–75). Both organisations have been active in ensuring the quality of services through the elaboration of norms and guidelines. For example, in 2006, the Royal Dutch Organisation of Midwives established a quality register for midwives certifying their training and education. The quality of services is also monitored externally by the Healthcare Inspectorate (Koninklijke Nederlandse Organisatie van Verloskundigen 2012).

Complaints can be referred by patients, their representatives, the superiors of the professionals in question and the Healthcare Inspectorate to regional branches of the Disciplinary Board for Medical Professions. Published reports suggest that there is no litigation culture in the Netherlands (De Vries 2005). Referrals are infrequent, although their total number (for all medical professions) has grown in the past decade from about 1,300 in 2005 to 1,640 in 2013. The referrals very rarely involve gynaecologists and even less frequently involve midwives (usually a few cases a year). If found guilty, professionals face caution, conditions of practice, suspension or a ban on practising in the profession (Tuchtcollege voor de Gezondheidszorg 2010, 2014).

Maternity entitlements

Between 1930 and 1990, Dutch leave policies were limited to a twelve-week maternity leave. Following changes in 1990 and 2001, this leave has been extended to a maximum of sixteen weeks (also after a multiple birth) during which employees receive 100 per cent salary, with a ceiling of €193 per day (OECD 2012b). Since 2008, self-employed women are also entitled to an allowance depending on the previous year's income, but not exceeding the statutory minimum wage (Kennisring 2013). The maternity leave is divided into a compulsory prenatal leave of four to six weeks and a postnatal leave of ten to twelve weeks. Since 1997, fathers are entitled to two days of paid paternal leave and, following 2014 legislation, paternal leave will be extended by another three days (unpaid). Unpaid six-month-long parental leave was introduced in 1991. Since January 2009, parents are entitled to a part-time (50 per cent) parental leave of fifty-two weeks per parent per child under the age of eight years, with compensation dependent on sectoral collective agreements and consequently not provided in all sectors (Plantenga and Remery 2009).

Thus the Netherlands offers among the shortest postnatal, paternal and parental leaves within the European Union (OECD 2012b). Figures on spending on maternity and parental leave payments per child born (as a percentage of the GDP per capita for 2005–2009) show that the Netherlands scores the fifth lowest within the OECD (OECD 2012b). Of the different childcare facilities, only day nurseries support working parents, but solely on a part-time basis. With no formal educational provision for small children, 98 per cent of children begin school at the age of four years, although the mandatory school age is five years (Thijs *et al.* 2009).

Childbirth in the Netherlands

Antenatal care

In recent years, about 84 per cent of pregnant women started pregnancy care in primary care and only the remaining 16 per cent started in secondary care (due to antenatal issues). The first contact with a primary care midwife is scheduled between eight and eleven weeks of pregnancy; however, 13 per cent of pregnant women initiate antenatal care after the completion of the first trimester (European Perinatal Health Report 2013). Depending on the level of risk established by the midwife, the women is further cared for in primary care or referred to secondary care, where she will be supervised by an obstetrician.

In primary care, ten to twelve consultations during the pregnancy are scheduled, lasting ten to forty-five minutes. Women in primary care are offered a blood test during the first contact with the midwife to check for infectious diseases and serological conflict, and a dating scan establishing the age of the pregnancy, performed in week twelve. Women aged thirty-six years or older are also offered a test for Down's syndrome consisting of amniocentesis or chorionic villus sampling. Since 2007, pregnant women older than thirty-six years have been entitled to a non-invasive combination test (maternal serum screening and nuchal translucency scan) for the probability of Down's, Edward's or Patau's syndromes (between nine and fourteen weeks). Women younger than thirty-six years have to pay for the combination test (around €130). Also since 2007, all pregnant women are entitled to an anomaly scan at twenty weeks of gestation (Rijksinstituut voor Volksgezondheid en Milieu 2013). The uptake of tests is low, which can be associated with the Dutch 'pregnancy culture' (Fransen *et al.* 2010), where prenatal testing and screening are seen as 'spoiling the pregnancy' (Katz Rothman 2001). The dating scan is actually offered to about 60 per cent of pregnant women (Wiegers 2009), while the uptake of the anomaly scan reaches 75 per cent (Rijksinstituut voor Volksgezondheid en Milieu 2013). The uptake of prenatal diagnostic tests for Down's syndrome has been below 30 per cent for invasive testing methods (Fransen *et al.* 2010) and 25 per cent for the non-invasive combination test (Rijksinstituut voor Volksgezondheid en Milieu 2013). In secondary care, the number of consultations and tests depends on the woman's medical condition. The level of risk might change during the pregnancy, which results in a referral to another echelon (upwards or downwards) at the rate of 40 per cent in recent years (Perinatale Registratie Nederland 2013).

Intrapartum

Dutch maternity care distinguishes between three types of delivery: a home birth and a 'policlinical' birth within primary care,[3] and a 'clinical' birth within secondary (and, in very complicated cases, tertiary) care. Women with low-risk pregnancies are only allowed to deliver in primary care and, in principle, they can choose between a home delivery and a policlinical delivery, although the choice is influenced by the midwife's positive or negative attitude towards policlinical delivery. The midwife's attitude can explain 64 per cent of the variation in home birth rates between midwifery practices (Wiegers *et al.* 2000). As a rule, a clinical birth is only allowed in the high-risk category. However, some women with a low-risk profile do deliver in obstetric-led care (Maassen et al., 2008), which suggests that low-risk patients with a strong preference for a secondary care delivery are not being refused (van Haaren-ten *et al.* 2012: 610).

Deliveries in primary care take course without the involvement of an obstetrician and without medical interventions such as medical pain relief, augmentation or continuous foetal monitoring (van Haaren-ten *et al.* 2012: 610). In a home birth, the midwife and a maternity care assistant assist the mother at home. The policlinical birth is a midwifery-led, short-stay hospital delivery. The woman rents a delivery room in the hospital. Low-risk women have to cover the costs of a policlinical birth (around €325); however, if there is a risk of intrapartum complications they might receive a medical indication for a policlinical delivery, in which case the costs are reimbursed. The delivery starts at home and the patient is only admitted to hospital once the cervix is halfway dilated (otherwise the women is sent back home), with regular contractions (or loss of amniotic fluid or blood loss) and only when having previously contacted the hospital by phone to check whether places are available (if not, another hospital has to be located because a delivery room cannot be booked in advance). The transfer to the hospital is organised by the patient (private car or taxi). In a policlinical delivery the midwife uses the same instruments and medication as in a home birth. If there are no complications, the mother and baby are discharged after two to four hours (also at night). The midwife visits the mother and baby at home during the first week (usually on days two, four and seven). In a clinical delivery, the patient travels to the hospital (by her own means) in the early stage of labour and spends the first day or two of the puerperium in the hospital. The delivery takes place under the responsibility of an obstetrician, but supervision is usually executed by a clinical midwife and/or a resident. After dismissal, puerperium care is provided by a primary care midwife.

The Dutch maternity care system has a high share of home births, although the rate has steadily decreased in the past few decades. Compared with 68.5 per cent in 1965 (Wiegers *et al.* 1998), the 2010 data show a home birth rate of 17.1 per cent, a policlinical birth rate of 11.7 per cent and a clinical birth rate of 71.2 per cent (Perinatale Registratie Nederland 2013). These statistics indicate where the delivery was completed. Many more women opt for a home delivery, but are transferred to secondary care intrapartum. For example, in 2010, 50.5 per cent of all deliveries started in primary care, but 43 per cent of these were referred to secondary care, mainly due to meconium-stained liquor, insufficiently progressing dilation and the need for analgesia (Perinatale Registratie Nederland 2013).

The decrease in the home birth rate can be explained by several factors, including the introduction of the policlinical delivery in 1965, access to hospital facilities for independent midwives, increased referral rates from primary to secondary care (Wiegers *et al.* 1998: 190) and the availability of epidural analgesia in secondary care only. The number of hospitals accepting deliveries has decreased (a decrease of 20 per cent between 1999 and 2010). This has implications for the home birth option which is only available in areas close to maternity wards.

As for pain relief in delivery, the rates of epidural analgesia have risen from 5.4 per cent in 2003 to 16.1 per cent in 2010 (Perinatale Registratie Nederland 2013). The limited use of epidural analgesia cannot be attributed to a high labour pain acceptance of Dutch women: Dutch and Belgian women giving birth in a hospital setting display similar labour pain acceptance (Christiaens *et al.* 2010) and pregnant women in the Netherlands have strong preferences for medical pain relief (Pavlova *et al.* 2009). Rather, the outcome can be explained by: (1) the physiological approach of midwives who declare analgesic drugs unnecessary for a normal birth (Abraham-van der Mark 1996: 4) and see labour pain as an ally in the birth process (Christaens *et al.* 2010); (2) high home birth rates (where epidural analgesia is not available); and (3) organisational and financial issues. As for the latter, until recently, epidural analgesia was available only on medical indication. Since the publication in 2008 of the Dutch guidelines for pharmaceutical pain relief during delivery, epidural analgesia should be available at a woman's request (Nederlandse

Vereiniging voor Anesthesiologie and Nederlandse Vereiniging voor Obstetrie en Gynaecologie 2008), which can explain the recent sharp increase in rates of epidural analgesia. The still low absolute levels of use of epidural analgesia can be related to hospital practice. In 2010, only 57 per cent of Dutch hospitals were able to provide epidural analgesia on a twenty-four hour, seven days a week basis due to staff shortages (Wassen *et al.* 2010). Midwives, while opposing easy access to epidural analgesia (*Algemeen Dagblad*, 27 September 2010), have promoted nitrous oxide and sterile water injections as pain relief methods that can be administered by primary care midwives themselves (*NRC*, 5 April 2013).[4] This suggests a concern with retaining the share of clients increasingly interested in pain relief, rather than with maintaining the physiological approach to childbirth.

The Netherlands has low intervention rates in childbirth, including low rates of caesarean section, induction of labour and episiotomy (Table 11.3). Despite a recent tendency towards more medical interventions in childbirth, the country is still unique in the West (Christiaens *et al.* 2013: e2).

Although in the 1960s the perinatal mortality rate in the Netherlands was among the lowest in Europe, since the mid-1990s it has been among the highest within the European Union (Graafmans *et al.* 2001; Buitendijk and Nijhuis, 2004; European Perinatal Health Report, 2008, 2013). Similarly, the infant mortality rate in the Netherlands scored among the lowest in Western Europe in 1980, but since the 1990s it has scored among the highest in the region (OECD, 2013a). Relatively high rates of multiple births and of mothers older than thirty-five years can only partly explain the poor birth outcomes in the Netherlands (Mohangoo *et al.*, 2008); other factors adversely affect the perinatal mortality. Eskes and Van Diem (2005) identified a possible relation with substandard care in 19 per cent of cases of perinatal mortality. With about half of deliveries occurring during the evening or at night, Visser and Steegers (2008) found that the risk of perinatal mortality in Dutch hospitals is 23 per cent higher at night and 7 per cent higher during weekends; De Graaf *et al.* (2010: 1098) concluded that, in the Netherlands, 'hospital deliveries at night are associated with increased perinatal mortality and adverse perinatal outcome', suggesting a relation with the lower availability of experienced care-givers. In the perinatal mortality of small-for-gestational-age babies in the Netherlands, more adequate action by care-givers, in particular adjustments in pregnancy monitoring, especially in low-risk pregnancies, could decrease the number of avoidable cases of perinatal mortality by nearly one-third (De Reu *et al.* 2010). A travel time from home to hospital of twenty minutes or longer has been associated with perinatal mortality in term births (Ravelli *et al.* 2011a). Ravelli *et al.* (2011b) detected increased perinatal mortality and mortality risk in non-Western women in the Netherlands. Regional data show increased perinatal mortality rates in the most

Table 11.3 Birth interventions and outcomes for selected years in the Netherlands

	1970	1980	1990	2000	2010
Maternal mortality per 100,000 live births	13.4	8.8	7.6	8.7	7[a]
Perinatal mortality per 1,000 live and stillbirths	18.6	11.1	9.6	11.4 (1999)[b]	8.5[c]
Neonatal mortality per 1,000 live births	9.5	5.7	4.8	4.0	3.3
Infant mortality per 1,000 live births	12.7	8.6	7.1	5.1	3.8
Induction[1]	–	–	15 (1993)[d]	15 (2002)[d]	20.9[e]
Forceps/vacuum/breech extraction (separate data not available)	–	–	–	10.3 (2003)[e]	10.2[e]
Caesarean section[2]	–	–	7.4[f]	14.8 (2003)[e]	17.1[e]

Sources: OECD (2013a); a WHO (2014); b Buitendijk and Nijhuis (2004); c European Perinatal Health Report (2013); d Kwee *et al.* (2007); e Perinatale Registratie Nederland (2013); f Patah and Malik (2011).

Notes
1 The increase in induction rates could be related to a campaign 'Preventive Support of Labour' launched in 2002, which has encouraged strict rules for the progression of the first stage of labour (Christiaens *et al*, 2013: e4).
2 Dutch doctors are relatively unwilling to perform an elective caesarean section without medical indications (Habiba *et al*, 2006). The 2010 rate of planned or elective caesarean sections was 7.7%, the second lowest in Europe (European Perinatal Health Report, 2013).

rural and least populated areas in the Netherlands and imply a role of health care factors. Among term births, regional mortality differences were the largest for births in women transferred intrapartum from primary to secondary care (Tromp *et al.* 2009). De Jonge *et al.* (2009) concluded that planned home births do not increase the risk of perinatal mortality and severe perinatal morbidity in low-risk women. However, Evers *et al.* (2010) found a higher risk of delivery-related perinatal death in babies born to low-risk women whose midwifery-led delivery started in primary care compared with babies of high-risk mothers whose labour started in secondary care. A higher risk of delivery-related perinatal death was also found in the babies of women who were referred intrapartum from primary to secondary care compared with infants of women who started and completed delivery in secondary care. Bonsel *et al.* (2010) found that the system of risk selection is failing as high risks are not properly recognised by primary care midwives (in 25 per cent of patients who are qualified as low risk, the actual risk is high).

Postnatal care

All new mothers in the Netherlands are entitled to postnatal maternity home care assistance, offered at home in the first eight to ten days after delivery (usually three to five hours a day) and covered by basic health insurance.

The maternal mortality rate in the Netherlands in the past decade has been among the highest in Western Europe, although recent years have seen some improvement, according to routine statistics (Table 11.3). However, confidential enquiries indicate a recent maternal mortality rate of around eight and suggest that almost half of maternal deaths are associated with substandard care (European Perinatal Health Report 2013). The main cause of maternal morbidity in the past decade has been postpartum haemorrhage (PPH)[5] (Perinatale Registratie Nederland 2013). No guidelines currently exist on the prevention and management of postpartum haemorrhage in primary maternity care in the Netherlands; an audit has shown 'considerable room for improvement of PPH management' (Smit *et al.* 2013: 2).

Despite the 'natural' approach to childbirth, the fact that 63 per cent of Dutch hospitals are 'Baby-Friendly'[6] (Save the Children Report 2012), and the legislated right to daily nursing breaks at work for the first nine months of the baby's life, the Netherlands displays poor breastfeeding practices. Although 81 per cent of babies are breastfed at the beginning of their lives, only 30 per cent of babies are exclusively breastfed during the first three months and only 37 per cent continue to be (exclusively or otherwise) breastfed until they are six months old (Save the Children Report 2012: 43). These rates are consistent with a historical trend. In 1850, 70–80 per cent of mothers initiated breastfeeding at the baby's birth, and since then, the number of mothers still breastfeeding their child at three months of age has never exceeded 50 per cent (Bulk-Bunschoten *et al.* 2001). In the early 1970s, breastfeeding initiation rates were 47 per cent (Lanting *et al.* 2005) and only 11 per cent of three-month-old babies were exclusively or partially breastfed (Bulk-Bunschoten *et al.* 2001). Lanting *et al.* (2005: 942) conclude that 'only a minority of infants in the Netherlands is fed in accordance with feeding recommendations for the first six months of life'. The obligation to resume work has been the main or second-main mother-related reason for discontinuing breastfeeding in the third and fourth months of the baby's life (Bulk-Bunschoten *et al.* 2001; Lanting *et al.* 2005), which is consistent with other sources attributing cross-country differences in breastfeeding duration to the duration of paid maternity leave (Lande *et al.* 2003; Save the Children Report 2012).

Consumer involvement

Patient satisfaction with health care providers has been measured by applying different methodologies and the results are difficult to compare (Schäfer *et al.* 2010: 49). The survey-based Consumer Quality Index, available since 2005, suggests that patients are, in general, satisfied with their health care. In 2008, about 91 per cent of patients rated the received health services 7 or higher on a scale of 0–10 and about 40 per cent of the population evaluated the functioning of the health care system positively (Schäfer *et al.* 2010: 49–50).

Sources focusing on satisfaction with maternity care offer divergent results. A study based on the Consumer Quality Index reports high satisfaction levels with service quality in different settings and by different care providers (3.75 on a scale of 1–4) (Wiegers 2009). However, Rijnders *et al.* (2008) showed that 16.5 per cent of women are unhappy or very unhappy about their delivery experience as a result of the related fear for their own or the baby's life during birth, no choice in pain relief, insensitive caregivers, obstetric interventions and referral during labour. Finally, compared with Belgian women, Dutch women seem less satisfied with childbirth (Christiaens and Bracke 2007).

Dutch women have never campaigned for hospitalisation or access to pain relief and, in the last quarter of the twentieth century, feminists were in favour of home deliveries (Abraham-van der Mark 1996: 4–5). In fact, '[t]he well-established position of Dutch midwives has resulted in a virtually non-existent consumer movement concerned with choice of maternity provider and birth place' (Benoit *et al.* 2005: 730). The interests of pregnant women have continued to be identified with the interests of the midwifery profession (De Vries 2005). Currently, there is no major consumer movement addressing issues related to maternity care (Christiaens and Bracke 2007: e13). Against heated debates between obstetricians and midwives on free access to pain relief during delivery and the quality of the Dutch maternity care, major women's groups and feminists have been silent.

Risk and rights

Pregnancy and birth in the Netherlands are perceived as normal phenomena for which family and home provide a natural and safe setting. For decades this approach has been visible in national regulations favouring home birth and the primacy of midwives within the Dutch maternity care system, in mainstream obstetric science and in the professional practice of primary care midwives striving to limit the medicalisation of pregnancy and birth, as well as in the original preference for home birth among a large share of pregnant women.

Although pregnancy and birth are not seen as risk-bearing events, the notion of 'risk' is fundamental in Dutch maternity care. First, the organisation and practical operation of the system is based on risk selection and the category of risk determines women's options and access to care. Second, numerous issues have been identified in the organisation and practice of maternity care in the Netherlands. The strict division between the two risk categories and the ensuing differences in entitlements, and the high rates of risk-related referrals in pregnancy and delivery, mean that only a minority of women experience continuity of care. Moreover, intrapartum referrals may generate an increased risk of perinatal mortality. The risk of perinatal mortality is unequally distributed across regions and ethnic groups. Another aspect of risk concerns inadequate risk assessment by primary care midwives, which generates further risks for women allocated to the inappropriate echelon of care and leads to adverse birth outcomes. Risk is also potentiated by a lack of adequate pregnancy monitoring, especially in low-risk pregnancies. Finally, increased risk is generated by organisational issues: inadequate staffing at hospitals at evenings, nights and during weekends, as well as delayed or protracted transfer from home to hospital.

The other pivotal notion within Dutch maternity care is the 'right,' understood in the context of women's self-determination, rather than related to the quality and adequacy of care. Midwives have been vocal about women's right to freely choose the place of delivery or, more precisely, to be able to choose home as the place of birth, and have used this argument in support of the existing system. This right is claimed to constitute the main advantage for women in the Dutch maternity care system. Home birth is also embedded in the fundamentals of the Dutch welfare state: the strengthened idea of family privacy and conducting one's life without government interference. Moreover, home birth without pain relief is also perceived as empowering women. The idea of empowerment through non-medicalised birth has been used by midwives opposing organisational change in maternity care (De Vries *et al.* 2001; Koninklijke Nederlandse Organisatie van Verloskundigen 2014a). However, the right to choose may actually be constrained by the preferences of the attending midwife, and by co-payments which may exclude the policlinical birth option for low-income, low-risk mothers. The right to access high-quality care, including up-to-date diagnostic techniques or pain relief, has not featured in midwives' narrative. Rather, these are seen as risks to the Dutch physiological paradigm of birthing.

In 1986, findings indicating that perinatal mortality in the Netherlands was declining at a slower pace than in other European countries (Hoogendoorn 1986) were dismissed by most professionals (Mackenbach 2006). However, in the last decade a series of studies has shown that consistently high Dutch perinatal mortality rates in international comparison are not due to registration artefacts. This has raised questions about the quality of Dutch maternity care. In this context, 'risk' and 'right', and the organisation of maternity care revolving around these two notions, have attracted attention.

The media has featured discussions on the peculiarities of Dutch maternity care, home births and the autonomous position of midwives as potential culprits (*NRC Next*, 3 November 2010; *NRC Handelsblad*, 3 November 2010; *Trouw*, 4 November 2010; *Vrij Nederland*, 20 November 2010; *NRC Handelsblad*, 27 November 2011) (Christiaens *et al.* 2013: e2). Coverage has included the issue of deliveries 'outside the book', where midwives are radical in their anti-medicalisation and advertise their assistance for home births in high-risk pregnancies (e.g. twin pregnancies, breech positions, a history of multiple caesarean sections) against the guidelines of the List of Obstetric Indications (*De Groene Amsterdammer*, 24 July 2013). In 2013, following the death of an infant and an almost fatal postpartum haemorrhage after a home birth in a high-risk woman, the three midwives involved were referred by the Healthcare Inspectorate to the Disciplinary Board for Medical Professions. One of them was banned from practising and the other two were cautioned. The sentences, which are under appeal (Regionaal Tuchtcollege voor de Gezondheidszorg Amsterdam 2013), provoked a discussion in the media. This included midwives claiming the superiority of the freedom of choice of birth location over the baby's right to safety, given that women have a legal personality while unborn babies do not (*EenVandaag*, 18 July 2013), and obstetricians accusing midwives of 'playing Russian roulette with the lives of mothers and babies' (*Volkskrant*, 29 April 2014). The official standpoint of the Royal Dutch Organisation of Midwives on the issue has been ambiguous (Koninklijke Nederlandse Organisatie van Verloskundigen 2013).

Midwifery care and home birth have also become agenda items for the Dutch Ministry of Health, Welfare and Sport and the Dutch parliament 'after decades of quiet acceptance' (Christiaens *et al.* 2013: e2; Klink 2008, 2010; Schippers 2010, 2012, 2013). The Dutch Ministry of Health, Welfare and Sport instituted an Advisory Committee on Pregnancy and Birth (Stuurgroep Zwangerschap en Geboorte), which published a report investigating the unsatisfactory perinatal outcomes in the Netherlands and concluding that the organisation and practice of the Dutch maternity care system were wanting (Stuurgroep Zwangerschap en Geboorte 2009). In 2014, the Perinatal Care Board (College Perinatale Zorg), funded by the Ministry of Health, Welfare and Sport, published guidelines on how to address system deficiencies (College Perinatale Zorg 2014) through the development of National Integrated Perinatal Care Standards. Specifically, every pregnant woman should be followed by a team consisting of professionals responsible for preconceptional, antenatal, natal and postnatal care, which will assess the risks and, considering patient's preferences, establishes a trajectory of care to minimise existing and prevent potential risks. A case manager will be selected within the team as the contact person responsible for the continuity of care. Should any of the team members identify new risks in the patient, the case has to be presented again to the team; the risk category might be adjusted and the case manager might change. The team will elaborate rules on how to address patients wishing to act outside the advised trajectory. Patient information will be contained in a single digital dossier available to the patient and all involved professionals. Any financial or organisational barriers to policlinical birth should be removed to avoid a forced choice of home birth. In the case of a preference for home delivery, an assessment of its possibility must be made by the team, including the distance to the hospital, access to birth location, living conditions and the family situation of the patient. As these solutions undermine the autonomy of primary care midwives and their position in the Dutch maternity care system, the reaction of the Royal Dutch Organisation of Midwives has been very negative (Koninklijke Nederlandse Organisatie van Verloskundigen 2014b, 2014c). At the time of writing, Ministry of Health, Welfare and Sport has not yet issued a decision on the implementation of the guidelines.

Conclusion

The unique Dutch maternity care system, strongly embedded in the sociocultural context and the Dutch welfare state, is changing from within as an increasing share of women deliver in obstetric-led care following medical indication or their desire to receive pain relief. Consequently, the rate of home births, the former cornerstone of the system, has been decreasing dramatically in the past few decades. At the same time, the system has been under pressure to change following unsatisfactory results reflected mainly in high perinatal mortality rates. The need to reach a consensus among groups with strongly vested interests renders maternity policy-making and reform extremely difficult. Increasingly, the debates seem to be developing into a conflict between safety and freedom of choice, reflecting to a large extent the different standpoints of obstetricians and midwives. The recently published guidelines – recommending the establishment of integrated perinatal care, facilitating access to policlinical birth and restricting the criteria for a safe home delivery – would produce a major shift in the balance of power between the two professions as the midwives would partly lose their professional autonomy, the responsibility for risk selection and their position as the exclusive providers in primary care.

Notes

1 However, in terms of net social expenditure, the Netherlands is ranked as 'one of the poorest performers' within OECD (Meulders and O'Dorchai 2007: 5).
2 The *primaat* has played a crucial role in the decrease in general practitioners' involvement in care at birth. Although in 1964 40 per cent of all births were still attended by a general practitioner, in 2002 the share dropped to 7.2 per cent and in 2013 was about 0.5 per cent of all births.
3 A third option for primary care deliveries has been gaining ground: an outpatient birth centre ('home birth away from home'). In 2013 there were twenty-six birth centres in the Netherlands, most in, or adjacent to, hospitals (European Perinatal Health Report 2013: 19).
4 The Dutch Association for Obstetrics and Gynaecology has criticised the Royal Dutch Organisation of Midwives for introducing the practice of sterile water injections. According to the Dutch Association for Obstetrics and Gynaecology, the evidence on the effects of injections is not sufficient to allow them to be used as a pain relief procedure and certainly not as a substitute for epidural analgesia as presented by the Royal Dutch Organisation of Midwives (*NRC*, 5 April 2013).
5 In the Netherlands, postpartum haemorrhage is defined at 1,000 ml or more of blood loss within twenty-four hours after childbirth, while most international sources define it as 500 ml.
6 The Baby-Friendly Hospital Initiative was launched in 1991 by UNICEF and WHO in an effort to ensure that all maternity wards become centres of breast-feeding support.

References

Abraham-Van der Mark, E. (ed.) (1996) *Successful Home Birth and Midwifery. The Dutch Model.* Amsterdam: Het Spinhuis.
Amelink-Verburg, M.P. and Buitendijk, S.E. (2010) 'Pregnancy and labour in the Dutch maternity care system: what is normal? The role division between midwives and obstetricians', *Journal of Midwifery and Womens Health*, 55: 216–225.
Andeweg, R.B. and Irwin, G.A. (2005) *Governance and Politics of the Netherlands*, 4th edn. Basingstoke: Palgrave Macmillan.
Arts, W. and Gelissen, J. (2010) 'Models of the welfare state'. In: F.G. Castles, S. Leibfried, J. Lewis, H. Obinger and C. Pierson (eds), *The Oxford Handbook of the Welfare State.* Oxford: Oxford University Press.
Benoit, C., Wrede, S., Bourgeault, I., Sandall, J., De Vries, R. and Teijlingen, E.R. van (2005) 'Understanding the social organisation of maternity care systems: midwifery as a touchstone', *Sociology of Health & Illness*, 27 (6): 722–737.
Böhm, K., Schmid, A., Götze, R., Landwehr, C. and Rothgang, H. (2013) 'Five

types of OECD healthcare systems: empirical results of a deductive classification', *Health Policy*, 113 (3), 258–269.

Bonsel, G.J., Birnie, E., Denktas, S., Poeran, J. and Steegers, E.A.P. (2010) *Signalementstudie Zwangerschap en Geboorte 2010* (Monitoring Report on Pregnancy and Delivery 2010) [in Dutch]. Rotterdam: Erasmum MC.

Buitendijk, S.E. and Nijhuis, J.G. (2004) 'Hoge perinatale sterfte in Nederland in vergelijking tot de rest van Europa' (High perinatal mortality in the Netherlands in comparison with the rest of Europe) [in Dutch], *Nederlands Tijdschrift voor Geneeskunde*, 148 (38): 1855–1860.

Bulk-Bunschoten, A.M.W., van Bodegom, S., Reering, J.D., Pasker-de Jong, P.C.M. and Groot, C.J. de (2001) 'Reluctance to continue breastfeeding in the Netherlands', *Acta Paediatrica*, 90, 1047–1053.

Christiaens, W. and Bracke, P. (2007) 'Place of birth and satisfaction with childbirth in Belgium and the Netherlands', *Midwifery*, 25 (2): e11–e19.

Christiaens, W., Nieuwenhuijze, M.J. and De Vries, R. (2013) 'Trends in the medicalisation of childbirth in Flanders and the Netherlands', *Midwifery*, 29 (1): e1–e8.

Christiaens, W., Verhaeghe, M. and Bracke, P. (2010) 'Pain acceptance and personal control in pain relief in two maternity care models: a cross-national comparison of Belgium and the Netherlands', *BMC Health Service Research*, 10 (268).

College Perinatale Zorg (CPZ) (2014) *Leidraden CPZ* (Guidelines of the College for Perinatal Care) [in Dutch] [online]. Available from: www.goedgeboren.nl/netwerk/Multimedia/Get/2458. Accessed 16 May 2014.

Daalen, R. van (2007) 'Paid mothering in the public domain: Dutch dinner ladies and their difficulties', *Journal of Social History*, 40 (3): 619–634.

De Graaf, J., Ravelli, A., Visser, G., Hukkelhoven, C., Tong, W., Bonsel, G. and Steegers, E. (2010) 'Increased adverse perinatal outcome of hospital delivery at night', *British Journal of Obstetrics and Gynaecology*, 117: 1098–1107.

De Jonge, A., Goes, B.Y. van der, Ravelli, A.C.J., Amelink-Verburg, M.P., Mol, B.W., Nijhuis, J.G., Bennebroek Bravenhorst, J. and Buitendijk, S.E. (2009) 'Perinatal mortality and morbidity in a nationwide cohort of 529 688 low-risk planned home and hospital births', *British Journal of Obstetrics and Gynaecology*, 116: 1177–1184.

De Reu, P.A.O.M., Oosterbaan, H.P., Smits, L.J.M. and Nijhuis, J.G. (2010) 'Avoidable mortality in small-for-gestational-age children in the Netherlands', *Journal of Perinatal Medicine*, 38: 311–318.

De Vries, R.G. (2005) *A Pleasing Birth: Midwifery and Maternity Care in the Netherlands*. Amsterdam: Amsterdam University Press.

De Vries, R.G. and Buitendijk, S.E. (2012) 'Science, safety, and the place of birth: lessons from the Netherlands', *European Obstetrics & Gynaecology*, 7: 13–17.

De Vries, R.G. and Lemmens, T. (2006) 'The social and cultural shaping of medical evidence: case studies from pharmaceutical research and obstetric science', *Social Science & Medicine*, 62: 2694–2706.

De Vries, R.G., Benoit, C., Teijlingen, E.R. van and Wrede, S. (2001) *Birth by Design. Pregnancy, Maternity Care, and Midwifery in North America and Europe*. New York and London: Routledge.

De Vries, R.G., Nieuwenhuijze, M. and Buitendijk, S.E. (2013) 'What does it take to have a strong and independent profession of midwifery? Lessons from the Netherlands', *Midwifery*, 29: 1122–1128.

Den Exter, A. (2010) 'Health system reforms in the Netherlands: from public to private and its effects on equal access to health care', *European Journal of Health Law*, 17 (3): 223–33.

Eskes, M. and Van Diem, M.T. (2005) *Landelijke Perinatal Audit Studie* (National Perinatal Audit Study) [in Dutch]. Diemen: College voor zorgverzekeringen.

Esping-Andersen, G. (1990) *The Three Worlds of Welfare Capitalism*. Princeton: Princeton University Press.

Esping-Andersen, G. (1996) *Welfare States in Transition. National Adaptations in Global Economies*. London: Sage.

European Commission (2014) *The Netherlands* [online]. Available from: http://ec.europa.eu/economy_finance/eu/countries/netherlands_en.htm. Accessed 25 June 2014.

European Perinatal Health Report (2008) *European Perinatal Health Report. EURO-PERISTAT Project in Collaboration with Surveillance of Cerebral Palsy in Europe (SCPE), European Surveillance of Congenital Anomalies (EUROCAT & EURONEOSTAT). Data from 2004 [online]*. Available from: https://docs.google.com/viewer?url=http%3A%2F%2Fwww.europeristat.com%2Fimages%2Fdoc%2FEPHR%2Feuropean-perinatal-health-report.pdf. Accessed 20 June 2014.

European Perinatal Health Report (2013) *European Perinatal Health Report. Health and Care of Pregnant Women and Babies in Europe in 2010* [online]. Available from: https://docs.google.com/viewer?url=http%3A%2F%2Fwww.europeristat.com%2Fimages%2Fdoc%2FPeristat%25202013%2520V2.pdf. Accessed 20 June 2014.

Evers, A.C.C., Brouwers, H.A.A., Hukkelhoven, C.W.P.M., Nikkels, P.G.J., Boon, J., Egmond-Linden, A., Hillegersberg, J., Snuif, Y.S., Sterken-Hooisma, S., Bruinse, H. and Kwee, A. (2010) 'Perinatal mortality and severe morbidity in low and high risk term pregnancies in the Netherlands: prospective cohort study', *BMJ*, 341: c5639.

Fransen, M.P., Essink-Bot, M.-L.,Vogel, I., Mackenbach, J.P., Steegers, E.A.P. and Wildschut, H.I.J. (2010) 'Ethnic differences in informed decision-making about prenatal screening for Down's syndrome', *Journal of Epidemiology and Community Health*, 64: 262–268.

Garssen, J. and Nicolaas, H. (2008) 'Fertility of Turkish and Moroccan women in the Netherlands: adjustment to native level within one generation', *Demographic Research*, 19 (33): 1249–1280.

Götze, R. (2010) 'The changing role of the state in the Dutch healthcare system', *TransState Working Papers*, 141: 1–46.

Graafmans, W.C., Richardus, J.H., Macfarlane, A., Rebagliato, M., Blondel, B., Verloove-Vanhorick, S.P. and Mackenbach, J.P. (2001) 'Comparability of published perinatal mortality rates in Western Europe: the quantitative impact of differences in gestational age and birthweight criteria', *British Journal of Obstetrics and Gynaecology*, 108: 1237–1245.

Haaren-ten Haken, T. van, Hendrix, M., Nieuwenhuijze, M., Bude, L., De Vries, R. and Nijhuis, J. (2012) 'Preferred place of birth: characteristics and motives of low-risk nulliparous women in the Netherlands', *Midwifery*, 28: 609–618.

Habiba, M., Kaminski, M., Da Frè, M., Marsal, K., Bleker, O., Librero, J., Grandjean, H., Gratia, P., Guaschino, S., Heyl, W., Taylor, D. and Cuttini, M. (2006) 'Caesarean section on request: a comparison of obstetricians' attitudes in eight European countries', *British Journal of Obstetrics and Gynaecology*, 113 (6): 647–656.

Hoogendoorn, D. (1986) 'Indrukwekkende en tegelijk teleurstellende daling van de perinatale sterfte in Nederland' (Impressive yet disappointing decrease in perinatal mortality in the Netherlands) [in Dutch], *Nederlands Tijdschrift voor Geneeskunde*, 130: 1436–1440.

Joumard, I., André, C. and Nicq, C. (2010) *Health Care Systems: Efficiency and Institutions*. OECD Economics Department Working Papers, No. 769. Paris: OECD Publishing.

Katz Rothman, B. (2001) 'Spoiling the pregnancy: prenatal diagnosis in the Netherlands'. In: R. De Vries, C. Benoit, E.R. van Teijlingen and S. Wrede (eds), *Birth by Design. Pregnancy, Maternity Care, and Midwifery in North America and Europe*. New York and London: Routledge, pp. 180–201.

Kennisring (2013) *Zwangerschaps – en bevallingsverlof. De uitkering* (Pregnancy and maternity leave. The allowance) [online]. Available from: www.kennisring.nl. Accessed 16 May 2014.

Klink, A. (2008) *Ketenzorg Zwangerschap en Geboorte* (Continuous care pregnancy and childbirth) [in Dutch]. Brief aan de 2e kamer, 16 July. The Hague: Ministry of Health.

Klink, A. (2010) *Antwoorden op de vragen van Kamerlid Arib (PvdA) over de noodzaak om de verloskundige zorg radicaal te veranderen*. [Answers to questions of MP Arib (Labour Party) about the necessity to radically change the maternity care sytem] [in Dutch], 22 July. The Hague: Ministry of Health.

Koninklijke Nederlandse Organisatie van Verloskundigen (2012) *Midwifery in the Netherlands* [online]. Available from: www.nurse.or.jp/nursing/international/icm/report/data/2012/icm-dutch.pdf. Accessed 16 May 2014.

Koninklijke Nederlandse Organisatie van Verloskundigen (2013) *Uitspraken tuchtrechter over verloskundig handelen* (Rulings of the Disciplinary Board related to midwives' professional performance) [online]. Available from: www.knov.nl/actueel-overzicht/nieuws-overzicht/detail/uitspraken-tuchtrechter-over-verloskundig-handelen/1213. Accessed 16 May 2014.

Koninklijke Nederlandse Organisatie van Verloskundigen (2014a) *KNOV lanceert campagne 'Zwanger op eigen kracht'* (KNOV launches a campaign 'Pregnant on your own strengths') [online]. Available from: www.knov.nl/actueel-overzicht/nieuws-overzicht/detail/knov-lanceert-campagne-zwanger-op-eigen-kracht/1396. Accessed 16 May 2014.

Koninklijke Nederlandse Organisatie van Verloskundigen (2014b) *Veel onrust over media-aandacht en CPZ leidraad* (A lot of turmoil over media attention and CPZ guidelines) [online] Available from: www.knov.nl/actueel-overzicht/nieuws-overzicht/detail/veel-onrust-over-media-aandacht-en-cpz-leidraad/1383. Accessed 16 May 2014.

Koninklijke Nederlandse Organisatie van Verloskundigen (2014c) *Onvoldoende draagvlak voor leidraad CPZ* (Missing support for CPZ guidelines) [online]. Available from: www.knov.nl/actueel-overzicht/nieuws-overzicht/detail/onvoldoende-draagvlak-voor-leidraad-cpz/1387. Accessed 16 May 2014.

Kwee, A., Elferink-Stinkens, P.M., Reuwer, P.J. and Bruinse, H.W. (2007) 'Trends in obstetric interventions in the Dutch obstetrical care system in the period 1993–2002', *European Journal of Obstetrics, Gynecology and Reproductive Biology*, 132 (1): 70–75.

Lande, B., Andersen, L.F., Baerug, A., Trygg, K.U., Lund-Larsen, K. and Veierod, M.B. *et al.* (2003) 'Infant feeding practices and associated factors in the first six months of life: the Norwegian infant', *Nutrition Survey*, 92: 152–161.

Lanting, C.I., Van Wouwe, J.P. and Reijneveld, S.A. (2005) 'Infant milk feeding practices in the Netherlands and associated factors', *Acta Paediatrica*, 94: 935–942.

Maassen, M.S., Hendrix, M.J. and VanVugt, H.C. (2008) 'Operative deliveries in low-risk pregnancies in The Netherlands: primary versus secondary care', *Birth*, 35: 277–282.

Mackenbach, J.P. (2006) 'Perinatale sterfte in Nederland: een probleem van velen, een problem van niemand' (Perinatal mortality in the Netherlands: everybody's problem, nobody's problem) [in Dutch], *Nederlands Tijdschrift voor Geneeskunde*, 150 (8): 409–412.

Manniën, J., Klomp, T., Wiegers, T., Pereboom, M., Brug, J., Jonge, A. de, van der Meijde, M., Hutton, E., Schellevis, F. and Spelten, E. (2012) 'Evaluation of primary care midwifery in the Netherlands: design and rationale of a dynamic cohort study (DELIVER)', *BMC Health Services Research*, 12 (69).

Meulders, D. and O'Dorchai, S. (2007) The position of mothers in a comparative welfare state perspective. In: D. Del Boca and C. Wetzels (eds), *Social Policies, Labour Markets and Motherhood. A Comparative Analysis of European Countries.* Cambridge: Cambridge University Press, pp. 3–27.

Mohangoo, A.D., Buitendijk, S.E., Hukkelhoven, C.W.P.M., Ravelli, A.C.J., Rijninks-van Driel, G.C., Tamminga, P. and Nijhuis, J.G. (2008) 'Hoge perinatale sterfte in Nederland vergeleken met andere Europese landen: de Peristat-II-studie' (High perinatal mortality in the Netherlands compared with other European countries: the Peristat II study) [in Dutch], *Nederlands Tijdschrift voor Geneeskunde*, 152: 2718–2727.

Nederlands Instituut voor Onderzoek van de Gezondheidszorg (2013) *Cijfers uit de registratie van Verloskundigen* (Data from Midwives' Registry) [in Dutch]. Utrecht: Nederlands Instituut voor Onderzoek van de Gezondheidszorg.

Nederlandse Vereiniging voor Anesthesiologie and Nederlandse Vereiniging voor Obstetrie en Gynaecologie (2008) *Richtlijn Medicamenteuze Pijnbehandeling tijdens de Bevalling* (Guidelines on pain relief medication during delivery) [in Dutch] [online]. Available from: www.nvog.nl/upload/files/definitief-richtlijn-pijnbehandeling-bij-de-partus_def-091208.pdf. Accessed 23 June 2014.

OECD (1993) *Employment Outlook.* Paris: OECD Publishing.

OECD (2012a) *OECD Economic Surveys: Netherlands* [online]. Available from: www.oecd-ilibrary.org/docserver/download/1012111e.pdf?expires=1403531472&id=id&accname=ocid53017056&checksum=C2D4AAB8A859BB05B04093AAFC3B77F6. Accessed 23 June 2014.

OECD (2012b) *Key Characteristics of Parental Leave Systems. OECD Family Database* [online]. OECD Social Policy Division, Directorate of Employment, Labour and Social Affairs. Available from: www.oecd.org/els/soc/PF2_1_Parental_leave_systems_1May2014.pdf. Accessed 23 June 2014.

OECD (2013a) *OECD Health Online Database* [online]. Available from: www.oecd.org/els/health-systems/health-data.htm. Accessed 16 May 2014.

OECD (2013b) *OECD Health Data 2013. How Does the Netherlands Compare?* [online] Available from: www.oecd.org/els/health-systems/Briefing-Note-NETHERLANDS-2013.pdf. Accessed 16 May 2014.

OECD (2013c) *Closing the Gender Gap: the Netherlands* [online]. Available from: www.oecd.org/gender/Closing%20the%20Gender%20Gap%20-%20Netherlands%20FINAL.pdf. Accessed 16 May 2014.

Oorschot, W.J.H. van (2009) 'The Dutch welfare system: from collective solidarity towards individual responsibility'. In: K. Schubert, S. Hegelich and U. Bazant (eds), *The Handbook of European Welfare Systems*. New York: Routledge, pp. 363–377.

Patah, L.E.M. and Malik, A.M. (2011) 'Models of childbirth care and cesarean rates in different countries', *Revista Saude Publica*, 45 (1), 1–9.

Pavlova, M., Hendrix, M., Nouwens, E., Nijhuis, J. and van Merode, G. (2009) 'The choice of obstetric care by low-risk pregnant women in the Netherlands: implications for policy and management', *Health Policy*, 93: 27–34.

Perinatale Registratie Nederland (2013) *Jaarboeken Zorg in Nederland* (Annual Report on Care in the Netherlands) [online] Available from: www.perinatreg.nl/jaarboeken_zorg_in_nederland?noCache=963;1410533532. Accessed 16 May 2014.

Pieters, A. (2013) 'Care and cure: compete or collaborate? Improving inter-organization designs in healthcare. A case study in Dutch perinatal care', PhD Thesis, University of Tilburg.

Plantenga, J. and Remery, C. (2009) *Parental Leave in the Netherlands*. CEifo DICE Report 2/2009, 47–51. Munich: IfO Institute.

Ravelli, A.C.J., Jager, K.J., Groot, M.H. de, Erwich, J.J.H.M., Rijninks-van Driel, G.C., Tromp, M., Eskes, M., Abu-Hanna, A. and Mol, B.W.J. (2011a) 'Travel time from home to hospital and adverse perinatal outcomes in women at term in the Netherlands', *British Journal of Obstetrics and Gynaecology*, 118 (4): 457–465.

Ravelli, A.C.J., Tromp, M., Eskes, M., Droog, J.C., van der Post, J.A.M., Jager, K.J., Mol, B.W. and Reitsma, J.B. (2011b) 'Ethnic differences in stillbirth and early neonatal mortality in The Netherlands', *Journal of Epidemiology and Community Health*, 65 (8): 696–701.

Reibling, N. (2010) 'Healthcare systems in Europe: towards an incorporation of patient access', *Journal of European Social Policy*, 20 (1): 5–18.

Regionaal Tuchtcollege voor de Gezondheidszorg Amsterdam (2013) *Cases 2012/357/V, 2012/358/V, 2012/359/V* [online]. Available from: http://tuchtrecht.overheid.nl/nieuw/gezondheidszorg/. Accessed 16 May 2014.

Rijksinstituut voor Volksgezondheid en Milieu (2013) *Nationaal Programma Bevolkingsonderzoek: de cijfers* (National Screening Programme: the numbers) [online]. www.rivm.nl/Onderwerpen/B/Bevolkingsonderzoeken_en_screeningen/Achtergrondinformatie/Bevolkingsonderzoek_de_organisatie/Nationaal_Programma_Bevolkingsonderzoek_de_cijfers#Down. Accessed 16 May 2014.

Rijnders, M., Baston, H., Schonbeck, Y., van der Pal, K., Prins, M., Green, J. and Buitendijk, S. (2008) 'Perinatal factors related to negative or positive recall of birth experience in women 3 years postpartum in the Netherlands', *Birth* 35 (2): 107–116.

Save the Children Report (2012) *Nutrition in the First 1000 Days. State of the World's Mothers 2012* [online]. Available from: www.savethechildren.org/atf/cf/%7B9def2ebe-10ae-432c-9bd0-df91d2eba74a%7D/stateoftheworldsmothersreport2012.pdf. Accessed 23 June 2014.

Schäfer W., Kroneman M., Boerma W., van den Berg, M., Westert G., Devillé, W. and van Ginneken, E. (2010) The Netherlands: health system review. *Health Systems in Transition*, 12 (1): 1–229.

Schippers, E. (2010) *Zwangerschap en geboorte* (Pregnancy and childbirth) [in Dutch]. Brief aan de 2e kamer, 14 December. The Hague: Ministry of Health.

256 *M.E. Kaminska*

Schippers, E. (2012) *Reactie Rapporten Acute Zorg en Verloskunde* (Reaction to the reports on emergency and obstetric care) [in Dutch]. Brief aan de 2de kamer, 1 March. The Hague: Ministry of Health.

Schippers, E. (2013) *Zwangerschap en Geboorte* (Pregnancy and childbirth) [in Dutch]. Brief aan de 2de kamer, 24 April, The Hague: Ministry of Health.

Smeenk, A.D.J. and Ten Have, H.A.M.J. (2003) 'Medicalization and obstetric care: an analysis of developments in Dutch midwifery', *Medicine, Health Care and Philosophy*, 6: 153–165.

Smit, M., Sindram, S.I.C., Woiski, M., Middeldorp, J.M. and van Roosmalen, J. (2013) 'The development of quality indicators for the prevention and management of postpartum haemorrhage in primary midwifery care in the Netherlands', *BMC Pregnancy and Childbirth*, 13 (194).

Statistics Netherlands (2014) Population: sex, age, origin and generation, 1 January. [online] Available from: http://statline.cbs.nl/StatWeb/publication/?VW=T&DM=SLEN&PA=37325eng&D1=0-2&D2=0&D3=0&D4=0&D5=0-1,3-4,139,145,210,225&D6=4,9,(l-1)-l&HD=090611-0858&LA=EN&HDR=G3,T&STB=G5,G1,G2,G4. Accessed 16 May 2014.

Structuurnota Gezondheidszorg (1974) *Structuurnota Gezondheidszorg* [in Dutch]. The Hague: Staatsuitgeverij.

Stuurgroep Zwangerschap en Geboorte (2009) *Een goed begin. Veilige zorg rond zwangerschap en geboorte. Advies Stuurgroep Zwangerschap en Geboorte.* (A good start. Safe care in pregnancy and delivery. Advice of the Steering Committee on Pregnancy and Delivery) [in Dutch]. Utrecht: Stuurgroep Zwangerschap en Geboorte.

Teijlingen, E.R. van (2004) 'Maternity home care assistants in the Netherlands'. In: E.R. van Teijlingen, G. Lowis, P. McCaffery and M. Porter (eds), *Midwifery and the Medicalization of Childbirth: Comparative Perspectives*. New York: Nova Science, pp. 163–172.

Thijs, A., Leeuwen, B. and van Zandbergen, M. (2009) *Inclusive Education in the Netherlands* [online]. Available from: www.slo.nl/downloads/2009/Inclusive_20Education_20Netherlands_20webversie.pdf/. Accessed 23 June 2014.

Tromp, M., Eskes, M., Reitsma, J.B., Erwich, J.J.H.M., Brouwers, H.A.A., Rijninks-van Driel, G.C., Bonsel, G.J. and Ravelli, A.C.J. (2009) 'Regional perinatal mortality differences in the Netherlands; care is the question', *BMC Public Health*, 9 (102).

Tuchtcollege voor de Gezondheidszorg (2010) *Jaarverslag 2009* (Annual Report 2009) [in Dutch] [online]. Available from: www.tuchtcollege-gezondheidszorg.nl/. Accessed 16 May 2014.

Tuchtcollege voor de Gezondheidszorg (2014) *Jaarverslag 2013* (Annual Report 2010) [in Dutch] [online]. Available from: www.tuchtcollege-gezondheidszorg.nl/. Accessed 16 May 2014.

Visser, J. and Hemerijk, A. (1997) *A Dutch Miracle. Job Growth, Welfare Reform and Corporatism in the Netherlands.* Amsterdam: Amsterdam University Press.

Visser, G.H.A. and Steegers, E.A.P. (2008) 'Beter baren. Nieuwe keuzen nodig in de zorg voor zwangeren' (Better delivery. New choices needed in the care of pregnant women) [in Dutch], *Medisch Contact*, 63 (3): 96–100.

Wassen, M.M.L.H., Buijs, C. and Nijhuis, J.G. (2010) 'Beschikbaarheid epidurale analgesie tijdens de bevalling in Nederland anno 2010' (Availability of epidural analgesia during delivery in the Netherlands in 2010) [in Dutch], *Nederlands Tijdschrift voor Obstetrie en Gynaecologie*, 10: 398–400.

(2010) *Dutch Health Care Performance Report 2010*. Bilthoven: Rijksinstituut voor Volksgezondheid en Milieu.

WHO (2014) *Global Health Observatory Data Repository* [online]. Available from: http://apps.who.int/gho/data/?theme=main. Accessed 20 June 2014.

Wiegers, T.A. (2009) 'The quality of maternity care services as experienced by women in the Netherlands', *BMC Pregnancy and Childbirth*, 9 (18).

Wiegers, T.A., Zee, J. van der and Keirse, M.J. (1998) 'Maternity care in The Netherlands: the changing home birth rate', *Birth*, 25: 190–197.

Wiegers, T., Zee, J. van der, Kerssens, J.J. and Keirse, M.J.N.C. (2000) 'Variation in home-birth rates between midwifery practices in the Netherlands', *Midwifery*, 16: 96–104.

World Bank (2013) *The World Bank Data* [online] Available from: http://data.worldbank.org/indicator/SM.POP.NETM. Accessed 23 June 2014.

Ziekenfondsraad (1987) *De Verloskundige Indicatielijst*. Amstelveen: Ziekenfondsraad.

12 Sweden

Jan Thomas and Ingegerd Hildingsson

Background

Sweden is a Scandinavian country in Northern Europe and is characterised by unspoiled natural beauty, technological innovation and a high level of spending on public services. This level of spending is designed to reduce inequality and provide a generous level of universal benefits for all citizens. Sweden has high levels of education and labour force participation and some of the best health outcomes in the world, including low infant mortality and high life expectancy (OECD 2014a). However, like other developed countries, Sweden's social safety net has become harder to sustain and changing demographics, such as an increasingly diverse and ageing population, are putting pressure on the social contract between the government and Swedish citizens.

Sweden has a population of approximately 9.7 million (Statistics Sweden 2014). Although comparable in size to the state of California in the USA, it is the third largest country in Western Europe, covering 450,294 square kilometres. The three largest cities are Stockholm (the capital), Gothenberg (on the west coast) and Malmö (in the south). The majority (85 per cent) of Swedes live in urban areas (Sweden.se 2014). In the past, most immigrants to Sweden came from the other Nordic countries; however, in recent years the largest immigrant groups have come from Iraq, Afghanistan and Poland (Sweden.se 2014a). In 2010, 16.8 per cent of the population was foreign-born (compared with 13.1 per cent in the USA) (OECD 2013a).

Sweden's government is based on a parliamentary democracy. For most of the twentieth century, the Social Democratic Party was in power and established the generous welfare state policies that Sweden is known for. At the core of Sweden's social democracy is a belief in solidarity and equality. Personal taxes are often considered to be high, but a system of income redistribution (cash transfers) helps to reduce inequality, especially for groups such as the elderly and single parents (Swedish Tax Agency 2012).

Sweden as a welfare regime

Sweden's high level of commitment to equality and the well-being of its citizens characterise it as an ideal type of a social democratic welfare state (Esping-Andersen 1990; Arts and Gelissen 2010). Universal rights are directed at the individual level, thus there is little dependency on the family or the market and the level of decommodification is fairly high. The Swedish welfare state, with its generous welfare programmes, considers the care needs of employees and increases women's autonomy, thus making it possible for women (and men) to be both workers and carers (Orloff 2010). Sweden's welfare state policies include benefits such as: generous paid parental leave; free education; heavily subsidised health care; subsidised childcare; five weeks of paid vacation for all employees; child allowances; sickness benefits; a pension; and a variety of other social insurance benefits. In addition, through policies such as paternal leave (480 days of paid leave, with sixty days reserved for the father), Sweden has actively engaged in altering gender relations (Orloff 1993). Sweden assumes all citizens are workers and care-givers (Fraser 2000) and welfare state policies send strong messages about autonomy and equality.

Since the election of a centre-right coalition government in 2006, taxes have been cut and transfers have been reduced. The government has also encouraged market competition for public services by allowing private companies to compete with government providers for public contracts. The impact of neoliberalism can be seen in the increased government interest in free markets, deregulation and privatisation (Ginsburg and Rosenthal 2006). Although these changes have resulted in some increases in inequality, universal access to high-quality public services, including health care, remains a core value in Sweden.

Health care system

According to the Ministry of Health and Social Affairs (2013), health care in Sweden should be of good quality, accessible, provide patients with freedom of choice of providers and be effective. The guiding principle of Swedish health care is that 'everybody has the same right to good quality care' (Anell *et al.* 2012). Responsibility for health care is shared by three levels of government (national, regional and local). The national government is responsible for the basic principles that guide the system and the overall health care agenda. At the regional level, the County Councils, whose members are elected every four years, are responsible for the organisation and delivery of care. Since the 1990s, local municipalities have been responsible for providing elder care, mental health services and care for the disabled.

All health care providers (e.g. nurses, doctors and midwives) receive their professional accreditation through the National Board of Health and

Welfare. There are seven university hospitals in Sweden that provide the most highly specialised care and medical training. There are also approximately seventy County Council hospitals and six private hospitals providing tertiary care (Anell *et al.* 2012). In 2010, there were 3.9 practising physicians per 1,000 inhabitants in Sweden (OECD 2013b). This is slightly higher than the OECD average of 3.1 per 1,000. University education is available following three years of high school education. Midwives in Sweden are registered nurses (three years of education at bachelor level) and registered midwives (1.5 years at advanced level). There are currently eleven midwifery schools in Sweden. Prior to applying for midwifery education, applicants must have worked for at least one year as a nurse. Table 12.1 provides additional data on the human and physical resources within the Swedish health care system.

The Medical Responsibility Board (Hälso- och Sjukvårdens Ansvarsnämnd), under the Ministry of Social Affairs, oversees disciplinary action against providers and complaints about possible malpractice. The system in Sweden for disciplining physicians is separate from the system that compensates patients. Patients who are dissatisfied with their care have mechanisms, through the health care system, to have their complaints investigated rather than filing a malpractice suit. In addition, the potential awards to patients are capped. In 2009, the average award in Sweden was US$20,000 (Mello *et al.* 2011).

Health spending in Sweden represents 9.5 per cent of GDP, which is just above the OECD average of 9.3 per cent (OECD 2013b). The health care system in Sweden is funded mainly through taxes levied by the County Councils and municipalities (amounting to about 80 per cent of expenditure on health). Various government grants, subsidies and user fees make up the remaining 20 per cent (Glenngård 2013). Health care in Sweden includes some cost-sharing with patients for most types of care. Children are exempt from any cost-sharing (up to the age of twenty years). In 2013, patients paid approximately SEK80 (US$11) per day for the first ten days of a hospital stay and SEK60 thereafter. Patients paid between SEK100 and 200 (depending on where they lived) for a primary care visit.

Table 12.1 Human and physical resources in Sweden

Physicians per 1,000 population	3.9
Nurses per 1,000 population	11
Medical graduates per 100,000 population	8.6 (2010)
Nursing graduates per 100,000 population	No reliable information
Total hospital beds per 1,000 population	2.7 (2011)
Curative (acute) care beds per 1,000 population	2.0 (2011)
Obstetricians and gynaecologists per 100,000 women	14
Registered midwives per 100,000 women	74

Sources: compiled from OECD (2014b, 2014c, 2014d); National Board of Health and Welfare (2014).

A maximum fee of SEK350 is charged for specialist visits. Cost ceilings are in place to control out-of-pocket expenses. Once a patient has paid between SEK900 and 1,000 during the year (depending on the place of residence), consultations are free. There is also an annual cost ceiling for pharmaceutical drugs (Sweden.se 2014b). Most hospitals are owned by the County Councils. Since 2000, Swedes have had 'free choice' of health care providers and hospitals, which now includes the choice of private or public providers (virtually all paid through contracts with the County Councils). Approximately 12 per cent of health care is financed by the County Councils, but carried out by private care providers (Sweden.se 2014b). In addition, about 10 per cent of employees have some kind of private health care insurance through their employer (Glenngård 2013).

The economic crisis in the early 1990s, and the election of centre-right governments in 1991, 2006 and 2010, led to cuts in some benefits and services and a shift towards more market-based policies, such as increasing competition, choice, the privatisation of providers and performance-based compensation models (Anell *et al.* 2012). In health care, the government has continued to increase the emphasis on a choice of providers and the growth of private providers. The greatest growth in private providers has been in the area of primary care; however, growth has clustered in a few highly populated areas, thus 'choice' is more available for some than for others (Anell *et al.* 2012).

Unlike other countries, Sweden has simply been adjusting its mix of public/private providers. The government remains the single-payer and providers (public and private) must contract with the local County Councils for payment. This system gives the government more opportunity to control health care resources.

Demographic profile

The number of births in Sweden in 2011 was 109,248. The number of births has fluctuated over the years, ranging from 121,981 births in 1991 to only 84,340 births in 1998. Table 12.2 shows the demographic characteristics for women giving birth in Sweden in 2011. In 1973, when the Swedish Medical Birth Register started, the mean age at first birth was 24 years (108,481 births). The mean age for women to have their first baby in 2011 was 28.5 years. The age at first birth for women living in the capital area of Stockholm is 30.0 years, whereas women living in areas with large industries, such as Södermanland, tend to be slightly younger than the national average (mean 26.9 years). Women in rural areas tend to have their first child around the national average (National Board of Health and Welfare 2013).

From a public health perspective, it is important to communicate the pros and cons of delayed childbearing (>35 years) as it has been found to be associated with maternal morbidity and mortality (Balasch and Gratacós 2012). The associated factors reported are higher rates of abortion and

Table 12.2 Demographic profile of Sweden

Population[a]	9,644,864
Women[a]	4,830,507
Population aged 0–14 yeas	1,646,101
Women of childbearing age (15–44 years)	1,807,851
Population aged 65 years or older	1,872,207
Population annual growth (%)[a]	95 (2013–2014)
Population density per square kilometre[b]	21.0 (2011)
Total fertility rate (births per woman)[a]	1.89
Crude birth rate per 1,000 people[a]	11.8
Crude death rate per 1,000 people[a]	9.4
Urban population (%)[b]	85
Ethnic groups (women aged 15–44 years) (breakdown)[a]	
Thailand	1,055
Iraq	9,795
Iran	5,048
Syria	4,594
Lebanon	635

Sources: a Statistics Sweden (2014); b UN Data (2014).

miscarriage, gestational diabetes, *in vitro* fertilisation, ectopic pregnancies, intrauterine foetal death, prematurity, multiple pregnancies and caesarean sections. For the baby there is an increased risk of chromosomal defects, cerebral palsy and neuro-developmental sequelae.

Since the early 1980s, assisted conception has been available in Sweden and in 2010 there were 14,500 treatments with *in vitro* fertilisation, resulting in 3,880 live babies. Since 2003, egg donation has been available in Sweden and, during 2010, seventy-four babies were born as a result of egg donation.

Pregnant women born in countries outside Sweden represented nearly 24 per cent of childbearing women in 2011, mainly from Iraq, Iran, Lebanon, Syria and Thailand. Data on women's level of education shows that 11 per cent of women giving birth in 2011 had primary school as their highest level of education, 37 per cent had completed high school and 51 per cent had a college or university level of education. A low level of education is over-represented in women born in countries outside Sweden (National Board of Health and Welfare 2013).

Maternity provision

Maternity care is situated within primary care in Sweden and there has also been growth in private providers of antenatal care (clinics staffed primarily by midwives) and, more recently, two private hospitals have developed labour and delivery wards. These 'private' wards are privately operated, but still contracted with the County Council for payments. These options tend to be concentrated in major urban areas.

Maternity care in Sweden reflects the country's overall guidelines that health care should be publicly financed and provided to all residents on the basis of medical need. Mothers have the right to choose which antenatal clinic to attend (publicly or privately run) and which hospital to give birth in. Midwives are the primary providers of maternity care. Virtually all births take place in hospital and obstetricians work with midwives to provide care when necessary. Midwives work in either community-based antenatal care clinics or in hospitals. In some cases, they may rotate between the labour ward and the postnatal ward. Continuity of care-giver through antenatal, intrapartum and postnatal care is rare in Sweden. Since the 1990s, a shift from inpatient to outpatient services and to primary care has resulted in an ongoing decrease in the total number of hospital beds (Anell *et al.* 2012). Most of the smaller maternity wards have been closed due to a concern that so few births might impact on safety (Wiklund *et al.* 2002). In the 2000s, restructuring led to the concentration of highly specialised care in university hospitals and additional reductions in beds. Between 1990 and 2005, almost half of all beds in acute care hospitals were eliminated (Wiklund *et al.* 2002). Since the mid-2000s, mergers between larger hospitals have continued the trend towards the consolidation of services.

Community-based midwives have played an important role in public health in Sweden for over 100 years. Since the early 1900s, physicians and midwives have worked together to keep maternal mortality rates low and government-supported midwifery training programmes have been in place since the early 1800s (Högberg 2004). Unlike other countries, physicians and midwives in Sweden have developed as complementary rather than competitive professions and both have important roles in patient care and health policy (Högberg 2004). The professional organisations (the Swedish Association of Midwives and the Swedish Association of Obstetricians and Gynaecologists) continue to work closely together in developing practice guidelines (Wiklund *et al.* 2012; Banke *et al.* 2008).

There is currently a growing shortage of midwives, particularly in the urban areas of Sweden. This is due, in part, to reductions in funding for higher education, including places in midwifery training programmes (Hedén 2014). There is also concern that the shortage has overburdened the midwives currently working in hospitals, is discouraging others from entering the profession and is encouraging current midwives to seek work in Norway (*The Local* 2014). A shortage of midwives is not only of concern for pregnant women, but also for the established balance of duties between midwives and physicians.

Maternity entitlements

Maternity care is free at the point of service to all legal residents in Sweden. Services include antenatal, intrapartum and postnatal care. In the

1970s, Sweden began a generous paid parental leave policy to encourage women to participate more as providers and men to participate more as care-givers (Chronholm 2007). Parents in Sweden are entitled to 480 days of parental leave on the birth or adoption of each child. For 390 of the days, parents receive 80 per cent of their regular pay up to a maximum (about US$5600/month in 2013). The remaining ninety days are paid at a lower flat rate. Parental leave benefits may be used until the child turns eight years of age (Sweden.se 2014c). Those not in employment are entitled to paid parental leave based on a flat rate. Employers must hold a parent's job open for them during this time, which encourages parents to return to work at the end of their leave. Subsidised daycare also facilitates the return to work for both parents.

Since the 1980s there has been a concerted effort to involve fathers more in childcare. Fathers have been encouraged to participate in all areas of pregnancy, birth and parenting, including: antenatal visits; parent education classes; labour and delivery; and parental leave. Government policy has been used to encourage fathers to become more involved in parenting and to promote equality between the sexes. Of the 480 days of paid parental leave, two months are reserved exclusively for the father. Fathers also have ten days of paid leave on the birth of the baby to help care for the newborn baby and other children. Most fathers take advantage of these ten days. Fathers took approximately 25 per cent of the total parental leave days used by couples in 2011 (Försäkringskassan 2012).

Childbirth in Sweden

Antenatal care

Swedish antenatal care takes place mainly in outpatient clinics. Antenatal care is funded by taxes and is free of charge to legal residents. Maternity care is considered a right that cannot be deferred, so it is also free to adult asylum seekers (Anell *et al.* 2012: 101). Sweden's emphasis on providing health care 'on equal terms' dictates that services are fairly standardised, regardless of where the care is obtained. Recently, private alternatives have become more common, but the care is still free of charge for pregnant women. The compliance rate is around 99 per cent. Parents usually meet the same midwife during their antenatal visits. During a normal pregnancy, women have between six and nine visits to a midwife. Since 2007, an early visit is recommended shortly after a positive pregnancy test. During this early visit health issues, such as the use of tobacco and alcohol, exercise and nutrition, are discussed. Women are offered an ultrasound around sixteen weeks of pregnancy. There is no routine visit to a medical doctor. If the midwife has concerns about the pregnancy, or the pregnant woman herself has a need or a wish to meet other professionals, the midwife will refer the woman to more specialised care. First-time parents

are offered parent education classes, typically in small groups and conducted by antenatal midwives. Prospective fathers are encouraged to participate during the antenatal visits and parent education (Banke *et al.*
2008).

Intrapartum care

Midwives are responsible for normal births and work in collaboration with
an obstetrician in complicated births. Even during complicated pregnancies, the midwife is in charge and assists all births, with the exception of
instrumental vaginal births (usually vacuum extractions) and caesarean
sections. Complicated pregnancies are defined by midwives, who continuously monitor pregnant women and refer to an obstetrician when necessary. The Swedish midwife has been educated, since 1829, to perform
instrumental vaginal births, but in reality these are carried out by obstetricians in hospitals.

Virtually all intrapartum care takes place in hospitals. Currently only a
few hospitals offer any type of alternative to traditional labour and delivery
wards. In one study, 25 per cent of women in early pregnancy expressed
an interest in alternative birth centre care (Hildingsson *et al.* 2003). These
are mainly described as 'alongside' midwifery units with more continuity
of care-giver during antenatal, intrapartum and postnatal care. In recent
years, the requirements of high technological environments, neonatal
intensive care and twenty-four hours a day, seven days a week obstetric and
paediatric competence are obstacles to initiating midwifery-led units.

Approximately 1 in 1,000 births take place at home (Lindgren *et al.*
2008). A national survey conducted in 1999–2000 found that, if Swedish
women were offered a choice regarding the place of birth, the home birth
rate would increase ten-fold (Hildingsson *et al.* 2003). Women who want to
give birth at home in Sweden have to find a midwife willing to assist them,
meet a stringent set of requirements and, in most areas, finance the midwife's attendance (Lindgren *et al.* 2008). There are around 25 Swedish
midwives that assist at home births and access depends on geographical
area. Most of them are also employed by the hospital labour wards, which
could make it difficult for the midwives to be available when a woman goes
into labour. In a national survey regarding home births in Sweden from
1992 to 2001, the transfer rate from home to hospital was 12 per cent.
Transfer was more common in first-time mothers. The main reason was
prolonged labour, followed by the unavailability of the midwife (Lindgren
et al. 2008).

Almost one-quarter of births in 2011 were to foreign-born women,
mainly from Asia (9.8 per cent), European countries outside Scandinavia
(7.4 per cent) and African countries (3.8 per cent). Since 2000, there have
been a number of studies examining the maternity care experiences and
outcomes of immigrant women in Sweden. Previous research has found

that immigrant women, particularly from Africa and the Middle East, are likely to delay antenatal care, have fewer antenatal visits, have higher perinatal mortality rates and more low birthweight babies (Ny *et al.* 2007; Råssjö *et al.* 2013), and have a higher age-adjusted risk of non-normal childbirth (Robertson *et al.* 2005).

Birth is increasingly becoming more medicalised in Sweden and younger midwives are becoming more comfortable with the use of technology during birth, and more dependent on written guidelines and doctor back-up, than previous generations of midwives (Larsson *et al.* 2007). Demands for safety and a fear of litigation have led to an increasing reliance on technology instead of the midwives' own judgement (Larsson *et al.* 2007).

Although most births occur vaginally after the spontaneous onset of labour, induction has increased over the years, from around 9 per cent in 1996 to nearly 15 per cent in 2011. The main reason for induction is that it is believed the pregnancy is overdue. Currently, many clinics induce labour before forty-two completed weeks of gestation. Caesarean section rates have also been increasing in Sweden, although slower than in some other technologically advanced countries. The proportion of caesarean sections is 17 per cent for all births. In full-term pregnancies there are similar proportions of elective and emergency caesarean sections. In 1973, the proportion of caesarean sections was 5.3 per cent and the highest percentage was in 2006: 17.7 per cent with regional variations between 12.6 and 20.5 per cent (National Board of Health and Welfare 2013).

In Sweden, a caesarean section is not an option women can 'order' themselves without medical reasons. In many hospitals, women who request a caesarean section without medical reasons, and who suffer from a fear of childbirth, are referred to the team dealing with fear of birth. These teams typically consist of specially trained midwives, obstetricians, social workers and psychologists and work with women to overcome their fears prior to the birth (Thomas 2009). As part of the maternity care system, these programmes are also available free to women who are referred by their prenatal midwife. After counselling, it is still an obstetrician who makes the decision about whether or not to grant the request (Wiklund *et al.* 2012). There are national guidelines for health care providers on how to deal with caesarean sections on maternal request and certain indications should be fulfilled before a request is granted (Wiklund *et al.* 2012). However, in practice, women who cannot be convinced to go through a vaginal birth, mainly because of previous negative experiences and/or childbirth-related fear, will generally have their request granted (Wiklund *et al.* 2012).

On the other hand, the proportion of episiotomies has been decreasing. In 2000, 12.6 per cent of births involved an episiotomy; in 2011 the percentage had fallen to 5.9. During this same period, the percentage of large perineal ruptures (grades III and IV) stayed about the same (3.9 per cent in 2000 and 3.5 per cent in 2011) (National Board of Health and Welfare 2013).

The proportion of premature births is around 6 per cent and similar proportions of pregnancies are overdue (6 per cent). Pre-eclampsia is found in around 3 per cent of pregnancies and is more common in primiparous women, whereas the opposite is found in gestational diabetes when multiparous women are more affected. Eighty-six per cent of women have a vaginal birth after the spontaneous onset of labour; the rate of instrumental vaginal births (vacuum extractions and forceps) is nearly 9 per cent.

Sweden has been collecting data on all pregnancies and births for approximately forty years through the Medical Birth Register. In addition, there are several other registers available for the quality assessment of care. Changing trends in pain relief methods can be documented through this resource. In the early 1970s there was a media debate in Sweden about a woman's right to pain relief during labour and birth. In 1973 (the year the Medical Birth Register was established), the percentage of women using epidural blockade was just less than 1 per cent. In 1975, a government recommendation was formulated giving women the legal right to have pain relief. However, due to the organisation of care, not all hospitals can offer round-the-clock access to all medication, such as epidural anaesthesia. The percentage of women using epidural anaesthesia has continued to climb. In 1983, it reached 15.1 per cent and, in 2011, almost one-third of women giving birth (32.7 per cent) used epidural anaesthesia (National Board of Health and Welfare 2013).

With the shift to centralised hospital care in larger hospitals, most women have access to whatever method of pain relief they prefer during labour and birth. Enthonox is the most popular method, used by around 80 per cent of all women, and has increased over time. Epidural anaesthesia is mainly used by first-time mothers and has become more popular over the years.

Sweden's rates of intervention are lower than many other countries, but the shift from natural birth to medical birth is well underway. Changes in health care services and practices reflect the confluence of changes in expectations and demands by patients, political and economic pressures, and medical practices.

Postnatal care

The length of postnatal stay is short (on average, 1.9 days after a normal birth and 3.2 days after a caesarean section) and postnatal care takes place in traditional postnatal wards, or family suites on hotel wards incorporated into the hospital (mainly available for parents with normal births and healthy babies). Hotel wards with family suites are designed for families and non-infectious patients who have extended stays (surgical patients,

patients undergoing radiation treatment or chemotherapy), or those who may need some type of transitional care from hospital to home. The hotel unit typically has a registration desk, private rooms and some type of restaurant or meal facility for staff and guests.

Because the hotel unit is usually attached to the hospital, health care providers can easily check on patients, but generally patients and their families are on their own, with the security of knowing care is readily available if needed. New mothers are officially discharged from hospital when they use the hotel ward, but have access to a midwife during the daytime. If there is a need for staff during the night, the parents call the traditional postnatal ward (Hildingsson *et al.* 2009). Parents pay a small fee for using the hotel ward. More hospitals are adding patient hotels, which provide more comfortable and private accommodation for new parents and aid in the transition from hospital to home. In some of the neonatal intensive care units, parents can stay in family rooms for co-care.

Early discharge (after six to seventy-two hours), with or without home visits, is recommended for healthy mothers and newborn babies. Different hospitals may have only some of the options available, usually depending on the hospital size. In some areas, midwives make home visits after discharge.

The mean weight of babies in 2011 was slightly over 3.5 kg. First-time mothers had smaller babies than mothers with previous children. Of the babies born in 2011, around 1 per cent had a low Apgar score. The proportion of infants small-for-gestational-age was 3.4 per cent in first-time mothers and 1.9 per cent in mothers with previous children. The opposite was found in infants large-for-gestational age, where 4.8 per cent of babies born to mothers with previous children were large, but only 1.5 per cent of babies born to first-time mothers. Four babies per 1,000 were stillborn and the rate of neonatal deaths was 0.9–1.4 in 1,000 live births, depending on the definition (first week after birth or in the first month) (National Board of Health and Welfare 2013). Table 12.3 summarises Sweden's maternal and neonatal mortality statistics from 1970 to 2010.

Sweden is the only industrialised country where all hospitals meet the WHO and UNICEF standards for Baby-Friendly Hospitals (Save the Children 2012). The Swedish government supported this initiative in the early 1990s and, by 1997, all Swedish hospitals were 'Baby-Friendly.' This designation helps insure support and encouragement for breastfeeding through trained staff, who support the mother in initiating breastfeeding within the first thirty minutes after birth, do not offer milk substitutes and provide clear articulations of the benefits of breastfeeding. Sweden has one of the highest rates of breastfeeding in the world, with 98 per cent of mothers having ever breastfed, 60 per cent exclusively breastfeeding at three months and 72 per cent with at least some breastfeeding at six months (Save the Children 2012). Sweden's lengthy paid parental leave policy is likely to be a significant factor in the high rates of breastfeeding.

Table 12.3 Birth interventions and outcomes for selected years[a] in Sweden

	1970	1980	1990	2000	2010*
Maternal mortality	–	–	–	–	4/100,000
Perinatal deaths per 1,000 live and stillbirths					
Stillbirths/1,000	7.2	4.3	3.5	3.8	3.7
Neonatal per 1,000 live births					
Early, 0–6 days	7	4	2.8	1.7	1.2
Late, 0–27 days	7.9	4.8	3.4	2.3	1.6
Infant mortality per 1,000 live births	–	–	–	–	2.4
Induction	No data	No data	No data	9.8	13.1
Forceps and vacuum together (instrumental vaginal)	4.5	7.1	6.1	8.6	9.2
Caesarean section	5.3	11.6	10.6	14.8	17

Source: a National Board of Health and Welfare (2013).

However, the rates of exclusive breastfeeding have been declining recently and the rate of exclusive breastfeeding at six months (recommended by WHO and the Swedish government) has decreased from 43.1 per cent in 1996 to 10.6 per cent in 2010 (National Board of Health and Welfare 2013). This decline may be due to shorter hospital stays (less time for breastfeeding to be established) women returning to work sooner, or hospitals may be increasing the use of formula (Holmberg *et al.* 2014).

Consumer involvement

There are few strong consumer groups in Sweden and, in contrast with other countries, they are seldom involved in discussions about the organisation of care. As health care is provided at the county level, citizens can take their concerns and complaints about the health care system to their elected representatives. Hospitals also have a process for patients to file complaints if they are dissatisfied with their care, or if there are concerns about injuries or complications resulting from their care. One home birth organisation was established in the 1970s and consisted of parents and midwives engaged in the issue. Although this organisation is still in existence, it is virtually invisible.

One reason for this lack of activism around maternity care may be because Swedish women are generally satisfied with the care they receive. A large national survey of childbearing women was conducted in Sweden in 1999–2000. All but fifteen of the 608 antenatal clinics in Sweden participated (97 per cent). In general, women were pleased with the care they received during pregnancy, birth and the postnatal period, with 87 per cent satisfied with their antenatal care overall (Hildingsson *et al.* 2005), 90 per cent satisfied with their intrapartum care and 74 per cent with their postnatal care (Hildingsson *et al.* 2005; Waldenström *et al.* 2006). In a regional study in the northern part of Sweden, where a one-year cohort of Swedish-speaking women and their partners were recruited during the year 2007, similar questions about satisfaction were asked and the responses showed similar results as in the national survey conducted in 1999–2000 (Hildingsson 2012).

Despite the fact that many issues in the provision of care have changed (e.g. a reduced number of antenatal visits, increased use of technology during labour and birth, and a reduced length of postnatal stay) between the years 2000 and 2008, when these women gave birth, fairly similar levels of satisfaction were found. Looking at the overall satisfaction, around 2 per cent were dissatisfied or very dissatisfied with their antenatal care, around 2.5 per cent were dissatisfied with their intrapartum care and 7–8 per cent were dissatisfied with their postnatal care.

The government has periodically made adjustments in the parental leave policy to incentivise fathers to become more involved in childcare and, while it is now much more common to see groups of fathers enjoying their parental leave with their babies in parks or coffee shops, fathers still feel that the maternity care system is not designed for them. Despite the fact that fathers are encouraged and invited to participate during episodes of care, research has consistently reported that fathers often feel excluded by health care professionals. Although they felt as though they were expected to attend antenatal visits, fathers often did not feel involved by the midwife when they did attend. Some fathers feel that they had been made invisible in midwives' narratives of being supportive to prospective parents during pregnancy (Hildingsson and Häggström 1999), but other fathers have also reported great satisfaction with antenatal care (Bogren Jungmarker *et al.* 2010). Studies on postnatal care also show that some men feel excluded, describing the experience as being 'still behind the glass wall' (Hildingsson *et al.* 2009).

Since the 1990s, the government has focused on giving patients more choices in health care. In 1992, the Patient Choice and Care Guarantee was enacted. This Act guaranteed individual choice of primary care provider, hospital, private clinics and second opinions, and advertised 'patient empowerment'. However, patients found that the rhetoric of choice did not always come with a mechanism for implementation. For example, women were guaranteed the right to choose their midwife, but the midwife they chose did not necessarily have room for new patients. Women were also guaranteed the right to choose the hospital they wanted to give birth in, but, if the hospital was full when they were ready to deliver, they were referred elsewhere. Little information was available to help women make informed choices.

Government policies to reduce costs and provide more choice may actually be helping to increase the rates of intervention and associated costs. With regard to maternity care, cut-backs in staff on labour wards, and hospital consolidations that closed some smaller labour units and reduced beds in others, were implemented to save costs and increase efficiencies. However, data from a Swedish national survey conducted in 1999–2000 found that pregnant women were worried about a shortage of staff, being referred to a hospital they had not planned for, and a general lack of resources in the health care system. Some women were concerned that the midwives would be overworked and not able to give them the attention they wanted and needed (Hildingsson and Thomas 2007). A recent study on burnout in Swedish midwives found that women's concerns may be justified. Just under a third of the midwives in the study had considered leaving their jobs, mainly due to conditions in the workplace, including a lack of staff, lack of resources and a stressful work environment. Working shifts or working in hospitals rather than in outpatient clinics was also related to stress (Hildingsson *et al.* 2013). As the authors concluded, the woman/family-centred care midwives are trained to provide has become increasingly difficult to offer as labour wards have 'become more technical and more obstetrician-driven despite evidence of benefits [of midwifery care]' (Hildingsson *et al.* 2013: 90).

Rights and risks

The 1982 Health and Medical Services Act guarantees all residents the same right to high-quality health care services (Anell *et al.* 2012). However, it guarantees them the services they need, not necessarily the services they want. In Sweden, rights and risks in health care are embedded in tensions between patient choice, cost control, professional practices and changing social norms about birth. Sweden's core values of universality and equality mean that all citizens should receive the same quality of care. Services such as maternity care should be consistent throughout the country. The facilities, hours and content of care (such as the number of visits, the number and timing of ultrasound scans, and parent education classes) should be the same, regardless of geography, type of provider (private or public), or even citizenship status, as maternity care is considered a type of care that cannot be postponed. All providers are paid the same rates by the government. However, private clinics are only available in certain urban areas and often offer extended hours and additional services, such as prenatal yoga (extra fee) and baby boutiques (Thomas 2009). Private options are not available to all women throughout the country.

More important than the inequalities that have been introduced by private providers are the ways in which the standardised package of maternity services is not meeting the needs of the increasingly diverse population of pregnant women in Sweden. As mentioned earlier, research in Sweden and elsewhere has shown that the needs and expectations of immigrant women are often not met by the standardised organisation of care. Western approaches to pregnancy are not necessarily shared by all cultures. Women unfamiliar with the Swedish system or uncomfortable with the structure of care may avoid using the services, or delay antenatal care even if it is available (Balaam *et al.* 2013). Bureaucratic rules, schedules, and childcare and transportation issues may also make it difficult for immigrant women to attend appointments (Wikberg and Bondas 2010). In addition to the structure of care, immigrant women may come with different mental and physical health needs, and different cultural norms around touching, interventions, diet and gender roles (Wikberg and Bondas 2010). Sweden's 'one size fits all' approach to equality in care must be adjusted to provide quality care for women from different cultures. Ongoing research continues to assess how to improve access and services for foreign-born pregnant women, but so far few changes have been made.

There has been a strong emphasis historically on birth as a natural process that should not be interfered with unless necessary but that has been changing in Sweden as well as in other high-income countries. A recent study from the Stockholm area showed that, in 1992, the main indications for a caesarean section were a problematic foetal position or uterine factors, whereas in 2005 the main indication was psychosocial, e.g. fear of giving birth and/or maternal request (Vladic 2007). A study of caesarean sections in Stockholm and four counties in northern Sweden found that the rates of caesarean section 'without medical indication' doubled between 1996 and 2007 (Karlström *et al.* 2009). The explanations for the rise in caesarean sections given by physicians and the media tended to focus on the changing demographic characteristics of patients, maternal request and a growing fear of birth (Karlström *et al.* 2009). However, also important are the changing norms of obstetric practice in which the definition of 'normal' has become narrower and providers' tolerances for deviation has become lower (Leeman and Plante 2006).

Until fairly recently, the cultural message that women received about birth emphasised the normality of birth rather than the pathology. Media stories and American TV shows such as *Birth Stories* have eroded this belief in recent years. Midwives report spending increasing time during prenatal visits dealing with women's fears, worries and psychological issues and trying to reinforce the view that generally everything goes just fine (Thomas 2009). In an effort to counter some of the increasing fears women have about birth, most hospitals now offer special programmes for women who are extremely fearful of birth and work with women to overcome their fears prior to birth, thus reinforcing the notion that birth is a normal and natural event.

There have certainly been changes in women's expectations and beliefs around pregnancy and birth. Although midwives have historically been the 'protectors of natural birth', they now report spending more time talking with women about what could possibly go wrong during childbirth and find women less willing to 'trust in nature'. Pregnancy has become a 'risk' instead of a natural process. Pregnant women want medical security and guarantees that everything will be fine (Thomas 2009).

A declining view of birth as a natural process, a narrowing of medical definitions of 'normal birth' and increased perceptions of risk have made both women and doctors more fearful of something going wrong and more willing to intervene during labour and birth. This has led to an increased use of interventions and technologies during the birth process, such as induction, electronic foetal monitoring, epidural, caesarean sections and instrumental births. For women who want and expect control over their lives, the 'risk' of birth must be controlled through technology and specialists. However, these are not necessarily evidence-based practices.

As Swedish women lose confidence in their ability to give birth naturally and begin to fear giving birth without medical assistance and intervention, the control shifts from the women to the providers. Some argue that women's empowerment has actually declined in the age of technology-assisted birth rather than increased (Larsson *et al.* 2007). The government's goals for ensuring that patients are given opportunities for participation, self-determination and care choices (Ministry of Health and Social Affairs 2013) are bumping up against the need to control costs and provide care based on patient need and professional best practice.

In addition to the increasing use of technology, caesarean section 'without medical indication' is also an example of the tensions between a patient's rights and medical risks. Doctors and midwives often cite increasing patient demand as one of the key reasons that caesarean section rates have increased over the years. Although guidelines are in place for deciding when a caesarean section is appropriate (Wiklund *et al.* 2012), providers lament the difficulties of respecting women's rights to choose and the expected professional practice (Karlström *et al.* 2010). The right to choose a provider is not the same as the right to choose a procedure, but as the government continues to pursue policies that give patients opportunities for participation and self-determination, it is going to be more difficult to draw the line between patients' rights to choice and evidence-based practices. The real dilemma for a country like Sweden is the 'cost' of choice. If women are allowed to see an obstetrician rather than a midwife for their antenatal care, or if they are allowed to choose a non-medically indicated caesarean section over a vaginal birth, or multiple ultrasound scans when not medically indicated, it will be increasingly difficult to control costs and continue to offer coverage to all.

How will the government change accepted professional practice that is not based on the most recent research? If it does not, it will be more challenging to hold costs down and to ensure the best quality of care for all residents. In Australia, rising costs in maternity care have been attributed to women's expectations of technology and interventions to protect them from perceived risk (McIntyre *et al.* 2011). In the absence of real (medical) risk, the government must decide how to deal with patients' demands for technological interventions, providers' practice routines, medical evidence that the intervention may be unnecessary and increasing costs.

Conclusion

A country's welfare state reflects its core values and Sweden is no exception. Sweden's welfare state is based on the values of solidarity, equality and redistributive social justice supported by a large public sector and high social spending. Universal social benefits, such as health care, are linked to citizenship rather than connected to an individual's labour market participation or family status. To support these benefits, government policies seek to make it possible for all adult citizens to be active participants in the labour market. Such policies include those that focus on health (health care, sick leave), education and job skills, support for children and families (child allowances, subsidised day care, elder care) and the reconciliation of work and family life (parental leave, shared parenting). With egalitarianism at its core, Swedish social welfare policies help provide women with individual autonomy and 'exit options' (Hobson 1990) and protect them from economic vulnerability.

Sweden is a very good place to have a baby, in large part due to the many welfare policies and services that help to create a secure and supportive environment for women and their children. As a social democracy, universal benefits are based on citizenship (defined as legal residence) and are directed at the individual level, thus increasing levels of decommodification. Attention to gender equity has been institutionalised in government policies since the 1970s and policies continue to support both men and women as earners and carers. Access to quality health care, including maternity care, is an important factor in developing citizens' human capital. Although Sweden's health outcomes, particularly in the areas of infant and maternal mortality, are some of the best in the world, Sweden also faces some significant challenges based on changing demographics and the development of health care policies based on patient choice, more private provision of care and market-based reforms. As maternity care becomes more medicalised, Swedish politicians will have to consider the 'cost' of choice and how to reconcile evidence-based knowledge regarding interventions with existing medical practice. In addition, the increasingly diverse population of pregnant women will also require a new conversation about how to provide equality in services and care for women coming with very different mental, physical and social needs. Old structures and services may no longer meet the needs of all Swedish citizens.

References

Anell, A., Glenngård, A. and Merkur, S. (2012) *Health Systems in Transition: Sweden Health System Review 2012*. Paris: OECD Publishing. Available from: www.euro.who. int/__data/assets/pdf_file/0008/164096/e96455.pdf/. Accessed 20 April 2014.

Arts, W. and Gelissen, J. (2010) 'Models of the welfare state'. In: F.S. Castles, S. Leibfried, J. Lewis, H. Obnger and C. Pierson (eds), *The Oxford Handbook of the Welfare State*. Oxford: Oxford University Press, pp. 569–583.

Balaam, M.-C., Akerjordet, K., Lyberg, A., Kaiser, B., Schoening, E., Fredriksen, A.-M., Ensel, A., Gouni, O. and Severinsson, E. (2013) 'A qualitative review of migrant women's perceptions of their needs and experiences related to pregnancy and childbirth', *Advanced Nursing*, 69: 1919–1930.

Balasch, J. and Gratacós, E. (2012) 'Delayed childbearing: effects on fertility and the outcome of pregnancy', *Current Opinions in Obstetrics and Gynecology*, 24 (3): 187–193.

Banke, G., Berglund, A., Collberg, P. and Ideström, M. (2008). *Mödrahälsovård, sexuell och reproduktiv hälsa* (Antenatal care, sexual and reproductive health) [in Swedish]. ARG-Rapport nr 59, Svensk Förening för Obstetrik & Gynekologi, Arbets & Referensgrupper rapportserie. Stockholm: Svensk Förening för Obstetrik & Gynekologi.

Bogren Jungmarker, E., Lindgren, H. and Hildingsson, I. (2010) 'Playing the second fiddle is ok – Swedish fathers' experiences of antenatal care', *Journal of Midwifery and Women's Health*, 55: 421–429.

Chronholm, A. *Fathers' Experience of Shared Parental Leave in Sweden* [online]. Recherches Sociologiques et Anthropologiques. Available from: http://rsa. revues.org/456. Accessed 20 April 2014.

Esping-Andersen, G. (1990) *The Three Worlds of Welfare Capitalism.* Cambridge: Polity Press.

Fraser, N. (2000) 'After the family wage: a postindustrial thought experiment'. In: B. Hobson (ed.), *Gender and Citizenship in Transition.* New York: Routledge.

Försäkringskassan (2012) *Analys och uppföljning av utvecklingen av föräldrapenninguttaget* (Analysis and monitoring of the evolution of parental leave) [in Swedish]. Report to Socialdepartmentet. Stockholm: Försäkringskassan.

Ginsburg, H. and Rosenthal, M. (2006) 'The ups and downs of the Swedish welfare state: general trends, benefits and caregiving' [online], *New Politics* XI (1). Available from: http://newpol.org. Accessed 3 November 2013.

Glenngård, A. (2013) 'The Swedish health care system, 2013'. In: S. Thomson, R. Osborn, D. Squires and M. Jun (eds), International Profiles of Health Care Systems, 2013. Publication No. 1717. Washington, DC: The Commonwealth Fund.

Hedén, D. (2014) *The State Must Ensure the Availability of Midwives* [online]. Available from: www.dagensmedicin.se/debatt/debattstaten-maste-sakra-utbildning-av-barnmorskor/. Accessed 3 May 2014.

Hildingsson, I. (2012) *Giving Birth in Västernorrland. Project Report* [in Swedish]. Sundsvall: Mid Sweden University.

Hildingsson, I. and Häggström, T. (1999) 'Midwives' lived experiences of being supportive to prospective mothers/parents during pregnancy', *Midwifery*, 15 (2): 82–91.

Hildingsson, I. and Rådestad, I. (2005) 'Swedish women's satisfaction with medical and emotional aspects of antenatal care', *Journal of Advanced Nursing*, 52: 239–249.

Hildingsson, I. and Thomas, J. (2007) 'Processes, problems and solutions: maternity services from women's perspectives in Sweden', *Journal of Midwifery and Women's Health*, 52 (2): 126–133.

Hildingsson I., Waldenström, U. and Rådestad, I. (2003) 'Swedish women's interest in homebirth and in-hospital birth center care', *Birth*, 30: 11–22.

Hildingsson, I., Engström-Olofsson, R., Thomas, J. and Nystedt, A. (2009) 'Still behind the glass wall? Fathers' experiences of postnatal care', *Journal of Obstetric Gynecological and Neonatal Nursing*, 38: 280–289.

Hildingsson, I., Westlund, K. and Wiklund, I. (2013) 'Burnout in Swedish midwives', *Sexual & Reproductive Healthcare*, 4 (3): 87–91.

Hobson, B. (1990) 'No exit, no voice: women's economic dependency and the welfare state', *Acta Sociologica*, 33: 335–350.

Högberg, U. (2004) 'The decline of maternal mortality in Sweden: the role of community midwifery', *American Journal of Public Health*, 94 (8): 1312–1320.

Holmberg, K., Peterson, U. and Oscarsson, M. (2014) 'A two-decade perspective on mothers' experiences and feelings related to breastfeeding initiation in Sweden', *Journal of Sexual & Reproductive Healthcare*, DOI: 10.1016/j.srhc.2014.04.001.

Karlström, A., Engström-Olofsson, R., Nysted, A., Thomas, J. and Hildingsson, I. (2009) 'Swedish caregivers' attitudes towards caesarean section on maternal request', *Women and Birth*, 22 (2): 57–63.

Karlström, A., Rådestad, I., Eriksson, C., Rubertsson, C., Nystedt, A. and Hildings-son, I. (2010) 'Cesarean section without medical reason, 1997 to 2006: a Swedish Register study', *Birth*, 37 (1): 11–20.

Larsson, M., Aldegarmann, U. and C. Aarts (2007) 'Professional role and identity in a changing society: three paradoxes in Swedish midwives' experiences', *Midwifery*, 25: 373–381.

Leeman, L. and Plante, L. (2006) 'Patient-choice vaginal delivery', *Annals of Family Medicine*, 4 (3): 265–268.

Lindgren, H., Hildingsson, I., Christensson, K. and Rådestad, I. (2008) 'Transfers in planned home births related to midwife availability and continuity: a nation-wide population-based study', *Birth*, 35: 9–15.

McIntyre, M., Francis, K. and Chapman, Y. (2011) 'Primary maternity care reform: whose influence is driving the change?', *Midwifery*, 28: 705–711.

Mello, M., Kachalia, A. and Studdert, D. (2011) 'Administrative compensation for medical injuries – lessons from three foreign systems' [online]. In: *Issues in International Health Policy, July 2011*. Commonwealth Fund Publication No. 1517, Vol. 14, pp. 1–18. Available from: www.commonwealthfund.org/~/media/Files/ Publications/Issue%20Brief/2011/Jul/1517_Mello_admin_compensation_ med_injuries.pdf.

Ministry of Health and Social Affairs (2013) *Objectives and Priorities for Health and Medical Care* [online]. Available from: www.government.se/sb/d/15472/a/184692. Accessed 28 November 2013.

National Board of Health and Welfare (2013) *Pregnancies, Deliveries and Newborn Infants. the Swedish Medical Birth Register 1973–2011 Assisted Reproduction, Treatment 1991–2010*. Official Statistics of Sweden – Health and Medical Care, Report. Stockholm: National Board of Health and Welfare.

National Board of Health and Welfare (2014). 'Statistics on health care personnel. Official statistics on the number of licensed practitioners (2013) and their labour market situation (2012)'. In: *Official Statistics of Sweden – Health and Medical Care*. Stockholm: National Board of Health and Welfare.

Ny, P., Dykes, A.-K., Molin, J. and Dejin-Karlsson, E. (2007) 'Utilisation of ante-natal care by country of birth in a multi-ethnic population: a four-year community-based study in Malmö, Sweden', *Acta Obstetricia et Gynaecologica Scandinavica*, 86 (7): 805–813.

OECD (2013a) *OECD Factbook 2013* [online]. Available from: http://www.oecd-ilibrary.org/sites/factbook-2013-en. Accessed 19 April 2014.

OECD (2013b) *OECD Health Data: How Does Sweden Compare?* [online]. Available from: www.oecd.org/els/health-systems/Briefing-Note-SWEDEN-2013.pdf. Accessed 19 April 2014.

OECD (2014a) *Better Life Index: Sweden* [online]. Available from: www.oecdbetterli-feindex.org/countries/sweden/. Accessed 19 April 2014.

OECD (2014b) 'Medical graduates'. In: *Health: Key Tables from OECD, No. 32*. doi: 10.1787/medgrad-table-2014-1-en.

OECD (2014c) 'Hospital beds'. In: *Health: Key Tables from OECD, No. 30*. doi: 10.1787/hosp-beds-table-2014-1-en.

OECD (2014d) 'Curative (acute) care beds' *Health: Key Tables from OECD, No. 34*. doi: 10.1787/curcarebed-table-2014-1-en.

Orloff, A. (1993) 'Gender and the social rights of citizenship: the comparative ana-lysis of gender relations and welfare states', *American Sociological Review*, 58: 303–328.

Orloff, A. (2010) 'Gender'. In: F.G.Castles, S. Leibfried, J. Lewis, H. Obnger and C. Pierson (eds), *The Oxford Handbook of the Welfare State*. Oxford: Oxford University Press.

Råssjö, E., Byrskog, U., Samir, R. and Klingberg-Allvin, M. (2013) 'Somali women's use of maternity health services and the outcome of their pregnancies: a descriptive study comparing Somali immigrants with native-born Swedish women', *Sexual & Reproductive Healthcare*, 4 (3): 99–106.

Robertson, E., Malmström, M. and Johansson, S.-E. (2005) 'Do foreign-born women in Sweden have an increased risk of non-normal childbirth?', *Acta Obstetricia et Gynaecologica Scandinavica*, 84 (9): 825–832.

Save the Children (2012) *Nutrition in the First 1,000 days: the State of the World's Mothers 2012* [online]. Available from: www.savethechildren.ca/document. doc?id=195. Accessed 20 April 2014.

Socialstyrelsen (2012) *Amning och föräldrars rökvanor. Barn födda 2010*. (Breastfeeding rates and tobacco use in Swedish parents 2010) [in Swedish] [online]. Sveriges officiella statistisk. Hälso -och sjukvård. Available from: www.socialstyrelsen. se/publikationer2012/2012-8-13. Accessed 19 April 2014.

Statistics Sweden (2014) [online] Available from: www.scb.se/en_/Finding-statistics/Statistics-by-subject-area/Population/Population-composition/Population-statistics/. Accessed 19 April 2014.

Sweden.se (2014a) *Sweden and Migration in Brief* [online]. Available from: https://sweden.se/society/sweden-and-migration-in-brief/. Accessed 19 April 2014.

Sweden.se (2014b) *Healthcare in Sweden* [online]. Available from: www.sweden.se/ eng/Home/Society/Health-care/Facts/Health-care-in-Sweden/www.sweden.se/ eng/Home/Society/Health-care/Facts/Health-care-inSweden/. Accessed 19 April 2014.

Sweden.se (2014c) *10 Things That Make Sweden Family Friendly* [online]. Available from: http://sweden.se/society/10-things-that-make-sweden-family-friendly/. Accessed 19 April 2014.

Swedish Tax Agency (2012). *Taxes in Sweden 2012: an English Summary of Tax Statistical Yearbook of Sweden* [online]. Available from: www.skatteverket.se/dow nload/18.3684199413c956649b57c0a/1361442608379/10413.pdf. Accessed 18 April 2014.

The Local (2014) *Midwives Quit Over Wages and 'Scared Mums'* [online]. Available from: www.thelocal.se/20140228/midwives-quit-over-wages-and-scared-mums. Accessed 3 May 2014.

Thomas, J. (2009) 'Trusting women, respecting birth: prenatal care in Sweden', *Journal of the Association of Research on Mothering*, 11 (1): 59–68.

UN Data (2014) *Country Profile: Sweden* [online]. Available from: https://data.un. org/CountryProfile.aspx?crName=SWEDEN. Accessed 6 September 2014.

Vladic, S. (2007) 'Increased number of caesarean sections without medical indications in spite of the risks', *Lakartidningen*, 104: 942–945.

Waldenström, U., Rudman, A. and Hildingsson, I. (2006) 'Intrapartum and postpartum care in Sweden. Women's opinions and risk factors for not being satisfied', *Acta Obstetricia et Gynaecologica Scandinavica*, 85: 551–560.

Wikberg, A. and Bondas, T. (2010) 'A patient perspective in research on intercultural caring in maternity care: a meta-ethnography', *International Journal of Qualitative Studies in Health and Well-being*, 5: 1–15.

Wiklund, I., Matthiesen, A.-S., Klang, B. and Ransjö-Arvidson, A.-B. (2002) 'A comparative study in Stockholm, Sweden of labour outcome and women's perceptions of being referred in labour', *Midwifery*, 18: 193–199.

Wiklund, I., Andolf, E., Lilja, H. and Hildingsson, I. (2012) 'Indications for cesarean section on maternal request: guidelines for counseling and treatment', *Sexual and Reproductive Healthcare*, 3: 99–106.

Index

Page numbers in *italics* denote tables.

For Product Safety Concerns and Information please contact our EU
representative GPSR@taylorandfrancis.com
Taylor & Francis Verlag GmbH, Kaufingerstraße 24, 80331 München, Germany

www.ingramcontent.com/pod-product-compliance
Ingram Content Group UK Ltd.
Pitfield, Milton Keynes, MK11 3LW, UK
UKHW052032210425
457613UK00033BA/1153